Occupational Analysis and Group Process

Occupational Analysis and Group Process

Jane Clifford O'Brien, PhD, OTR/L

Program Director
Occupational Therapy Department
Westbrook College of Health Professions
University of New England
Portland, Maine

Jean W. Solomon, MHS, OTR/L

Occupational Therapist
Berkeley County School District
Charleston, South Carolina

Illustrator: Morgan Midgett Taylor

3251 Riverport Lane
St. Louis, Missouri 63043

OCCUPATIONAL ANALYSIS AND GROUP PROCESS   ISBN: 978-0-323-08464-2
Copyright © 2013 by Mosby, an imprint of Elsevier Inc.

Notices

Knowledge and best practice in this field are constantly changing. As new research and experience broaden our understanding, changes in research methods, professional practices, or medical treatment may become necessary. Practitioners and researchers must always rely on their own experience and knowledge in evaluating and using any information, methods, compounds, or experiments described herein. In using such information or methods they should be mindful of their own safety and the safety of others, including parties for whom they have a professional responsibility.

With respect to any drug or pharmaceutical products identified, readers are advised to check the most current information provided (i) on procedures featured or (ii) by the manufacturer of each product to be administered, to verify the recommended dose or formula, the method and duration of administration, and contraindications. It is the responsibility of practitioners, relying on their own experience and knowledge of their patients, to make diagnoses, to determine dosages and the best treatment for each individual patient, and to take all appropriate safety precautions.

To the fullest extent of the law, neither the Publisher nor the authors, contributors, or editors, assume any liability for any injury and/or damage to persons or property as a matter of products liability, negligence or otherwise, or from any use or operation of any methods, products, instructions, or ideas contained in the material herein.

Library of Congress Cataloging-in-Publication Data (in PHL)
Library of Congress Cataloging-in-Publication Data
O'Brien, Jane Clifford.
Occupational analysis and group process / Jane Clifford O'Brien, Jean W. Solomon.–1st ed.
    p. ; cm.
  Includes bibliographical references and index.
  ISBN 978-0-323-08464-2 (pbk.)
  I. Solomon, Jean W. II. Title.
  [DNLM: 1. Occupational Therapy--methods. 2. Group Processes. WB 555]
  615.8'515–dc23   2012032408

Vice President and Publisher: Linda Duncan
Content Manager: Jolynn Gower
Publishing Services Manager: Rajendrababu Hemamalini
Project Manager: Siva Raman Krishna Moorthy
Cover Designer: Brian Salisbury
Text Designer: Brian Salisbury
Illustrator: Morgan Taylor

Printed in United States

Last digit is the print number: 9 8 7 6 5 4 3 2 1

Dr. Gary Kielhofner was dedicated to making a difference in the lives of those with disability. He encouraged practitioners and scholars to engage in meaningful practice and provided an evidence-based model to guide practice. Throughout his impressive career, Dr. Kielhofner mentored faculty, students, and practitioners by empowering them to succeed. His work and vision profoundly influenced the occupational therapy profession. This book is dedicated to the memory and contributions of our dear friend and mentor, Dr. Gary Kielhofner.

Contributors

Nancy Carson, PhD, MHS, OTR/L
Acting Program Director
Occupational Therapy Educational Program
College of Health Professions
Medical University of South Carolina
Charleston, South Carolina

Judith Clifford Cohn, MS Ed
Certified Elementary School Teacher
Pet Assisted Therapy Intern
The D.J. Pet Assisted Therapy University Certificate Program
Providence, Rhode Island

Kate McLean Hanrahan, MSOT
University of New England
Portland, Maine

Deborah Hyman, OTR/L
Occupational Therapy Assistant Program
Santa Ana College
Santa Ana, California

Lisa Mahaffey, MS., OTR/L
Assistant Professor
Occupational Therapy Program
College of Health Sciences
Midwestern University
Downers Grove, Illinois

Elizabeth A. Moyer, MS, OTR/L, FAOTA
Assistant Clinical Professor
Occupational Therapy Department
Westbrook College of Health Professions
University of New England
Portland, Maine

Michelle Parolise, MBA, OTR/L
Program Director
Occupational Therapy Assistant Program
Santa Ana College
Santa Ana, California

Regula H. Robnett, PhD, OTR/L
Professor
Occupational Therapy
Westbrook College of Health Professions
University of New England
Portland, Maine

Renée R. Taylor, PhD
Professor
Department of Occupational Therapy
University of Illinois
Chicago, Illinois

Laura VanPuymbrouck, MS, OTR/L
PhD Student in Disability Studies
University of Illinois
Chicago, Illinois

Kerryellen Vroman, PhD, OTR
Associate Professor
Occupational Therapy
College of Health and Human Services
University of New Hampshire
Durham, New Hampshire

Preface

This textbook provides readers with practical information on two key components of occupational therapy practice: occupational analysis and group process. Occupational analysis is essential to the occupational therapy process. Practitioners engage in occupational analysis by carefully examining the many features of occupations so that they can better understand how to intervene with a variety of clients. This process allows practitioners to help clients return to meaningful activities and occupations that provide them with identity. This textbook is designed to provide practitioners with strategies and guidelines for analyzing occupations across the lifespan. The authors provide case scenarios, clinical examples, and suggestions for working with different populations. This serves as the foundation for intervention planning.

Occupational therapy practitioners often provide interventions in groups. This textbook provides readers with an understanding of the group process, strategies to lead groups and guidelines for group interventions. The authors describe the communication process and therapeutic relationships in regards to working in groups.

The book is organized into 14 chapters (covering content regarding occupational analysis and group process), perforated pages, and a glossary of terms. The perforated pages include forms presented throughout the manuscript (tables and boxes) which may be copied and used to promote student learning or to assist practitioners in planning, implementing, and evaluating group work. The authors of each chapter have provided an outline, objectives, key terms, and review questions. Each chapter includes case examples, tables, and boxes to highlight key content. Clinical pearls are provided as tips gained in practice.

The first chapter provides an overview of the *Occupational Therapy Practice Framework*[1] (2nd edition) in regards to occupational analysis and group process. The author describes how practitioners use the framework to analyze activities and develop groups addressing clients' occupational needs. The process of activity analysis is further examined in Chapter 2. This chapter provides readers with a description of various types of analyses, such as task-focused, biomechanical, and *Model of Human Occupation*.[2] This helps readers understand the complexities of occupational analysis. Numerous tables, boxes, and forms help to illustrate the concepts. Chapter 3 describes the skills for successful interpersonal relationships and communication necessary to be an effective group leader. Leadership styles, group models, and stages of group development are presented along with a discussion on the components of communication. The author provides strategies for establishing rapport with clients and many examples and clinical pearls. Chapter 4 describes how to apply the *Intentional Relationship Model*[3] in a group setting. The authors present an overview of the model and specific examples of its use in practice. A description of inevitable events of therapy and the reasoning process helps readers apply concepts. Chapter 5 helps readers understand the complexities of teaching clients in occupational therapy by describing the concepts of teaching and learning, modes or pathways of learning, and universal design to learning. Chapters 6 and 7 explain the specifics of managing groups, including planning, designing, and facilitating groups. These chapters outline the process for developing group and individual goals. Chapters 8 through 11 convey the intricacies of occupational and group analysis across the lifespan. Chapter 12 explores emerging areas of occupational therapy practice in regards to group work. The authors give community examples in alignment with AOTA's Centennial vision. Chapter 13 examines AOTA's ethical standards and the ethical reasoning process. Chapter 14 gives examples of potential difficult groups and offers solutions to managing difficult groups.

Each chapter presents readers with practical examples. The forms in the chapters are completed using examples (and may be found in tables or boxes), while those in the perforated section provide headings only. Readers are urged to refer back to the chapters for examples.

Acknowledgments

We would like to acknowledge and express our appreciation to Jolynn Gower, Content Manager, Health Professions for her support, guidance, and gentle nudging while writing this manuscript. We appreciate Sara Alsup's administrative support throughout the process. We thank Sivaraman Moorthy for his editorial skills and turn-around deadlines. Thank you to Brian Salisbury for the cover and text design expertise. We are grateful to Morgan Taylor for being so talented and adept at turning our words into beautiful illustrations. We express our gratitude to the contributing authors for the knowledge they shared. We feel honored to have worked with such an impressive group of colleagues.

JOB and JWS

I would like to thank Sylvia and Gordan for allowing Jane and I to brainstorm and write in their home. I acknowledge the students enrolled in Berkeley County School District who helped me gain knowledge and skills in working with children in small groups. I thank special education teachers, Ashley, Avis, Bassanya, Kristen, and Laura, for opening their classroom doors and allowing me to design and implement a variety of different groups for the past two school years. Finally, I acknowledge and thank my friend and colleague, Jane O'Brien. We did it!

JWS

Thank you to Mike who stands by me consistently. My children, Scott, Alison and Molly serve as a source of inspiration daily. Kara Beal and Judy Cohn listened to many renditions of book chapters. My colleagues and students at the University of New England supported, encouraged, and served as writers and consultants. I would like to acknowledge Kate Hanrahan, MSOT Class 2012 for her careful attention to details and positive spirit. I am grateful for my friend and colleague Jean Solomon for our numerous collaborations.

JOB

Contents

Occupational Analysis and Group Process

Jane Clifford O'Brien

KEY TERMS

activity analysis	objects
adjourning	occupation
areas of occupation	performance skills
blocking role	performance patterns
body functions	performing
body structures	preparatory methods
client factors	purposeful activity
cohesiveness	required actions
contexts	sequencing and timing
environment	social demands
forming	space demands
functional group	storming
interest group	task group
maintenance role	worker role
norming	values, beliefs, and spirituality

OBJECTIVES

1. Understand how the occupational therapy practice framework (OTPF) may structure activity analysis for intervention.
2. Define terms from the OTPF as they are used in activity analysis.
3. Describe the stages of groups.
4. Identify the types of groups.
5. Differentiate between occupation, task, and activity.
6. Discuss the basic concepts of group process and acuity analysis.

This chapter provides an overview of occupational analysis and group process. The author describes how practitioners use the occupational therapy practice framework (OTPF) to develop and lead groups addressing occupational needs. An overview of how the OTPF assists practitioners in analyzing activities for clinical application is presented. This chapter defines groups and describes the basic concepts of group processes and dynamics in the context of occupational therapy intervention.

OCCUPATIONAL THERAPY PRACTICE FRAMEWORK

Practitioners use the OTPF to structure the analysis of activities for intervention. The following scenario illustrates how a practitioner might use concepts from the OTPF when designing group activities.

Lila is an OT student who is assigned to develop a group activity for retired veterans.

The OTPF provides guidance for developing therapeutic group activities. First, the practitioner examines the **area of occupation** important to address within the group (Box 1-1).

In the previous example, the OT student decides to design a group activity to increase the veterans' independence in community mobility (Figure 1-1). The occupational area of community mobility includes moving around in the community and using transportation, such as driving, walking, bicycling, or accessing public transportation (i.e., buses, subway). Other areas of concern that could be the focus of the intervention include the areas of self-care, leisure, or social participation. The student (Lila) may decide group activities should target areas of home management or financial management. It may be that the members' goals focus on different areas of occupation during group sessions.

Examining the group members' **values, beliefs, and spirituality** is useful for motivating clients, addressing key areas of concern, and helping members understand themselves. Periodically, group sessions focus on values clarification exercises or exercises to identify one's belief systems (Table 1-1). In this example, the veterans acknowledged that increased independence in community mobility will enhance their feelings of self-worth and believe that this group activity will be of value to them.

BOX 1-1 Areas of Occupation

Activities of Daily Living
- Bathing, showering
- Bowel and bladder management
- Dressing
- Eating
- Feeding
- Functional mobility
- Personal device care
- Personal hygiene and grooming
- Sexual activity
- Toilet hygiene

Instrumental Activities of Daily Living
- Care of others (including selecting and supervising caregivers)
- Care of pets
- Child rearing
- Communication management
- Community mobility
- Financial management
- Health management and maintenance
- Home establishment and management
- Meal preparation and cleanup
- Religious observance
- Safety and emergency maintenance
- Shopping

Rest and Sleep
- Rest

- Sleep
- Sleep preparation
- Sleep participation

Education
- Formal education participation
- Informal personal educational needs or interests exploration (beyond formal education)
- Informal personal education participation

Work
- Employment interests and pursuits
- Employment seeking and acquisition
- Job performance
- Retirement preparation and adjustment
- Volunteer exploration
- Volunteer participation

Play
- Play exploration
- Play participation

Leisure
- Leisure exploration
- Leisure participation

Social Participation
- Community
- Family
- Peer

From the American Occupational Therapy Association: Occupational therapy practice framework: domain and process, *Am J Occup Ther* 62:635-637, 2008.

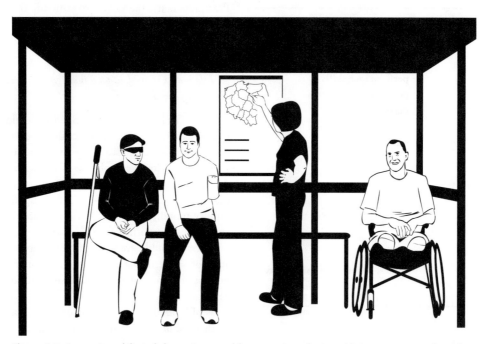

Figure 1-1 Community mobility includes moving around the community and using public transportation, such as a bus. Instrumental activities of daily living is an area of occupation that includes community mobility.

Importantly, the practitioner identifies the **client factors** and **body functions** considered when developing the community mobility group activity. Such factors as impaired attention, memory, or perception may interfere with a person's ability to engage in the activity. Additional client factors are neuromusculoskeletal, sensory and pain, and mental (specific and global) functions. The practitioner may work on multiple client factors within a group session. Understanding the individual's strengths and weaknesses in terms of client factors allows the practitioner to design

TABLE 1-1	Values, Belief, and Spirituality
Category and Definition	**Examples**
Values: Principles, standards, or qualities considered worthwhile or desirable by the client who holds them	**PERSON** ■ Practices honesty with self and with others. ■ Adheres to personal religious convictions. ■ Exhibits commitment to family. **ORGANIZATION** ■ Feels an obligation to serve the community. ■ Practices fairness. **POPULATION** ■ Values freedom of speech. ■ Values equal opportunities for all. ■ Practices tolerance toward others.
Beliefs: Cognitive content held as true	**PERSON** ■ He or she is powerless to influence others. ■ Hard work pays off. **ORGANIZATION** ■ Profits are more important than people. ■ Achieving the mission of providing service can effect positive change in the world. **POPULATION** ■ People can influence government by voting. ■ Accessibility is a right, not a privilege.
Spirituality: The "personal quest for understanding answers to ultimate questions about life, about meaning, and the sacred"[1]	**PERSON** ■ Pursues a daily search for purpose and meaning in one's life. ■ Actions guided by a sense of value beyond the personal acquisition of wealth or fame. **ORGANIZATION AND POPULATION** ■ See "Person" examples related to individuals within an organization and population.

From the American Occupational Therapy Association: Occupational therapy practice framework: domain and process, *Am J Occup Ther*, 62:634, 2008.

appropriate activities. The goal of the group activities is for all participants to benefit. Therefore, the practitioner examines how client factors enable or hinder a person's performance (Table 1-2). For example, the practitioner may modify activities for clients who are unable to read or follow multiple-step directions.

The practitioner determines the individual's goals as well as the group's goals (see Chapters 6 and 7). After determining the goals, the practitioner creates activities to address these needs. **Activity analysis** involves examining the aspects of activities required to carefully plan how to work with clients and help them meet their goals. Spending time doing this provides the practitioner with the information needed to adjust activities quickly during intervention sessions. Therefore, practicing analyzing activity in multiple situations benefits students and practitioners. This text provides numerous examples of activity analyses. Box 1-2 provides a sample analysis for a community mobility group.

The OTPF provides examples and definitions of activity demands that may be used for analyzing activities (Table 1-3). Understanding the activity demands in relationship to the group goals allows practitioners to problem solve prior to leading the group. Preparation and reflection help the practitioner plan and determine if and how tasks may be

modified for specific individuals to meet multiple goals. For example, the practitioner may need to provide bus schedules in large print.

Understanding the **objects** used for an activity helps practitioners decide if the client or group members are able to carry out the activity. One of the objects necessary for bus transportation is the bus schedule. The client who is visually impaired in Lila's community mobility group may also benefit from a portable magnifier.

Practitioners use clinical reasoning and experience to determine if the activity is appropriate to meeting the individual and group goals. For example, when working with children who have handwriting difficulties, the practitioner may decide that paint-by-numbers requires too much fine motor precision and holding a small paint brush will not be successful. After careful review of each individual's occupational profile, Lila may decide that this group of men enjoy working with their hands to complete wood projects such as bird houses.

Practitioners make note of the **space demands** required for activities. The practitioner may decide that space is a limiting factor for a specific activity. For example, some groups do not have access to public transportation and have a fixed space for groups. Practitioners may need to consider if the space requires a large gym, small quiet room, area to walk around, or private

Text continued on page 6

TABLE 1-2 Client Factors: Body Functions and Structures

BODY FUNCTIONS

Categories	Body Functions Commonly Considered by Occupational Therapy Practitioners (Not All-Inclusive)
MENTAL FUNCTIONS (AFFECTIVE, COGNITIVE, PERCEPTUAL)	
Specific Mental Functions	
Higher-level cognition	Judgment, concept formation, metacognition, cognitive flexibility, insight, attention, awareness
Attention	Sustained, selective, and divided attention
Memory	Short-term, long-term, and working memory
Perception	Discrimination of sensations (e.g., auditory, tactile, visual, olfactory, gustatory, vestibular-proprioception), including multisensory processing, sensory memory, spatial, and temporal relationships[2]
Thought	Recognition, categorization, generalization, awareness of reality, logical and coherent thought, and appropriate thought content
Mental functions of sequencing complex movement	Execution of learned movement patterns
Emotional	Coping and behavioral regulation[3]
Experience of self and time	Body image, self-concept, self-esteem
GLOBAL MENTAL FUNCTIONS	
Consciousness	Level of arousal, level of consciousness
Orientation	Orientation to person, place, time, self, and others
Temperament and personality	Emotional stability
Energy and drive	Motivation, impulse control, and appetite
Sleep (physiologic process)	
SENSORY FUNCTIONS AND PAIN	
Seeing and related functions, including visual acuity, visual stability, visual field functions	Detection and registration, modulation, and integration of sensations from the body and environment
	Visual awareness of environment at varying distances
Hearing functions	Tolerance of ambient sounds; awareness of location and distance of sounds such as an approaching car
Vestibular functions	Sensation of securely moving against gravity
Taste functions	Association of taste
Smell functions	Association of smell
Proprioceptive functions	Awareness of body position and space
Touch functions	Comfort with the feeling of being touched by others or touching various textures, such as food
Pain (e.g., diffuse, dull, sharp, phantom)	Localized pain
Temperature and pressure	Thermal awareness
NEUROMUSCULOSKELETAL AND MOVEMENT-RELATED FUNCTIONS	
Functions of Joints and Bones	
Joint mobility	Joint range of motion
Joint stability	Postural alignment (the physiologic stability of the joint related to its structural integrity as compared with the motor skill of aligning the body while moving in relation to task objects)
Muscle power	Strength
Muscle tone	Degree of muscle tone (e.g., flaccidity, spasticity, fluctuating)

TABLE 1-2   Client Factors: Body Functions and Structures—cont'd

Muscle endurance	Endurance
Motor reflexes	Stretch, asymmetrical tonic neck, symmetrical tonic neck
Involuntary movement reactions	Righting and supporting
Control of voluntary movement	Eye-hand-foot coordination, bilateral integration, crossing the midline, fine and gross motor control, and oculomotor (e.g., saccades, pursuits, accommodation, binocularity)
Gait patterns	Walking patterns and impairments such as asymmetric gait, stiff gait. (Note: Gait patterns are considered in relation to how they affect ability to engage in occupations in daily life activities.)
CARDIOVASCULAR, HEMATOLOGIC, IMMUNOLOGIC, AND RESPIRATORY SYSTEM FUNCTIONS	
Cardiovascular system function	Blood pressure functions (hypertension, hypotension, postural hypotension) and heart rate
Hematologic and Immunologic System Function	
Respiratory system function	(Note: Occupational therapy practitioners have knowledge of these body functions and understand broadly the interaction that occurs between these functions to support health and participation in life through engagement in occupation. Some therapists may specialize in evaluating and intervening with a specific function as it is related to supporting performance and engagement in occupations and activities targeted for intervention.)
Additional functions and sensations of the cardiovascular and respiratory systems	Rate, rhythm, and depth of respiration Physical endurance, aerobic capacity, stamina, and fatigability
VOICE AND SPEECH FUNCTIONS	
Voice Functions	
Fluency and rhythm	
Alternative vocalization functions	
DIGESTIVE, METABOLIC, AND ENDOCRINE SYSTEM FUNCTIONS	
Digestive system function	
Metabolic system and endocrine system functions	
GENITOURINARY AND REPRODUCTIVE FUNCTIONS	
Urinary functions	
Genital and reproductive functions	
SKIN AND RELATED STRUCTURE FUNCTIONS	
Skin functions	Protective functions of the skin—presence or absence of wounds, cuts, or abrasions
Hair and nail functions	Repair function of the skin—wound healing
BODY STRUCTURES	
Categories	Examples are delineated in the "Body Structures" section of this table.
Structure of the nervous system Eyes, ears, and related structures Structures involved in voice and speech Structures of the cardiovascular, immunologic, and respiratory systems Structures related to the digestive, metabolic, and endocrine systems Structures related to the genitourinary and reproductive systems Structures related to movement Skin and related structures	(Note: Occupational therapy practitioners have knowledge of body structures and understand broadly the interaction that occurs between these structures to support health and participation in life through engagement in occupation. Some therapists may specialize in evaluating and intervening with a specific structure as it is related to supporting performance and engagement in occupations and activities targeted for intervention.)

From the American Occupational Therapy Association: Occupational therapy practice framework: domain and process, *Am J Occup Ther* 62:635-637, 2008.

BOX 1-2   General Group Activity Analysis: Community Mobility

Group Activity: Learning to take the bus
Goal: Members will be able to take the bus to a community
    destination

Steps
1. Decide on destination.
2. Secure bus schedule.
3. Determine time and location of the bus stop.
4. Get to the bus stop.
5. Pay correct fee.
6. Get off at destination.
7. Identify correct bus and return to take bus back to original location at designated time.
8. Take correct bus back.
9. Return as scheduled.

Preparation
- Decide on destination.
- Gather adequate money for fees.
- Secure bus schedule.
- Determine time and location of the bus stop.

Client Factors
Cognitive
- Read schedule.
- Tell time.
- Understand bus system.
- Count money.

Social
- Interact with others in the community.
- Ask questions if needed.
- Use polite social conversation.
- Understand body space.

Motor
- See the bus schedule.
- Walk to bus stop.
- Climb up stairs onto bus.
- Sit in seat or stand and hold railing.
- Climb down stairs off bus.
- Walk to destination.
- Have endurance for activity (1 hour).
- Motor planning to walk around people and to destination.

Physical and Environmental Contexts
- Uneven side walks
- Many distractions
- Weather
- Unfamiliar location
    Precautions: Members should bring written addresses for the destination, bus schedule, and contact phone numbers in case they get lost. Members who are taking medications may need to avoid sun (or put on sunscreen).

---

setting. They should decide if the activity requires members to navigate within the community. While analyzing the space demands, the practitioner considers the ability of individuals and group members to be successful in these settings.

Often the goal of a group activity is to improve the social participation of members. Understanding the **social demands** of activities is the first step in developing activities to address socialization. Practitioners determine the rules of the interactions, expectations of the activity and other participants, and cultural expectations. For example, the social demands involved in a small game of cards with friends differ from a formal dinner party with strangers. Clients may be comfortable in familiar one-on-one activities with a practitioner, although they are challenged when attending a social event in the community (such as an art fair).

Once the practitioner has determined the activity (often in collaboration with group members), a review of the **sequence and timing** of tasks is required. Understanding the order of each step and the timing involved allows the practitioner to completely understand the activity and use clinical reasoning to determine if the activity can be successfully completed by members in the desired time frame. The practitioner who understands the order of the key tasks is able to lead the group more effectively.

For example, Lila must first help members decide on the destination of the community trip. Members must find a destination that is close enough that they can get there and back within the designated time frame. The destination should be interesting to the members but not require complicated bus changes for this first trip. The group must time how long it will take them to walk to the bus stop and determine how long they will stay

at the destination. Timing and sequencing the steps is key to the success of this activity. Therefore, Lila teaches the group members the order of the steps, reviews it, and asks them to repeat it before they go on the trip. Lila is hoping that engaging members in the planning will help them to do this independently.

Another important component to the activity analysis involves understanding the **required actions** and **performance skills** necessary for the activity. Occupational therapy practitioners become skilled at analyzing all actions and performance skills necessary for clients to successfully engage in purposeful activities and occupations. By understanding the actions required, practitioners are able to modify or adapt activities so members can complete them. Spending time in advance of the group activity, determining the required actions and performance skills, allows practitioners to preplan and decide in which aspects of the activity the members may have difficulty.

OT practitioners examine **client factors** and determine how they support or interfere with a client's ability to complete the required action or performance skill.

For example, a client who exhibits difficulty with endurance may need to take frequent breaks when walking to the bus stop. The client may need extra time for this step or Lila may decide that the member should use a wheelchair in the community. It may be that this member needs to build up his or her endurance by walking more prior to the event. The group may decide to adapt the activity by requiring only a short trip with minimal walking. There are many ways to change the activity to accommodate or remediate for client factors that interfere with the required actions and performance skills necessary (Figure 1-2).

TABLE 1-3 Activity Demands		
Activity Demand Aspects	**Definition**	**Examples**
Objects and their properties	Tools, materials, and equipment used in the process of carrying out the activity	Tools (e.g., scissors, dishes, shoes, volleyball) Materials (e.g., paints, milk, lipstick) Equipment (e.g., workbench, stove, basketball hoop) Inherent properties (e.g., heavy, rough, sharp, colorful, loud, bitter tasting)
Space demands (relates to physical context)	Physical environmental requirements of the activity (e.g., size, arrangement, surface, lighting, temperature, noise, humidity, ventilation)	Large, open space outdoors required for a baseball game Bathroom door and stall width to accommodate wheelchair Noise, lighting, and temperature controls for a library
Social demands (relates to social environment and cultural contexts)	Social environment and cultural contexts that may be required by the activity	Rules of game Expectations of other participants in activity (e.g., sharing supplies, using language appropriate for the meeting)
Sequence and timing	Process used to carry out the activity (e.g., specific steps, sequence, timing requirements)	Steps to make tea: Gather cup and tea bag, heat water, pour water into cup, and so forth. Sequence: Heat water before placing tea bag in water. Timing: Leave tea bag in cup to steep for 2 minutes. Steps to conduct a meeting: Establish goals of meeting, arrange time and location for meeting, prepare meeting agenda, call meeting to order. Sequence: Have people introduce themselves before beginning discussion of topic. Timing: Allot sufficient time for discussion of topic and determination of action items.
Required actions and performance skills	The usual skills that would be required by any performer to carry out the activity Sensory, perceptual, motor, praxis, emotional, cognitive, communication, and social performance skills should each be considered. The performance skills demanded by an activity will be correlated with the demands of the other activity aspects (e.g., objects, space).	Feeling the heat of the stove Gripping the handlebar Choosing the ceremonial clothes Determining how to move limbs to control the car Adjusting the tone of voice Answering a question
Required body fuctions	"[P]hysiological functions of body systems (including psychological functions)"[4] that are required to support the actions used to perform the activity	Mobility of joints Level of consciousness
Required body structures	"Anatomical parts of the body such as organs, limbs, and their components [that support body function]"[4] that are required to perform the activity	Number of hands Number of eyes

From the American Occupational Therapy Association: Occupational therapy practice framework: domain and process, *Am J Occup Ther* 62:635-637, 2008.

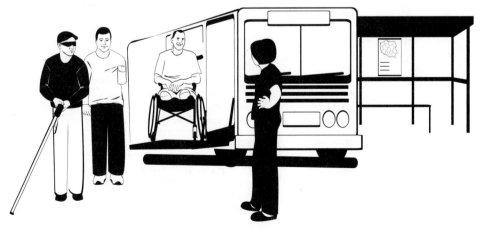

Figure 1-2 The occupational therapy practitioner evaluates how group members will perform an activity such as getting on a bus. Members may need extra time or adaptations (e.g., wheelchair lift) to accomplish the tasks.

Performance skills include motor and praxis, sensory-perceptual, emotional-regulation, cognitive, communication, and social. These skills require a variety of actions and tasks to complete them. See Table 1-4 for definitions and examples of specific performance skills.

Performance skills necessary for active participation in Lila's community mobility group include motor planning to walk around obstacles (e.g., people, things on sidewalks, stairs) and perceptual skills to read the bus schedule and identify the correct bus. Members must be able to communicate with others, including asking the bus driver for change, interacting with people on the bus, and asking for directions if needed. Members must demonstrate emotional-regulation skills by responding to others in an acceptable manner and adhering to social norms.

TABLE 1-4 Performance Skills

Skill	Definition	Examples
Motor and praxis skills	Motor: Actions or behaviors a client uses to move and physically interact with tasks, objects, contexts, and environments[5]; (Includes planning, sequencing, and executing new and novel movements.) Praxis: Skilled purposeful movements[6]; ability to carry out sequential motor acts as part of an overall plan rather than individual acts[7]; ability to carry out learned motor activity, including following through on a verbal command, visual-spatial construction, ocular and oral-motor skills, imitation of a person or an object, and sequencing actions[8,9]; organization of temporal sequences of actions within the spatial context, which form meaningful occupations[1]	Bending and reaching for a toy or tool in a storage bin Pacing tempo of movements to clean the room Coordinating body movements to complete a job task Maintaining balance while walking on an uneven surface or while showering Anticipating or adjusting posture and body position in response to environmental circumstances, such as obstacles Manipulating keys or lock to open the door
Sensory-perceptual skills	Actions or behaviors a client uses to locate, identify, and respond to sensations and to select, interpret, associate, organize, and remember sensory events based on discriminating experiences through a variety of sensations that include visual, auditory, proprioceptive, tactile, olfactory, gustatory, and vestibular	Positioning the body in the exact location for a safe jump Hearing and locating the voice of your child in a crowd Visually determing the correct size of a storage container for leftover sound Locating keys by touch from many objects in a pocket or purse (i.e., stereognosis) Timing the appropriate moment to cross the street safely by determining one's own position and speed relative to the speed of traffic Discerning the distinct flavors in foods or beverages
Emotional regulation skills	Actions or behaviors a client uses to identify, manage, and express feelings while engaging in activities or interacting with others	Responding to the feelings of others by acknowledgment or showing support Persisting in a task despite frustrations Controlling anger toward others and reducing aggressive acts Recovering from a hurt or disappointment without lashing out at others Displaying the emotions that are appropriate for the situation Using relaxation strategies to cope with stressful events
Cognitive skills	Actions or behaviors a client uses to plan and manage the performance of an activity	Judging the importance or appropriateness of clothes for the circumstance Selecting tools and supplies needed to clean the bathroom Sequencing tasks needed for a school project Organizing activities within the time required to meet a deadline Prioritizing steps and identifying solutions to access transportation Creating different activities with friends that are fun, novel, and enjoyable Multitasking—doing more than one thing at a time, necessary for tasks such as work, driving, and household management
Communication and social skills	Actions or behaviors a person uses to communicate and interact with others in an interactive environment[5]	Looking where someone else is pointing or gazing Gesturing to emphasize intentions Maintaining acceptable physical space during conversation Initiating and answering questions with relevant information Taking turns during an interchange with another person, verbally and physically Acknowledging another person's perspective during an interchange

From the American Occupational Therapy Association: Occupational therapy practice framework: domain and process, *Am J Occup Ther* 62:635-637, 2008.

Along with the previously described demands, practitioners consider the members' body functions and **body structures** when determining how a member will perform in a given activity. *Body functions* include such things as mobility of joints and level of consciousness, whereas *body structures* include the number of hands and body parts.

Lila considers body functions of the members by determining how quickly members walk, move, and respond to verbal directions. She considers their awareness and attentiveness to their surroundings. Furthermore, Lila also considers that two members are amputees and they must use wheelchairs to be mobile. However, these members are adept at maneuvering through obstacles and thus will benefit from learning that public transportation is accessible to them.

The practitioner considers the **performance patterns** of the person, organization, and population. This includes the members' habits, routines, rituals, and roles. The practitioner considers what the person does daily and the sequence of behaviors. Understanding members' roles (e.g., mother, father, worker) helps practitioners design meaningful activities.

The **context** and **environment** in which the activity occurs are central to the analysis. The OTPF describes six contexts: cultural, personal, temporal, virtual, physical, and social (Table 1-5). Practitioners consider the culture of the client and activity. For example, the demands of the activity may differ if it is performed as part of one's culture. Cooking a special holiday meal may hold more meaning for clients than making an everyday meal. The requirements to perform may change when the activity is part of one's culture. The following example highlights the role of contexts.

Lila examines the contexts of her group activity, realizing that this may place additional demands on group members. For the first trip into the community, the group agreed to go to a local coffee shop that requires no bus transfers.

Cultural: *The coffee shop is quiet and slow paced. Many retired veterans frequent this coffee shop, and the owners are kind and supportive. Patrons are allowed to spend time in the shop. There are comfortable couches and reading materials available. Local college students also frequent this coffee shop. The atmosphere is relaxed and comfortable.*

Personal: *Some of the group members are familiar with the setting. Others are open to the new experience. Some members have used the bus system in the past but others have never tried. They prefer driving (although many have no license or car). Some members are reluctant about this form of transportation,*

Temporal: *All members are retired veterans who are 65 to 80 years old and are living in the community.*

Virtual: *Members are reluctant to use computers, although the bus schedule is available to them on the computer. Computers are available to them at the coffee shop and day treatment center. There is no virtual aspect to this activity because members will use printed schedules (enlarged print).*

Physical: *Members must have 1½ hours of endurance for activity. They must walk to and from the bus stop (approximately 1½ mile total) with frequent breaks. They must move around objects and people and climb stairs as needed. Members*

must be able to walk on uneven surfaces. Once at the coffee shop, they must be able to bring their hand to their mouth to eat and drink.

Social: *Members must be able to engage in light conversation with peers, ask directions, and show socially acceptable behaviors in the community. Once at the coffee shop, members may sit quietly with one or two peers.*

OCCUPATIONAL ANALYSIS

Completing an occupational analysis using the OTPF as a guide involves considering the activity demands associated with an occupation. **Occupations** are the activities in which people find meaning and provide them identity. Consequently, occupations differ among people. For example, Nancy enjoys gardening. She spends time on the weekend looking for new plants and reads up on the gardening tips. She attends workshops and enjoys receiving plants for gifts. Her house holds contains many gardening references, such as a beautiful gardening calendar. During breaks at work, Nancy talks to others about her latest gardening adventure. Nancy defines herself as a "gardener." For Nancy, gardening is an occupation (Figure 1-3).

Kristin, on the other hand, enjoys having flowers surrounding her house. She weeds her flower beds begrudgingly. She knows she needs to weed and water her flowers to have the beautiful flowers and make her home look nice. However, she completes the gardening activities for the end product alone. For Kirstin, gardening is a **purposeful activity** in that it allows her to enhance her sense of "home." Purposeful activities help individuals develop skills that assist them in occupational engagement[13].

Margo has suffered a mild stroke and is unable to use her right hand. Because she was an avid gardener prior to the injury, the practitioner decides to help Margo return to gardening. Before engaging in purposeful activity, Margo needs to begin to use her right hand as an assist. The practitioner provides some **preparatory methods** to help her regain function, consisting of range of motion, applying an orthosis, and hand-over-hand assistance. Following the preparatory activities, Margo plants herb seeds in small containers for her window garden. (Figure 1-4).

The practitioner begins by determining the occupation or activity that will help a group member achieve the desired occupational goal. This involves getting to know the person and his or her identity. Understanding what someone values is key to successful occupational therapy intervention.[14] Some important questions to consider include:

- What gives you meaning?
- How do you spend your days?
- What types of activities do you enjoy?
- How would you describe yourself?
- What types of things make you excited?
- What would you like to get back to doing?
- What would you like to accomplish in therapy?

Appendix 1 in the back of the book provides a sample template of an occupational analysis based on the OTPF.

TABLE 1-5	Contexts	

Context and Environment	Definition	Examples
Cultural	*Cultural* context includes customs, beliefs, activity patterns, behavior standards, and expectations accepted by the society of which the client is a member. Includes ethnicity and values as well as political aspects, such as laws that affect access to resources and affirm personal rights. Also includes opportunities for education, employment, and economic support	**PERSON** ■ Shaking hands when being introduced **ORGANIZATION** ■ Employees marking the end of the work week with casual dress on Friday **POPULATION** ■ Celebrating Independence Day
Personal	*Personal* context refers to "features of the individual that are not part of a health condition or health status."[4] Personal context includes age, gender, socioeconomic status, and educational status. Can also include organizational levels (e.g., volunteers and employees) and population levels (e.g., members of society).	**PERSON** ■ 25-year-old unemployed man with a high school diploma **ORGANIZATION** ■ Volunteers working in a homeless shelter **POPULATION** ■ Teenage women who are pregnant or new mothers
Temporal	*Temporal* context refers to "location of occupational performance in time"[10] and the experience of time as shaped by engagement in occupations. The temporal aspects of occupation that "contribute to the patterns of daily occupations" are "the rhythm . . . tempo . . . synchronization . . . duration . . . and sequence."[11,12] Includes stages of life, time of day or year, duration, rhythm of activity or history.	**PERSON** ■ A person retired from work for 10 years **ORGANIZATION** ■ Annual fundraising campaign **POPULATION** ■ Engaging in siestas or high teas
Virtual	*Virtual* context includes the environment in which communication occurs by means of airways or computers and an absence of physical contact. Includes simulated or real-time or near-time existence of an environment via chat rooms, e-mail, video conferencing, radio transmissions.	**PERSON** ■ Text message to a friend **ORGANIZATION** ■ Video conference, telephone conference call, instant message, interactive whiteboards among all the members **POPULATION** ■ Virtual community of gamers
Physical	*Physical* context includes natural and manufactured nonhuman environments and the objects in them: Natural environment includes geographic terrain, sensory qualities of environment, plants, and animals. Manufactured environment and objects include buildings, furniture, tools, or devices.	**PERSON** ■ Individual's house, apartment **ORGANIZATION** ■ Office building, factory **POPULATION** ■ Transportation system
Social	The *social* context is constructed by presence, relationships, and expectations of persons, organizations, populations. Includes availability and expectations of significant individuals, such as spouse, friends, and caregivers; relationships with individuals, groups, or organizations; relationships with systems (e.g., political, legal, economic, institutional) that are influential in establishing norms, role expectations, and social routines.	**PERSON** ■ Friends, colleagues **ORGANIZATION** ■ Advisory board **POPULATION** ■ City government

From the American Occupational Therapy Association: Occupational therapy practice framework: domain and process, *Am J Occup Ther* 62:635-637, 2008.

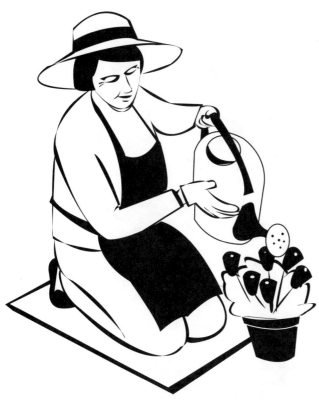

Figure 1-3 Nancy enjoys gardening. She spends time planning her garden, discusses it with friends, and finds it rewarding. For Nancy, gardening is an occupation.

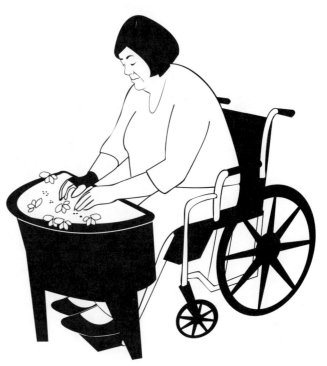

Figure 1-4 Margo likes to have flowers around her home. She is proud of her decorating. For Margo, gardening is an activity.

GROUP PROCESS

A group consists of two or more people who meet to address a specific task or goal. In occupational therapy, groups are formed to address intervention goals. Members are generally grouped according to those with similar goals. Often this means that members have similar issues (such as motor, psychological, or cognitive processes). Members may share similar experiences (e.g., veterans, mothers, school-aged children). They may be of a similar age cohort (e.g., children, teens, adults, older adults). Groups may be formed according to specific diagnoses (e.g., stroke, hip fracture, arthritis).

The occupational therapy (OT) practitioner may elect to lead a group session as a way to facilitate interaction among members or to help members find support from each other. Group sessions may help members learn from each other. The positive experience from group relationships helps members achieve success. Group interactions and relationships form when members work together to achieve tasks. This often results in creative solutions and more productivity. Groups may allow practitioners to work with multiple clients in an effective way.

Practitioners carefully design groups to benefit all clients. Thus, practitioners must understand the stages and types of groups possible. Chapters 8 through 11 in this text provide suggestions on how to facilitate the group process across the lifespan.

STAGES OF GROUPS

Each group progresses through different stages. Tuckman[15,16] theorized five stages of group development: forming, storming, norming, performing, and adjourning. The OT practitioner generally leads the groups, but in certain situations the practitioner may allow a group member to take the lead. This may be particularly helpful in psychosocial group sessions as a way to enable members to assert leadership skills.

When **forming** a group, the practitioner may invite participants or select members based on their goals.[15,16] For example, the practitioner may decide to conduct a prewriting group with children or explore leisure opportunities with teens. A practitioner may design a group for persons who have psychosocial issues by grouping a variety of clients who are trying to become more independent in the community. Other groups may focus on living skills such as cooking meals, eating healthy, and developing healthy habits (Figure 1-5). When forming groups practitioners consider:

- Group and individual goals
- Ages, genders, characteristics of members
- Common interests of members
- Settings of groups
- Contexts (cultural, personal, temporal, physical, social, virtual)
- Needs of members
- Strengths and weaknesses of individuals
- Number of members
- Types of possible activities
- Duration

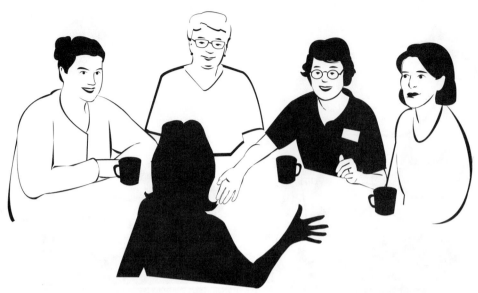

Figure 1-5 During the forming stage, the occupational therapy practitioner explains the purpose of the group to participants.

- Associated costs
- Personnel needed
- Length of membership and how it is established

Once the group is formed and the membership established, the practitioner develops an agenda for meetings and activities that fit the group goals.[15,16] The practitioner may decide to ask the group to develop the agenda in the **storming** stage (Box 1-3 and Figure 1-6). This is an effective way to establish the rules and allow members to resolve conflict. The OT practitioner helps the group negotiate and work through differences respectfully. During this stage, members may need redirection and information to stay on course.[15,16] They may need to be reminded of the rules. Practitioners may need to engage members in values clarification exercises or trust activities.

During the **norming** stage, the group engages in activity together and begins to feel an identity. Members divide responsibilities and begin to cooperate to produce results.[15,16] The practitioner may help group members contribute to the success of the group, develop skills in areas in which they are weak, and engage in the group process equally. The OT practitioner may have to delegate responsibilities to those members who may not be engaging completely. Sometimes giving members extra responsibilities or chores may be enough to help them engage and feel more identity in the group.

This feeling allows the group to **perform** and accept one another. At this point, the group members work together and begin to realize group and individual goals.[15,16] The OT practitioner may have to encourage members to perform together. During this stage, members who have physical limitations may require assistance in performing tasks. Members with psychosocial limitations may require support and guidance to continue to perform. Practitioners remain aware of the physical, psychosocial, or cognitive difficulties members face and provide necessary activity modifications to ensure success of all members within the group context.

> **BOX 1-3   Developing a Group Agenda**
>
> An effective way to develop an agenda for a psychosocial day treatment group is to present the group with a variety of activities (books, flyers, community events) and ask the group to prioritize activities. This allows members to take ownership of the events and engage in the planning. Planning activities provides members with important life skills and facilitates problem solving and community independence.

Group members may **adjourn** at different times, depending on the groups. Some members leave as they meet their goals, move on to different groups, or no longer benefit from the group. The practitioner helps members deal with possible sadness from leaving the group and helps remaining group members experience feelings of closure.[15,16]

TYPES OF GROUPS

OT groups are designed to address goals. Therefore, the groups include members who may be working toward similar outcomes. Perhaps the most common type of OT group is the **task group**. Task groups have specific outcomes and tasks to be accomplished. Task groups may include cooking groups with the goal of teaching members how to prepare low-cost meals, community mobility groups teaching members how to get around the community, or teen support groups with the task of helping teens find positive role models. Some task groups allow members to complete projects, such as a children's group that makes a craft item for Mother's Day.

Functional groups are created to accomplish specific goals within an unspecified time frame.[2] A functional OT group includes a publicity group or fundraising group. These groups serve a purpose to the institution.

Interest groups are formed around common interests. These informal groups may include support groups, such as veteran's

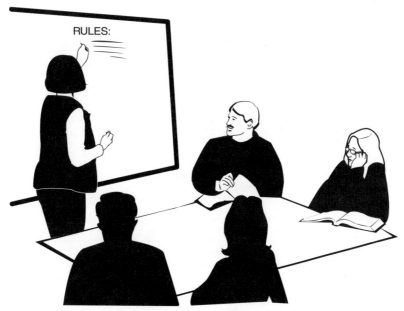

Figure 1-6 Group members try to determine the rules and expectations of the group during the storming phase.

support groups, parenting groups, or teen groups. Groups may form around leisure interests as well, such as walking groups. Many OT practitioners develop groups to help parents, caregivers, or clients find support around a particular diagnosis.

GROUP STRUCTURE

The *structure* of a group refers to the size, roles, norms, and cohesiveness. Group size may vary from two or more. OT practitioners generally prefer smaller groups so that they can assist clients more easily in reaching their individual goals. Depending on the needs of the group, practitioners may require extra help when leading groups. Group size affects participation and satisfaction.

The roles of group members can be divided into worker roles, maintenance roles, and blocking roles.[15,16] **Worker roles** include initiator, informer, clarifier, summarizer, and reality tester (Box 1-4). **Maintenance roles** are important to the group because they help members commit to the group and stay involved. **Blocking roles** are disruptive to the group process and include aggressor, blocker, dominator, comedian, and avoidance behaviors (Box 1-5). These members resist group ideas, interrupt others, and can be manipulative.

The norms of the group are the established guidelines and expectations for behaviors. OT practitioners often begin groups by establishing the rules and expectations. This helps members organize their behavior and address the tasks and functions of the group. The **cohesiveness** of the group refers to how the members bond or interact. Understanding how members contribute to the group helps the practitioner change the activity to facilitate different roles. For example, asking someone who acts as an "initiator" to allow someone else to contribute before stepping in changes the group dynamics and may empower another member. The OT practitioner can try to encourage those who are "blocking" by asking them to take the lead periodically.

BOX 1-4 **Worker Roles**[2,9]

- Initiator—Takes the lead, volunteers first, tries to organize group.
- Informer—Provides information on rules, data, or procedures.
- Clarifier—Makes sense of things for the group, asks questions to make things more understandable.
- Summarizer—Asks for simple conclusions or brief outlines of meetings, findings, or tasks.
- Reality tester—Considers pragmatic aspects of ideas.

BOX 1-5 **Blocking Roles**[2,9]

- Aggressor—Challenges the leader and other group members.
- Blocker—Negative about other's ideas, resists group ideas.
- Dominator—Takes over group, forces his or her ideas on group, does not listen.
- Comedian—Makes jokes instead of getting work done, derails conversations.
- Avoidance behaviors—Manipulates direction of group, changes focus, interrupts process.

CASE APPLICATION

Ingrid is an OT working in a psychosocial day treatment center. She is responsible for helping clients with a variety of psychosocial issues regain independence in the community. Ingrid is new to the position and has been asked to design a month's worth of group activities for the day treatment group.

Background Information: Ingrid begins her task by researching the types of clients who participate in the day treatment center. She finds out that the groups consist of clients with a variety of diagnoses (e.g., bipolar, anxiety disorder, depression, schizophrenia). The clients show no signs of psychosis and are mobile. Most of these clients live in supported

TABLE 1-6 Schedule of Activities for June

		Monday	Tuesday	Wednesday	Thursday	Friday
Week 1		Schedule events	Trip to fresh-air market	Hike	Art museum	Downtown movie
		Gym games	Cooking with fresh food	Board games	Crafts and painting	Project from home (bring in and work on something you want finished)
Week 2		Walk around town	Shopping affordably	Audubon Society	Arts and crafts	Picnic on waterfront
		Budgets	Yoga	Gym games	Yoga	Weekend projects
Week 3		Arts and crafts	Trip to mall	Beauty secrets (grooming, makeovers)	Lunch ideas	Picnic
		Music games	Yoga	Gym games	Yoga	Old-fashioned games
Week 4		Arts and crafts	Help at animal shelter	Transportation: Using the bus	Help at animal shelter	Trip to grocery store
		Music games	Yoga	Gym games	Yoga	Fast and healthy snacks

residential homes. They show poor problem solving and difficulty regulating emotions, and most are unemployed. Many have been involved in the day treatment program in the past. They will attend for at least three months, three days a week. Some clients attend all day, whereas others attend morning or afternoon sessions only. Groups must be arranged for 12 clients. A certified occupational therapy assistant (COTA) will help Ingrid lead the group sessions.

Context: The group sessions will take place in the OT room at the center. The large room houses a round table that seats 15, and there are many arts and crafts activities and supplies. The room has a kitchen area, with sink, stove, oven, and refrigerator. The center has a gym and is close to the downtown area of a small city. Public transportation is easily accessible.

Group Goals: The goals of the day treatment group are to develop independence in community mobility, leisure, and instrumental activities of daily living (IADL; e.g., budgeting, meal management) for clients who have psychosocial difficulties. Morning groups focus on helping clients develop community mobility and leisure skills. Afternoon groups focus on helping clients develop IADL skills, such as home maintenance, budgeting, meal preparation, and socialization.

Development of Group Activities: Ingrid engaged the entire group in the development of the group activities. She began by bringing in last month's schedule and a template of the month. She asked group members to consider the environment and brainstorm activities they might find enjoyable. She brought a variety of catalogs and ideas. Members were informed that they must decide on two activities a day: one in the community and one at the center. Ingrid gave them a tour of the center and described past events.

Format of Group: All 12 group members were present. The members had doctor's orders to attend occupational therapy. The group consisted of four men and eight women; ages ranged from 35 to 70 years old. Diagnoses ranged from schizophrenia, bipolar disorder, depression, anxiety disorder, borderline personality disorder, and obsessive compulsive disorder.

Rules and Expectations: Ingrid reviewed the rules and expectations of the group prior to beginning the session.

Because this was the first meeting, the group members were invited to add rules or expectations. Ingrid asked one member to write down the changes in the rules and expectations and to be reviewed at the following meeting. Allowing members ownership of the rules and expectations early in the process helps them feel that the group belongs to them and may promote feelings of belongingness. The group agreed on the following rules and expectations:

- Be on time to group meetings.
- Be polite with peers.
- Try all activities before refusing them.
- Members who are having a "bad day" will move to a quiet area if they desire.
- Help with set up and clean up.
- Speak softly to one another. No foul language.
- Adhere to the agreed-on schedule.
- Work on agreed-on goals.
- Do not discuss other's issues outside of the group.
- Help each other meet goals.

Sample Group Sessions: After discussion, the group decided on the schedule of activities outlined in Table 1-6. Ingrid reviewed the list and will complete an activity analysis (see Chapter 2) for each activity.

ACTIVITY PREPARATION

Now that the schedule is complete, Ingrid must determine the cost and pragmatics of each activity. She must schedule rooms, space, and order supplies. She must figure out the logistics of transportation and arrange for extra personnel to assist her. The timing of each activity must be calculated so that members can complete the activity in the scheduled times.

Ingrid clearly analyzes the individual's goals to decide how the group activity will enable members to work toward their goals. She clinically reasons how to best facilitate and challenge each member to succeed. This requires that she completely understand each member's strengths and weaknesses. She hypothesizes how members may respond to each other. It may be that some members work well in one-on-one sessions, but become overwhelmed in group sessions. Furthermore, Ingrid remains aware of changes in members' status because this may influence their behavior in the group. Careful observation and experience reading people's nonverbal and verbal cues can prove beneficial for group work.

Ingrid must secure all materials for each activity. Gathering needed materials can also be the activity. For example, the group will be going to the grocery store one morning and preparing healthy snacks in the afternoon. Encouraging group members to participate in preplanning teaches them how to plan, organize, and carry out activities.

The OT practitioner evaluates how each member functions and progresses toward his or her individual goals. The practitioner may need to prepare members differently for each activity. For example, a practitioner may review "appropriate" social behaviors

with a client prior to going into the community. The member may need close supervision during a community outing or activity at the center. The OT practitioner preplans for these types of events and observes clients during the events (see Chapter 14).

SUMMARY

Occupational analysis and group process are key elements to occupational therapy practice. The OTPF helps practitioners structure activity analysis for intervention when working with individuals and groups. This chapter provides an overview of group process, including the stages and types of groups. A case application illustrates the complexities of occupational analyses and the dynamic nature of groups. Activity analysis is presented in Chapter 2.

REVIEW QUESTIONS

1. What are the areas of occupation delineated in the OTPF?
2. How does a client's values, beliefs, and spirituality affect the active participation in group activities?
3. What is activity analysis? How is activity analysis used by OT practitioners in the occupational therapy process?
4. What are performance skills?

5. What are the differences among preparatory activities, purposeful activities, and occupations?
6. What are the stages and types of groups?
7. What roles can group members assume?
8. How does a practitioner prepare for group activities?

REFERENCES

1. Blanche EI, Parham LD: Praxis and organization of behaviour in time and space. In Smith Roley S, Blanche EI, Schaaf RC, editors: *Understanding the nature of sensory integration with diverse populations*, San Antonio, TX, 2002, Therapy Skill Builders, pp 183–200.
2. Calvert G, Spence C, Stein BE, editors: *The handbook of multisensory processes*, Cambridge, MA, 2004, MIT Press.
3. Schell BAB, Cohn ES, Crepeau EB: Overview of personal factors affecting performance. In Crepeau EB, Cohn ES, Schell BAB, editors: *Willard and Spackman's occupational therapy*, ed 11, Baltimore, 2008, Lippincott Williams & Wilkins, pp 650-657.
4. World Health Organization: *International classification of functioning, disability, and health (ICF)*, Geneva, 2001, World Health Organization.
5. Fisher A: Overview of performance skills and client factors. In Pendleton HM, Schultz-Krohn, W: *Pedretti's occupational therapy: practice skills for physical dysfunction,* St Louis, Elsevier, pp 372-402, 2011.

6. Heilman KM, Rothi LJG: *Clinical neuropsychology*, ed 3, New York, 1993, Oxford University Press.
7. Leipmann H: *Apraxie: ergebnisse der gesamten medizin* 1:516-543, 1920.
8. Ayres AJ: *Developmental dyspraxia and adult onset apraxia*, Torrance, CA, 1985, Sensory Integration International.
9. Filley CM: *Neurobehavioral anatomy*, Boulder, CO, 2001, University of Colorado Press.
10. Neistadt ME, Crepeau FB, editors: *Willard and Spackman's occupational therapy*, ed 9, Philadelphia, 1998, Lippincott Williams & Wilkins, p 292.
11. Larson E, Zemke R: Shaping the temporal patterns of our lives: the social coordination of occupation, *J Occup Sci* 10:80-89, 2004.
12. Zemke R: Time, space, and the kaleidoscopes of occupation (Eleanor Clarke Slagle Lecture), *Am J Occup Ther* 58:608-620, 2004.

13. American Occupational Therapy Association: Occupational therapy practice framework: domain and process, *Am J Occup Ther* 62:625-683, 2008.
14. Kielhofner G: *Model of human occupation: theory and application*, ed 4, Philadelphia, 2008, Lippincott Williams & Wilkins.
15. Smith MK, Bruce W: *Tuckman: forming, storming, norming and performing in groups, The encyclopaedia of informal education*, http://www.infed.org/thinkers/tuckman.htm.
16. Tuckman BW: Citation classic: developmental sequence in small groups, *Current Concerns*, http://www.garfield.library.upenn.edu/classics1984/A1984TD25600001.pdf.

2 Activity Analysis

Jane Clifford O'Brien

KEY TERMS

activity	grading
activity analysis	Model of Human Occupation
activity configuration	(MOHO)
activity match	occupations
activity synthesis	psychosocial aspects
adapting	tasks
biomechanical approach	therapeutic media
cognitive aspects	

OBJECTIVES

1. Describe the process of activity analysis.
2. Describe the process of activity configuration and activity synthesis.
3. Discuss the process of activity match.
4. Differentiate between *occupation, activity,* and *tasks.*
5. Compare and contrast a variety of activity analyses.
6. Discuss how Model of Human Occupation (MOHO) theory helps practitioners conduct activity analyses.
7. Identify a variety of therapeutic media and how they are used in practice.
8. Identify ways to "grade" and adapt activities.

Activity analysis is central to occupational therapy (OT) practice. Practitioners use knowledge of the steps and actions required to perform activities to design interventions for a variety of clients. Practitioners evaluate the specific steps, movements, and processes involved in an activity so they can help clients compensate, remediate, or adapt to be successful. The process of activity analysis is ongoing throughout intervention; OT practitioners continually grade or change the activity requirements to help clients engage in their desired occupations. This chapter provides a description of activity analysis and the process of activity configuration and synthesis. A review of types of activity analyses, including task-focused, biomechanical, and Model of Human Occupation (MOHO), is presented. The chapter concludes by describing the use of therapeutic media in activities and grading and adapting activities.

OVERVIEW OF THE PROCESS OF ACTIVITY ANALYSIS

OT practitioners use activity to help clients regain function for their occupations. By thoroughly understanding all the steps, actions, and skills required to complete a given activity, practitioners clinically reason how they might adapt or change the demands for a given client. This process is ongoing. As clients develop skills and abilities, the practitioner adjusts the activity demands for success. Designing activities that challenge clients allows them to be successful without overwhelming them. Sometimes the practitioner wants to show the client that he or she can be successful and enjoy past activities. In this case, the practitioner may decide to adapt the activity completely so that the person is able to engage in this familiar pastime.

CASE STUDY

For example, Juan enjoyed fishing with his family before he had a stroke (Figure 2-1). His motivation for therapy is low and he does not seem invested in group activities. The practitioner, Raven, decides to help Juan take a field trip with his family (on the hospital grounds) to a small fishing pond. Prior to the event, Raven analyzes the activity and decides that Juan will need to use an adapted fishing pole and a supported seat, and will require help getting the bait on the hook. Raven concludes that Juan should participate in the activity in the morning when he is rested (and the fish are jumping). She reviews the steps with Juan and his son. As an added touch, Raven brings a camera and takes a photo

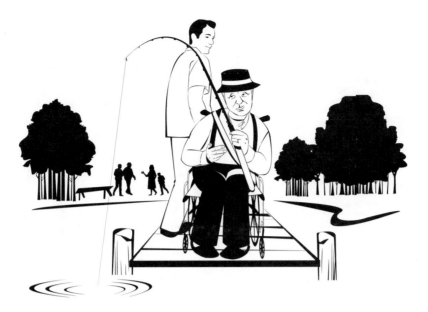

Figure 2-1 Juan is able to enjoy fishing using an adapted pole and sitting in his wheelchair at an accessible dock.

of Juan and his family and their "catch." She posts the photo in Juan's room to remind him of the event. In therapy, they discuss how the activity went and decide to continue to work on his motor skills for fishing. Her careful analysis of the activity and its demands allowed her to make the adaptations needed so that Juan could be successful.

By thoughtfully analyzing the activity of fishing, the OT practitioner is able to make appropriate accommodations and plans so the client can be successful. On another day, the practitioner works with the client to improve his ability to hold objects. As Juan increases his ability to effectively hold objects in his right hand, the practitioner reasons that he will be better able to fish without the use of the adapted pole. This activity is close to the occupation of fishing, which Juan enjoyed with his family prior to his stroke. By reminding Juan (through the picture) that he may be able to reengage in this familiar past-time, the practitioner is helping to motivate him to continue with therapy and reestablish his identity. Understanding the demands of the activity through activity analysis sets the stage for many aspects of the OT intervention.

The process of activity analysis allows practitioners to consider many elements of the activities. For example, the practitioner considers the motor tasks involved in each step. When examining the requirements, the practitioner contemplates how the individual will perform each step and often questions:

- Are there aspects of the activity that may be motorically difficult for the client?
- How does the person's sight, hearing, and sensory processing influence the movement?
- Does the activity require endurance?
- How long does the person need to stand or sit?
- Are there alternative ways to motorically perform the activity?

The practitioner examines the **cognitive aspects** of the activity and determines how things may need to be changed

BOX 2-1   Analysis of Cognitive Skills
Judging distance, location, force   **Selecting** items, choosing preferences   **Identifying** materials and supplies   **Counting** items as needed   **Organizing** materials and process to meet deadlines   **Problem solving** how to arrange items, make corrections   **Using** materials and supplies in intended manner   **Sequencing** steps for success   **Prioritizing** time for each step   **Understanding** the relationships of items or persons   **Being aware** of safety issues and foreseeing possible difficulties

for success (Box 2-1). For example, the practitioner explores how the directions are relayed to the client.

- Will the client have to read?
- Are there multiple steps to the directions?
- Does this activity require a high or low degree of concentration?
- How much problem solving is required?
- What is the level of difficulty of the activity?
- Can the directions be demonstrated?
- What might interfere with the client's ability to comprehend the activity demands?

Practitioners also consider the **psychosocial aspects** to activities (Box 2-2). Understanding the client's previous level of performance is important in determining the acceptable performance level for the activity. For example, if the client was a professional dancer prior to the injury, he or she may feel it is condescending to be asked to learn a few dance steps. Other clients may enjoy this activity as a way to reengage in leisure. The OT practitioner uses the process of activity analysis to explore all angles of the activity to be sure it is the right fit for the client. This process includes both the science and art of therapy. The science of therapy involves understanding the components and parts of activities, such as range of motion

---

BOX 2-2 | **Psychosocial Skills Considered for Activity**

Responding to other's questions and requests
Reading cues from others
Persisting with the activity to completion
Controlling one's frustration level
Displaying satisfaction or pleasure with product
Coping with changes in activity
Problem solving to complete activity
Recovering from disappointment
Listening and responding to feedback
Engaging in conversation appropriate to setting
Relaxing and engaging in process
Responding to others

BOX 2-3 | **Occupational Profile**

Name of client:
Reason for seeking services:
Concerns related to occupational therapy:
   Why are you here?
   What do you find meaningful in your life?
Client's goals (what would you like to do differently?):
   Describe your priorities.
   What do you enjoy doing?
   What would you like to learn in occupational therapy?
Describe your life experiences.
   What types of leisure activities do you like?
   What are your interests?
   What is important to you?
How would you define yourself?
Where do you live and with whom do you interact?

(Adapted from the American Occupational Therapy Association: Occupational therapy practice framework: domain and process, *Am J Occup Ther* 62:650, 2008.)

or movement required to perform. The art of therapy requires understanding how to deliver the directions, work with the client, and use one's self therapeutically (see Chapter 4).

STEPS TO ACTIVITY ANALYSIS

OT practitioners engage in activity analysis to identify goals and to develop intervention plans. As such, activity analysis is an important tool for OT practitioners. The following steps describe the process involved:

- Understand the client's story (occupational profile).
- Define the client's goals and objectives.
- Describe the elements of the activity (activity configuration).
- Develop activities that match the client's needs (activity synthesis).
  - Modify and adapt activity to match needs

Understand the Client's Story: The Occupational Profile

Understanding the client's story is the first step in designing effective intervention and conducting an activity analysis. This involves gathering information on the types of occupations in which the person has interest, routines, roles, family history, and medical history. Understanding the client's desires and motivations (or what Kielhofner[6] terms *volition*) is essential when designing individualized intervention. The occupational profile provides the first step in the activity analysis process. See Box 2-3 for sample questions that help to gain information for an occupational profile.[1]

Define the Client's Goals and Objectives

After developing an understanding of the client through the occupational profile and an initial evaluation, the practitioner works with the client to define the goals and objectives for therapy. The goals and objectives may be specific to the setting in which the client is receiving intervention. Developing goals that are occupation-based ensures that the client will be invested in the outcomes.[2,5,7,8] Consequently, practitioners are most effective when they develop occupation-based goals. The following questions may help practitioners develop these goals:

- What would you like to accomplish before you leave?
- What types of activities did you do before coming here?
- What provides you with meaning in your life?
- What are the three most important things to you?
- What types of things would you like to do when you leave?
  Once the client answers these questions, the practitioner decides on specific goals and objectives for therapy. After

drafting some samples, the practitioner often shares these with the client to get feedback on how well these goals meet the client's needs. By observing the client's expression as he or she hears the goal, practitioners can determine if the client believes the goal is meaningful and appropriate. Asking the client for feedback and adjusting the goal to represent that feedback encourages "buy-in" from the client, which suggests better follow through and motivation.[3,5-7] (See Chapter 7 for more details on documentation of individual goals.)

OCCUPATIONAL THERAPY CONCEPTS OF OCCUPATION, ACTIVITY, AND TASK

OT practitioners work to help clients return to their occupations.

- **Occupations** are the meaningful and everyday things in which people engage that give them meaning and identity.[1] Occupations are defined by the person. These events are important to one's sense of self.
- **Activity** is purposeful and meaningful, but it may not be central to one's identity. Activity frequently results in an end product. People engage in a variety of activities each day.
- **Tasks** are the basic actions required to complete activities or occupations.

The following example differentiates between *occupation, activity,* and *task.*

CASE STUDY

Kara loves to run. She runs every day rain or shine. She buys the newest running shoes and clothes and searches for new trails. Kara enjoys finding new routes. She travels to different locations to run and enjoys running in local races. She eats well and goes to bed early so she can run in the morning. When traveling, she seeks running routes. When she misses a run, Kara feels like something is "missing" in her day (Figure 2-2).

For Kara, running is an occupation because it gives her meaning and she identifies herself as a "runner." This occupation holds certain expectations and responsibilities. The activities that help her achieve this occupation include buying

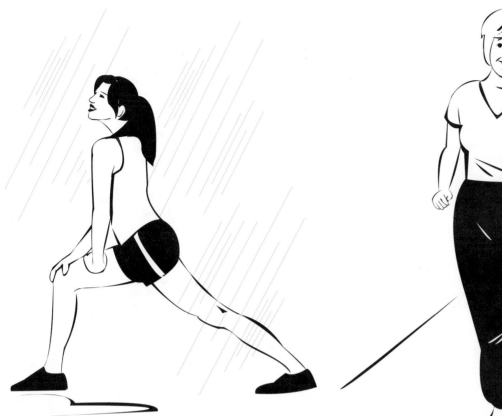

Figure 2-2 For Kara, running is an occupation in which she finds identity.

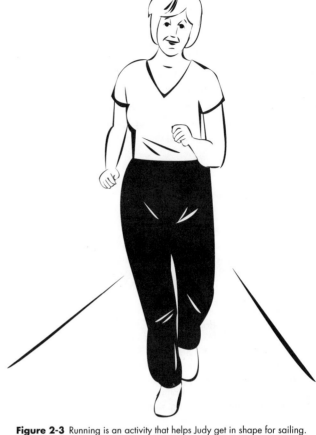

Figure 2-3 Running is an activity that helps Judy get in shape for sailing.

running shoes, signing up for races, and eating well. All these activities support her occupation. The tasks needed for her to accomplish the occupation include postural control, strength, endurance, and flexion and extension of the lower extremities.

CASE STUDY

Judy does not like to run, but she values being in shape for sailing. She is training for a sailing race and decides to run to increase her endurance and strength (Figure 2-3).

For Judy, running is an activity, a way to allow her to be more successful in her occupation of sailing. Judy does not identify herself as a "runner" but rather as a "sailor." In this example, running is a purposeful activity.

OT practitioners analyze occupations, activities, and tasks. Understanding the components allows the practitioner to design effective intervention.

ELEMENTS OF THE ACTIVITY: ACTIVITY CONFIGURATION

Activity configuration refers to designing, arranging, or shaping with a view for use. It includes the arrangement of parts or elements, the way the components are arranged, the steps involved, and the relationships present.[10] Subsequently, activity configuration involves examining the arrangement, parts, components, and relationships between elements in a given task or activity. OT practitioners analyze activity to determine all the steps, actions, contexts, and demands. By understanding the configuration of the activity, the practitioner is able to modify and change steps

or how the tasks are performed so that clients can be successful while working toward their individual goals. Understanding the many parts to an activity allows the practitioner to work with group members effectively. Activity configuration involves analyzing all aspects of the activity (Box 2-4). This is a comprehensive approach to activity analysis. For example, consider all the elements involved in a simple card game (Box 2-5 and Figure 2-4).

Once the practitioner has considered the elements and parts to the activity, the practitioner begins to individualize the activity for specific members. This involves activity synthesis.

ACTIVITIES THAT MATCH THE CLIENT'S NEEDS: ACTIVITY SYNTHESIS

Activity synthesis refers to combining separate elements to form a coherent whole specific to the person[10]. The OT practitioner considers all the elements required in the activity, the client's goals, the contexts of the activity, and the client's strengths and weaknesses, along with knowledge of OT practice, scientific knowledge of the client's condition, and group process when developing activities for an intervention plan. Activity synthesis involves considering all known information to develop the best plan for a client within the given context. Activity synthesis requires that practitioners understand all aspects of the activity and the dynamic nature of practice. Although preparation is key, the practitioner must also observe and intervene during the activity to ensure that all clients are working toward their goals (see Chapter 7).

Activity Match

OT practitioners use their knowledge of clients' performance to design activities to target their selected goals. Understanding the client's motivations, interests and previous habits and routines in the context of his or her environment provides the foundation for matching the activity with the client for successful intervention.[5,6] The **activity match** begins with identifying activity that will interest the client and serve to motivate the client to achieve. Clients will engage in more repetitions of activities they find meaningful or purposeful.[2,3,7,8] Furthermore, research shows that more areas of the brain are stimulated when clients are engaged in meaningful versus rote activities.[11]

Once the practitioner determines the activity for the intervention, the practitioner analyzes the requirements in relation to the client's goals. The practitioner matches the client's

---

BOX 2-4   Activity Configuration

Name: Mr. Smith

Occupational profile summary: Mr. Smith is a 75-year-old veteran who expressed an interest in card playing, bowling, and attending sports events. Mr. Smith is married and enjoys his grandchildren. He has lost complete use of his right side secondary to a stroke, although he is beginning to use his right arm as an assist.

Goals: Mr. Smith will show improved use of his right arm and hand to perform daily activities.

Objectives: Mr. Smith will exhibit 45 degrees of shoulder adduction AROM to use his arm as an assist. Mr. Smith will be able to hold objects in his right hand using a gross grasp.

Suggested activities: Card playing, cooking activities, sports board games, adapted golf game, Wii games

Rationale: Games involving sports may be motivating to Mr. Smith. He also expressed some interest in cooking activities with his wife, and the OT may be able to show him simple tasks he can do with his grandchildren. Mr. Smith can play cards with the men at the VA center or cards with his grandchildren. Therefore, starting with a card game may be the best to engage him quickly in the OT process. Once the OT has engaged him, the activities may involve dressing, feeding, and bathing. The OT practitioner sensed Mr. Smith felt most comfortable with cards versus dressing, feeding, and bathing activities. Furthermore, Mrs. Smith is invested in "caring" for her husband and the practitioner will serve to provide assistance with strategies. The activities promote the goals and objectives (use of the right arm and hand) while considering the individual profile of Mr. Smith.

AROM, Active range of motion; *OT,* occupational therapy; *VA,* United States Department of Veterans Affairs.

BOX 2-5   Activity Analysis: Card Game

Activity:	Card game
Materials:	Deck of cards
Equipment:	Table, chairs, relatively quiet room
Group members:	4 years to adult, depending on type of card game (best with fewer than eight members)
Precautions:	None
Sequence:	1. Decide on card game.
	2. Review rules (written or oral).
	3. Deal the cards.
	4. Follow the rules.
	5. Each member responds.
	6. Game ends when a "winner" emerges.
	7. Return all cards to center, shuffle.
	8. Redeal the cards.
Requirements:	■ Maintain sitting posture in chair.
	■ Bilateral upper extremity: Hold cards, grasp one card at time.
	■ Vision: Must see cards and discriminate numbers.
	■ Cognitive: Understand meaning on the card and how it relates to the game.
	■ Sequence: Identify who is next and how the game progresses.
	■ Socialization: Take turns, manage frustration, interact with peers.
Contexts:	Card game with peers, family members or teaching a card game to a child.
Activity Demands:	■ Posture: Sit upright in chair.
	■ Timing: Wait turn, follow rules.
	■ Endurance: Sit and concentrate for 30 minutes.
	■ Cognition: Decide strategy, play by rules, remember, identify numbers, math skills, remember rules to game.
	■ Social-emotional: Interact with others, take turns, respond to questions.
	■ Motor: Hold cards in hand.

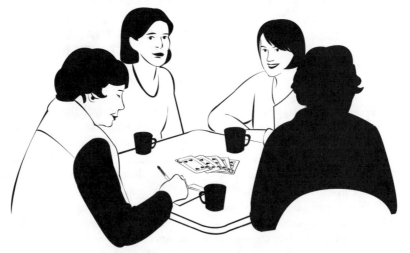

Figure 2-4 Adults may enjoy socializing while playing a card game. This activity helps clients because it requires many skills, such as memory, problem-solving, timing, postural control, bilateral hand use, and social participation.

goals with how the activity will be modified or adapted to best address the individual's needs. In this way, one activity may meet several person's goals when it is adjusted accordingly. This allows for group activities. Addressing multiple individual goals in a group session requires practice and intention (see Chapters 6 and 7).

TYPES OF ACTIVITY ANALYSES

Understanding activity analysis is essential to OT practice. Students complete many types of activity analyses. The process of detailing activity requirements helps students solidify a basic OT skill. This chapter presents three types of activity analyses (occupation, activity, and task-focused; biomechanical; and MOHO) that may be useful while planning OT interventions.

OCCUPATION, ACTIVITY, TASK-FOCUSED

OT practitioners help clients reengage in occupations. Intervention that is occupation-based requires that the client complete the steps in the actual context. For example, baking a birthday cake for a loved one in one's own kitchen is an occupation performed in the natural context. Frequently, the practitioner instead decides to measure the client's ability by engaging him or her in the same activity within a different context. For example, baking a birthday cake in the clinic kitchen is an occupation performed in a simulated context. Whereas baking in one's own kitchen is an occupation, baking in the clinic is an activity. The task or basic actions involved to perform the activity or occupation are often the same.

BOX 2-6 | **Understanding Occupation, Activity, and Task**

Occupation analysis includes examining the contexts, meaning, and steps included in completing the actions. Emphasis is on how performing provides the person with a sense of identity.
Activity analysis refers to examining the steps, sequences, and demands included in completing the actions. Emphasis is placed on the skills required to successfully complete the activity.
Task analysis examines the basic units of action required to complete a given activity.

Practitioners can analyze occupations, activities, and tasks. The analysis involves detailing each of the steps involved. The most basic level of analysis is the task-focused analysis. A task-focused analysis describes the basic actions required to perform each step, such as flexing fingers around the spoon to stir. Box 2-6 provides an overview of the occupation, activity, and task-focused analysis (Figure 2-5).

Activity analysis involves understanding key sequences and steps of activity and determining what is required to complete it. Once a practitioner determines the steps, the practitioner examines the client's abilities to perform these steps (considering motor, cognitive, psychological, and communication requirements).

- Is the client able to stand?
- Is the client able to grasp with two hands?
- Is the client able to hold the cup?
- What is interfering with the client's success?
- How could the activity be made easier or harder?
- How does the client communicate?
- What might be frustrating for the client?
- How will the directions be relayed to the client?

BIOMECHANICAL

OT practitioners are frequently concerned about the **biomechanical** aspects of movement. This includes range of motion, muscle strength, and endurance. A biomechanical analysis details the movements required for a given activity. It details how much strength is needed to perform the activity and the type and amount of endurance. The following scenario illustrates this analysis.

CASE STUDY

Jill recently was diagnosed with carpel tunnel syndrome. Her hand specialist referred her for outpatient OT for intervention. Amy, her assigned OT practitioner, completes the initial evaluation. Jill has 45 degrees of active wrist flexion and 60 degrees of extension. She has 0 degrees of active movement for radial and ulnar deviation (Figure 2-6).

The practitioner, using a biomechanical approach, targets goals to increase active range of motion (AROM) for radial ulnar movement so that the client can perform activities.

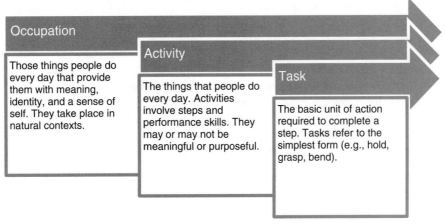

Figure 2-5 Relationship between occupation, activity, and task-focused analysis.

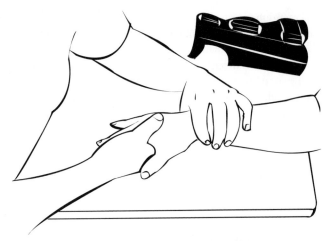

Figure 2-6 Occupational therapy practitioners help clients regain physical range of motion, strength, and endurance to use their hands for activities of daily living.

The practitioner will facilitate AROM of the wrist and adapt activities to help the client succeed. Once AROM has been achieved, the practitioner will focus on strength and endurance for activity.

MODEL OF HUMAN OCCUPATION

Kielhofner[6] conceptualized the **Model of Human Occupation (MOHO)** as a way to organize one's thinking and practice. By understanding clients using this model as a framework, practitioners are able to focus on the occupations that give people meaning. Furthermore, many assessments designed with practitioners have been developed following MOHO theory. It is the most evidence-based model in OT practice.[4,9]

MOHO emphasizes the dynamic nature of individuals and the numerous practice settings. As such, MOHO strives to provide structure and organization to evaluation and intervention so that practitioners can more easily address issues of importance. Kielhofner[6] and colleagues developed easy to administer, flexible, reliable, and valid assessments (Table 2-1). Practitioners use these assessments to understand the client's strengths and weaknesses to develop activities. Furthermore, the assessments clearly describe and operationalize the components of the model, so the process of using the assessments in practice also helps practitioners understand human occupation more clearly.

MOHO acknowledges the dynamic nature of human occupation. The model helps practitioners understand clients in terms of volition, habituation, performance capacity, and environment. Volition includes understanding one's values, interests, and personal causation, and is key to designing occupation-based activity. One's habits, roles, and routines are important when determining OT intervention. *Performance capacity* refers to a person's abilities (physical, social-emotional, or cognitive) and skills needed for the given occupation. Finally, MOHO examines the influence of the environment (considered the space, objects, social, or occupational tasks) in which the occupation occurs.[6]

The following example illustrates how MOHO might inform practice and activity choice.

TABLE 2-1 Model of Human Occupation Assessments

Assessment*	Target Population
Assessment of Communication and Interaction Skills	All
Assessment of Motor and Process Skills	All
Assessment of Occupational Functioning	Adolescents to older adults
Child Occupational Self-Assessment	Children to adolescents
Interest Checklist	Adolescents to older adults
Model of Human Occupation Screening Tool	Adolescents to older adults
NIH Activity Record	Adolescents to older adults
Occupational Circumstances Assessment—Interview and Rating Scale	Adolescents to older adults
Occupational Performance History Interview—II	Adolescents to older adults
Occupational Questionnaire	Adolescents to older adults
Occupational Self-Assessment	Adolescents to older adults
Occupational Therapy Psychosocial Assessment of Learning	Children
Pediatric Interest Profile	Children to adolescents
Pediatric Volitional Questionnaire	Children to adolescents
Role Checklist	Adolescents to older adults
School Setting Interview	Children to adolescents
Short Child Occupational Profile	Children to adolescents
Volitional Questionnaire	Adolescents to older adults
Worker Role Interview	Adults
Work Environment Impact Scale	Adults

NIH, National Institutes of Health.

*Assessments are available through the MOHO Clearinghouse (www.mohoclearinghouse.uic.edu)

CASE STUDY

Maylene is a 21-year-old woman who has experienced a stroke, leaving her right side weak. She completed her sophomore year in a nursing program at a local college. Maylene is showing signs of recovery but she is concerned that she will not be able to continue her education. The OT practitioner in a rehabilitation center decides to use MOHO to organize the intervention.

- **Volition:** Maylene identifies herself as a college student. The practitioner observes many cards with school logos and references, and pictures of college students in Maylene's room. Maylene values her helping role as a nursing student and smiles when she sees a nurse and points to a sign that reads "I love nurses." She also has many pictures of her family in her room and her brother and sister (both younger) visit her every day.
- **Habituation:** Prior to Maylene's stroke, she attended school every day, worked evenings at a local restaurant,

and engaged in many social events with friends. May-lene was a diligent student and responsible worker. She enjoyed nice clothes and was physically active (attending yoga classes three times a week). Maylene visited her family frequently and enjoyed spending time with her younger brother and sister.

- **Performance capacity:** Maylene currently has difficulty speaking since the stroke. She uses her right extremity as an assist and is beginning to bear weight on the right side. Maylene sits leaning to the left. She tires after 30 minutes of activity. She follows multistep directions, but her movements are slow and inaccurate. She was an excellent student, scheduled to begin her junior year in college in the fall.
- **Environment:** When at school, Maylene lives close to her parents. Her mother is a nurse who works part time; her father works at the local paper mill. Her younger brother and sister are both in high school (senior and freshman, respectively). The rehabilitation center is located close to Maylene's college.

Using this information, the practitioner decides to engage Maylene in activities that support her returning to college. As time progresses, the practitioner may help Maylene modify her goals. The practitioner involves Maylene's family in activities and incorporates yoga into sessions. Knowing that Maylene was busy and enjoyed an active lifestyle, the practitioner arranges a busy rehabilitation schedule with many therapists of Maylene's age working with her. This helps Maylene continue to socialize and reinforces her goals.

As they progress in therapy, the practitioner becomes concerned that Maylene may not be able to attend college in the fall. She decides to administer the Occupational Self-Assessment, a MOHO-based assessment that looks at one's performance capacity and values. The practitioner also administers the Interest Checklist to help Maylene consider new interests. Together, they discuss the findings and develop suggestions and strategies suitable for Maylene.

This brief example illustrates how understanding MOHO concepts strengthens the intervention sessions and can help a practitioner determine suitable activities for Maylene. The practitioner considers this information in determining the therapeutic media beneficial for the client.

USE OF THERAPEUTIC MEDIA

Kielhofner writes, "The enjoyment of doing things ranges from the simple satisfaction derived from small daily rituals to the intense pleasure people feel in pursuing their driving passions."[6]

OT practitioners recognize the value of media in helping clients achieve their goals. *Media* refers to the materials and items used in therapy. **Therapeutic media** involves choosing materials and activities that will help the client achieve, regain ability, and perform and learn new skills. OT practitioners use media to help people return to their occupations. The objects and materials used in intervention can help clients return to previous levels of function. The act of interacting with media serves as the intervention. The media selected by practitioners vary and can include arts and crafts, cooking, online games, interactions with others, and exercise.

BOX 2-7   **Properties of Media**

Texture: hard, soft, rough
Consistency: fluid vs. solid
Size: large (requiring two hands to hold) or small (hold in one hand)
Purpose: flexible vs. structured
Shape: spherical, cylindrical, square, triangular
Color
Sensory properties: texture, consistency, color, feel

OT practitioners often use arts and crafts as therapeutic media. Helping clients manipulate and work with media can help clients achieve many goals. Practitioners consider the types of material and requirements needed to work with this material. Understanding the properties of the media is necessary when designing activities for clients (Box 2-7).

GRADING AND ADAPTING ACTIVITY

Practitioners may decide to change the requirements of an activity to help a client be successful or to provide the "just-right" challenge. The "just-right" challenge is one that is neither too easy nor so difficult that it overwhelms a client. The difficulty of an activity can be changed by altering the requirements. **Grading** an activity refers to changing the requirements of the activity by changing the task requirements or steps involved. For example, the practitioner may grade an activity by requiring the client to complete only the last step. In a painting activity, the practitioner may allow the client to paint without any constraints. The activity could be graded to be more difficult by requiring the client to stay within the lines. Requiring that clients do things with greater precision or speed is considered grading an activity. Grading activities is used to provide clients with successful experiences. For example, the practitioner may choose an activity with little precision requirements for a client who is experiencing difficulty with hand skills.

Adapting an activity changes the degree of difficulty by using alternative materials or steps. A practitioner may change the type of medium to allow the client more ease in handling it. For example using thicker paint and a built-up paintbrush may allow the client to succeed. As the client improves hand skills, the practitioner can provide a smaller brush and thinner paint. The practitioner can also grade the activity to make it more challenging by requesting a more detailed painting.

For another client, the practitioner may use painting to explore relaxation strategies. In this case, the practitioner provides warm and soothing colors and a calming environment. The focus of the session is for the client to relax while expressing feelings on paper. This example shows the range of therapeutic intervention that can be accomplished with one activity. Table 2-2 provides examples of how activities can be changed to allow clients to succeed.

All activities start with a purpose or goal. The practitioner must first understand the client and develop goals that show an understanding of the client's needs and developmental stage. By understanding the client's personal story and history,

TABLE 2-2 Adapting and Grading Tasks

Task	Easier	Harder
Grasping objects	Larger objects with better gripping surfaces	Smaller objects with slippery surfaces
Following directions	One-step verbal directions	Multistep written directions
Walking to kitchen or living room	Short distance, no obstacles, rest allowed	Longer distance, obstacles, no rest allowed
Socializing	Small group of familiar people, nonemotional topics	Large group of unfamiliar people, emotional topics
Preparing lunch	Sitting down, all materials placed in front of person, one-on-one supervision, familiar recipe	Client must locate supplies, intermittent supervision, complicated recipe

practitioners are able to match the activity to best address the goals. *Activity match* refers to the process of finding the appropriate activity that allows the client to be successful and motivated. Understanding the client helps the practitioner find interesting and meaningful activities that encourage clients to succeed and challenge themselves. For example, helping a competitive runner who has lost the use of his legs return to a competitive sport (such as adapted sailing, swimming, or wheelchair basketball) allows the athlete to regain a sense of self. The client can return to competition although in a different form. Finding the

activity that fulfills the client is essential to OT practice. Once the practitioner finds the match, the practitioner works with the client to adapt or modify the activity so the client is successful. This may involve changing how the activity is performed, providing the client with specialized equipment to allow success, or changing the activity completely. In the previous example, the client could continue to run competitively through wheelchair racing. The client may decide to experience a new form of competition in wheelchair basketball. The client may decide to modify the activity by using a different wheelchair for racing.

SUMMARY

Activity analysis forms the foundation for OT practice. The process of activity analysis involves activity configuration (determining the components of the activity), activity synthesis (considering all the information to develop an activity plan), and activity match (finding the right activity to meet the client's goals). Understanding the client's story is key to developing client-centered goals and matching activity to specific clients. The OT practitioner carefully analyzes the aspects of activities before determining how they will be used in practice. A variety of activity analyses were presented in this chapter: the occupation, activity, and task-focused approach; biomechanical; and MOHO. Each type of analysis provides practitioners with the tools to understand all aspects of activity for intervention. An overview of therapeutic media and grading and adapting activity are discussed, leading to Chapter 3, which examines therapeutic communication when carrying out group activity.

REVIEW QUESTIONS

1. What are the components of an activity analysis?
2. How do activity configuration, activity synthesis, and activity match relate to each other?
3. What is the difference between *occupation, activity,* and *tasks*?
4. How would a practitioner analyze an occupation in terms of the MOHO analysis? Biomechanical analysis? Or task-focused analysis?
5. How are therapeutic media used in practice?
6. What is meant by *grading* and *adapting activity*?
7. What are some ways activity can be changed to ensure success?

REFERENCES

1. American Occupational Therapy Association: Occupational therapy practice framework: domain and process, *Am J Occup Ther* 62:625-683, 2008.
2. Bakshi R, Bhambhani Y, Madill H: The effects of task preference performance during purposeful and non purposeful activities, *Am J Occup Ther* 45:912-916, 1991.
3. Bloch MW, Smith DA, Nelson DL: Heart rate, activity, duration, and affect in added-purpose versus single-purpose jumping activities, *Am J Occup Ther* 43:25-30, 1989.
4. Haglund L, Ekbladh E, Thorell LH, Hallberg IR: Practice models in Swedish psychiatric occupational therapy, *Scan J Occup Ther* 7:107-113, 2000.
5. Fisher AG: Uniting practice and theory in an occupational framework, *Am J Occup Ther* 52:509-519, 1998.
6. Kielhofner GW: *Model of human occupation,* ed 4, Philadelphia, 2008, Lippincott Williams & Wilkins.
7. Kircher MA: Motivation as a factor of perceived exertion in purposeful versus nonpurposeful activity, *Am J Occup Ther* 38:165-170, 1984.
8. Miller L, Nelson DL: Dual-purpose activity versus single-purpose activity in terms of duration on task, exertion level, and affect, *Occup Ther Ment Health* 7:55-67, 1987.
9. National Board for Certification in Occupational Therapy: A practice analysis study of entry-level occupational therapists registered and certified occupational therapy assistant practice, *OTJR* 24(Suppl 1):S3-S31, 2004.
10. Pickett JP: *American Heritage dictionary of the English language,* ed 4, Boston, MA, 2000, Houghton Mifflin Company.
11. Ray WJ, Cole HW: EEG alpha activity reflects attentional demands, and beta activity reflects emotional and cognitive processes, *Science* 228:750-752, 1985.

Interpersonal Relationships and Communication

Nancy Carson

KEY TERMS

active listening	non-verbal communication
activity groups	norming
adjourning	open group
authoritarian style	participative style
closed group	paternalistic style
democratic style	performing
developmental groups	psychoanalytic groups
evaluation groups	social systems groups
forming	storming
functional group model	task-oriented groups
group protocol	thematic groups
growth groups	topical groups
instrumental groups	verbal communication
involuntary group	voluntary group
laissez faire style	

CHAPTER OBJECTIVES

1. Identify components of communication.
2. Define groups and components of group structure.
3. Identify and give examples of different group models.
4. Identify the stages of group development.
5. Discuss methods of establishing rapport within a group.
6. Explain how to plan and lead an effective occupational therapy group.

The interpersonal relationship and the communication between an occupational therapy practitioner and client are important factors for satisfactory intervention outcomes. Knowing how to treat a client requires more than knowledge of the client's medical diagnosis and treatment protocols; an understanding of personal psychosocial, environmental, cultural, socioeconomic, and occupational factors affecting the client's level of function is also required. The practitioner must be able to communicate effectively to gather this information and a positive interpersonal relationship facilitates the therapeutic process. Good communication is a key factor in establishing the interpersonal relationship. Therapeutic use of self is also an essential element in the interpersonal relationship and will be addressed in Chapter 4.

Increased awareness of the interpersonal communication of the health care provider–client relationship has evolved in recent years. Mutual respect, trust, and collaborative decision-making will result in positive outcomes for the client. Respect, or regard for the client, can be demonstrated to the client through communication that is caring and compassionate; in doing so, trust develops and collaborative decision-making is encouraged. The client needs to know that the health care provider cares and is committed to his or her well-being. Whether providing services individually or within a group context, the occupational therapy practitioner needs to have excellent communication skills for this to occur. Communication can be described by verbal components, nonverbal components, and the use of skills such as active listening. For many clients, just having the opportunity to express their concerns and state their goals in a supportive environment is the most important to them.

COMPONENTS OF COMMUNICATION

Components of **verbal communication** include written and spoken words. In both instances, the practitioner considers the characteristics of the audience. For written communication, the reading and comprehension levels of the reader should be assessed. Plain-language literature suggests that verbal communication be written at a sixth-grade comprehension level. Some clients may be embarrassed at their inability to read and may not wish to disclose this to the practitioner. Careful observation of the client's skills is necessary to ensure that any written information provided to the client is appropriate. Practitioners should consider the use of simple explanations of health information versus medical jargon to ensure understanding in both written and verbal communication. They must be aware of the client's environment and influence of culture, spiritual beliefs, and socioeconomic status. These influences may affect the ways health information and treatment are perceived by the client.

Verbal communication includes formality and complexity of language used, content of the message, tone and volume of voice, and speed and length of presentation. It is generally respectful to initially refer to an adult by his or her last name or professional title unless otherwise instructed by the client. Following the lead of the client in regard to how he or she prefers to be addressed is best in most situations. Assumptions should not be made regarding the level of complexity in verbal communication. When communicating, the language should be simple and direct. Observing the client to assess level of understanding and asking if the client needs clarification can allow for assessment of the level of understanding. Care should be taken to avoid talking down to the client or making the client feel uncomfortable. Content should be concise and clearly express the message that the practitioner is conveying. Providing the client with large amounts of information at one time can be overwhelming. Providing information in short and direct messages increases the likelihood that the client will understand and retain the information. Tone of voice should match the content of the message and be appropriate to the person. Talking to an older adult in a childlike voice is never appropriate. Likewise, talking in a loud voice when not required for the client to hear you can be over stimulating and distressing to clients. Most times, individuals who are hard of hearing do better with a moderate tone of voice and the opportunity to look directly at the practitioner to read lips and nonverbal cues to understand what is being said. The speed of the verbal message is also important. Care should be taken to speak at an average rate. In a busy health care setting it can be easy to speak quickly to move the therapy session along at a faster rate; however, this can result in the client misunderstanding the intended message.

Components of **nonverbal communication** include eye contact, facial expression, and body language such as positioning of self and use of gestures. Looking the client in the eye conveys interest and attention to the conversation. Consistently looking away from the client and demonstrating behaviors such as frequently checking the time indicate a lack of interest and caring. Facial expression should be consistent with the verbal message being provided. Smiling when talking about a serious topic is not appropriate and it does not portray compassion. Body language should be appropriate to the situation as well. Placing your hand on the client's arm when he or she is speaking or providing a hug can be comforting to a client coping with the stress of illness or injury (Table 3-1).

Active listening is another essential component of effective communication. It is through listening to the client that the practitioner becomes aware of the client's goals and concerns. Critical information for effective intervention may be missed if the practitioner fails to engage in active listening. The practitioner must convey to the client a willingness to listen to what the client has to say and allow the client adequate time to express his or her needs and concerns. Strategies for active listening include maintaining eye contact with the other person, use of nonverbal gestures such as nodding your head and smiling appropriately to indicate you are listening, actively avoid distractions, concentrating on what the person is saying instead of other aspects of the person such as appearance or gestures, and avoiding thinking ahead or trying to finish the other person's statements. Asking questions to clarify what the person is saying can be useful as well.

Clinical Pearl

Paraphrasing is an effective way to ensure that active listening has occurred and that an understanding of what the client has said is accurate. The practitioner can summarize the content of the client's message and ask the client if this summary is an accurate understanding of what was said to validate that active listening has occurred.

TABLE 3-1	Components of Communication	*Examples Related to Collage Group with Teenage Girls*		
Verbal Communication	**Examples**	**Nonverbal Communication**	**Examples**	
Tone of voice	Use friendly tone to welcome a new member.	Eye contact	The practitioner makes eye contact with each teen.	
Volume	Lower voice to calm the group.	Facial expression	As one teen starts to use improper language, the practitioner makes a disapproving expression and the teen stops.	
Speed	Slow speech to ensure everyone can follow.	Body positioning	Sitting close to a few teens who are having difficulty paying attention.	
Length of message	Keep the directions short.	Use of gestures	Pointing to the materials as one provides directions.	
Formality of language	Use plain language to describe project in the group with adolescents, but do not use slang.	Use of touch	Gently placing one's hand on the teen's forearm to provide positive support.	
Use of medical jargon	Avoid medical jargon and use plain language that teens will understand.	Active listening	Making eye contact, nodding as one listens, being comfortable with silence.	

There are many techniques for improving communication skills. By carefully evaluating one's verbal and nonverbal communication skills and one's ability to engage in active listening, areas for improvement can be identified. Self-evaluation along with objective feedback from peers can provide insight into communication strengths and weaknesses and how one is perceived by others. The best way to improve communication skills is to practice. Identifying a specific technique and establishing a plan for practicing this skill are suggested. Specific skills for nonverbal communication may include use of appropriate eye contact and facial expressions, whereas skills for verbal communication may include use of language that is appropriate for the client and awareness of speed and tone of voice. Feedback from others is essential in evaluating improvement in skills.

When therapy is provided in the context of a group format, the occupational therapy practitioner must be aware of the interpersonal relationships with all group members individually and as a whole, and be aware of the interpersonal relationships that exist among group members. An understanding of the interpersonal communication that is needed within the context of the group dynamics is necessary for a therapeutic group process to occur. People are instinctively social beings. They naturally form relationships with other people and are part of groups through these relationships or as part of their work, family, or leisure pursuits. Interpersonal communication as related to group processes is discussed in this chapter.

DEFINITION OF A GROUP

A group can be defined as individuals who share a common purpose that can be attained only by group members interacting and working together.[4] All occupational therapy groups can be described as consisting of content and process. The content of a group includes the occupational activity that the group completes during the group time and includes what is said, written, or produced during the course of the group. The *process* of a group refers to the manner in which the occupational activity is conducted and the emotional tone of the verbal and nonverbal content that occurs during the group. Although the occupational activity content of a group may remain constant for a series of groups, the process may vary greatly, depending on the interpersonal communication that occurs and the facilitation skills of the group leader during the group process.

GROUP STRUCTURE

Many elements describe **group structure**. The organization and procedures of the group may be well developed and formal or may be loosely developed with no specific format. The **setting** of the group refers to the environment in which the group is conducted. The type of facility and the type of room can influence the group process in many ways. Elements of the environment include aesthetic properties such as color scheme and use of art and decoration in the meeting space, comfort of the environment such as type of seating provided and temperature, and ability to attend well by minimizing auditory and visual distractions. Attention to the environment can have a significant effect on the ability of the group to attend to the activity and engage in interpersonal communication.

Logistical factors can also affect the group. Factors include time of day, length of group, frequency of group meetings, and number of participants per group. Whether the group is open or closed can significantly affect participation. If group membership remains the same over time for groups that meet regularly, then the group is considered a **closed** group. **Open** groups allow for new participants to join the group so the membership changes over time. With closed groups there is more opportunity to establish interpersonal relationships with other group members and greater rapport with the group leader as opposed to open groups.

Group participation may also be **voluntary** or **involuntary**. If members are attending based solely on their personal desire to attend the group, they will be more invested in engaging in the group process. Some group members may be participating at the advice of their physician or because of pressure from family and friends. Group participation may even be court ordered or required for obtaining other services. In these cases, the participant may not be as invested in the group process.

Group **size** can influence the amount of interpersonal interactions that occur during the process of the group; the larger the number of participants, the less opportunity there will be for interactions. Up to 10 members will allow for members to participate and interact as desired or as facilitated by the group leader. More than 10 members can impede the opportunity for participation of all members. The frequency of group meetings can increase the comfort levels of participants and increase participation as well, particularly for groups that have more consistent membership and attendance.

Time of day and **length** of groups can also affect participation. Some members may have more difficulty concentrating and participating later in the day. Planning groups with awareness of the participants' schedules can facilitate greater attentiveness and involvement. The length of the group should be appropriate for the type of group. Groups that are enjoyable and relaxing can be implemented for longer periods, whereas groups that are more cognitively intense or physically or emotionally stressful may need to be limited to what the clients are able to tolerate.

ⓞ Clinical Pearl

When planning for a stress-management group designed to increase the group members' ability to relax, the setting should be conducive to enabling relaxation. Elements to consider include providing comfortable seating, using soft colors and calming visual stimuli, eliminating outside or distracting noises, providing background music or sounds that are pleasing to the group members, and other elements such as room temperature and tone of voice of the group leader.

GROUP MODELS

Occupational therapy practitioners have the opportunity to engage clients in a variety of different groups based on purpose, group goals, and setting. The theoretical basis for group design and the purpose of the group dictates how the group is structured and implemented. Occupational therapy groups may be classified into different categories: activity groups, psychoanalytic or intrapsychic, social systems, and growth groups.[6]

ACTIVITY GROUPS

Schwartzberg, Howe, and Barnes write, "Activity groups are small, primary groups in which members are engaged in a common activity or task that is directed toward learning and maintaining occupational performance."[6] **Activity groups** can be further classified into six different types of groups as described by Mosey.[5] These include evaluation, task-oriented, developmental, thematic, topical, and instrumental groups. **Evaluation groups** allow for assessment of both interpersonal and activity skills. **Task-oriented groups** allow for the focus to be on both self-awareness and interactions with other group members through the activity process. **Developmental groups** focus on teaching group interaction skills that are considered developmental stage–specific. There are five stages, ranging from parallel groups in which clients work on individual projects in shared space to mature groups in which the group's needs take priority over the individual's needs. **Thematic groups** focus on the clients learning the knowledge, skills, and activities for a specific activity. **Topical groups** are similar to thematic groups, with the difference being the focus of implementing the group activity in the community. **Instrumental groups** focus on clients maintaining their current level of function and meeting health needs.[5]

PSYCHOANALYTIC GROUPS

Psychoanalytic or intrapsychic groups are focused on increasing insight into the self and increasing understanding of personal behavior. These groups can be thought of as traditional group therapy sessions led by a trained psychiatric professional in which the primary means of accomplishing the goal is talking about personal issues and sharing these with the group. Occupational therapy groups may have the same outcome, but are structured with the focus on occupation to achieve insight into the self and to increase understanding of personal behavior. Projective occupational therapy groups and groups that use therapeutic media as a means to understanding behavior are examples of **psychoanalytic groups**. Therapeutic media may include any form of art such as painting or working with clay, other forms of media such as wood or leather, or creative media such as music or dance.

Shatara is an occupational therapist who works in an acute psychiatric hospital on the adolescent unit. She provides group interventions to her clients. Shatara facilitates improved communication skills by having a small group of teenage girls make individual collages of their favorite activities. Although the teenagers are making individual projects, all of the materials and supplies to make the collages are shared. There is one pair of scissors, one glue stick, and only three magazines available during the group activity. Each client explains her individual collage at the end of the group session (Figure 3-1).

SOCIAL SYSTEMS GROUPS

Social systems groups focus on the group and learning about group dynamics; an example is team-building groups. Occupational therapy practitioners working in long-term settings may lead these types of groups. An example may be a residential setting for adolescents with emotional and behavioral problems in which the occupational therapy practitioner designs occupational therapy groups to focus on team building and group dynamics. Team building can be a lengthy process and require many sessions, ideally with a closed-group membership. The purpose of a team-building group is for the group members to learn how to work together productively to achieve a group goal. Learning to trust others and to communicate effectively

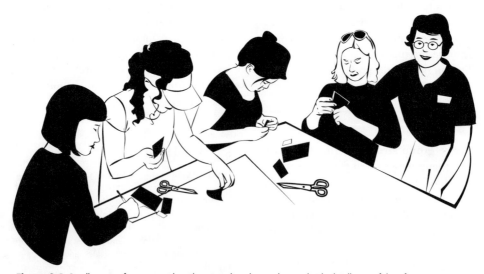

Figure 3-1 Small group of teenage girls with eating disorders making individual collages of their favorite activities.

are the primary goals of the group process. Examples include activities during which members have to depend on others to achieve the outcome of the group. An example is being blindfolded while completing an activity and relying on other group members for guidance.

Benjamin is an occupational therapist who works in a long-term facility that provides interventions for young boys who have emotional and behavioral disorders. All of his clients have issues with trusting their peers and adults. Most of the boys have been in and out of foster care, which has given them a sense of abandonment. Benjamin plans a trust-building group activity. He randomly pairs off six boys. Each pair of two boys stands tandem at a distance of two feet apart on a mat. The boy in front is asked to close his eyes and to fall backward into the extended arms of the boy standing behind him. On another day the practitioner plans a community outing to engage the boys in a rock-climbing activity (Figure 3-2).

GROWTH GROUPS

Growth groups focus on increasing self-awareness and sensitivity to others; an example is self-help groups. Most self-help groups are organized and led by clients who share the diagnosis or behavior that is the focus of the group. An example is Alcoholics Anonymous or a support group for a particular diagnosis. Occupational therapy practitioners may be invited to participate in self-help groups to share knowledge or insight related to the behavior but do not lead or organize the group.

FUNCTIONAL GROUP MODEL

The **functional group model** was initially developed by Howe and Schwartzberg[2] and subsequently refined "to incorporate the use of purposeful activity and meaningful occupation into the process and dynamics of group work."[6]

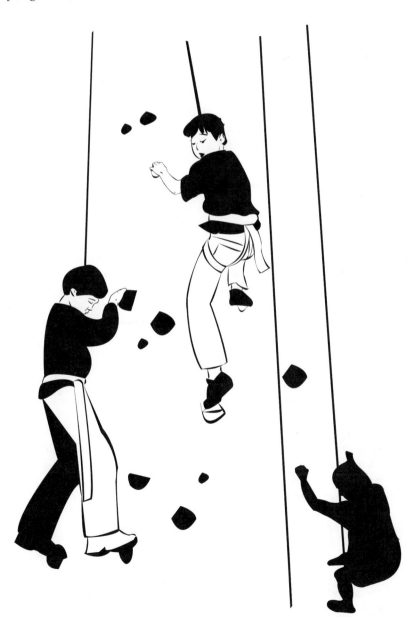

Figure 3-2 Adolescents boys engaged in trust-building activity.

The frame of reference for this model is based on research in group dynamics, effectance, needs hierarchy, purposeful activity, and adaptation. Based on a literature review of the research, a variety of assumptions related to people, health, occupation, therapy, social systems, change, function, and action were formed. Some of these assumptions related to people include people as action-oriented and social beings who exist in groups that are models of the social behavior patterns of society. Health assumptions include the support of purposeful activity for the health of the mind and the body, whereas occupation assumptions stress the use of purposeful activity and active doing for skill development in self-care, work, and leisure. Therapy assumptions include elicitation of adaptive responses in groups, and change assumptions assert that functional groups provide a supportive environment for practicing the skills of living.[3]

The assumptions provide the foundation for this model and for the structure of the group. Schwartzberg, Howe, and Barnes write, "The ultimate goal of the functional group is to promote health or adaptation through purposeful, self-initiated, spontaneous, and group-centered action. A functional group can have multiple goals, incorporating the specific needs and goals of individual members as well as more general goals and needs shared by all members."[6] A wide variety of groups may be designed using the functional group model because this model provides a method of designing occupational therapy groups that are theory-based in the use of occupation and purposeful activity to support goal achievement.

STAGES OF GROUP DEVELOPMENT

As groups engage in the group process, they typically progress through stages of development. The most well-known explanation of group development is provided by Tuckman and Jenson.[7] Tuckman, an educational psychologist, first described four stages of group development in 1965: forming, storming, norming, and performing.[8] In 1977, the final stage, adjourning, was added to the model of group development.

The first stage, **forming**, may also be referred to as the *orientation stage*. Group members are focused on understanding the nature of the group task and bonding with group members. They may be eager and have positive feelings about the group process and group members or they may have some anxiety about what they are expected to accomplish in the group and how they are expected to interact with other members. Establishing relationships with others during this stage is important for facilitating positive growth through the rest of the stages. It is important that the group's purpose be clarified as well.

The second stage, **storming**, may also be referred to as the *conflict* or *dissatisfaction stage*. Group members may experience differences in their expectations of how to proceed with the group task and become aware of differences in opinions, personalities, and values. Interpersonal communication may be difficult to establish and members may feel frustration and possibly even anger with other members as well as the group leader. For some groups, this will be a short stage if the group members are homogenous and similarly focused on the group task and process. Other groups may not proceed past this stage in the initial group meeting and require a subsequent group to deal with the conflict appropriately.

The third stage, **norming**, may also be referred to as the *resolution* or *structure stage*. Issues are resolved and positive interpersonal communication increases. The group becomes more unified and focused on establishing group procedures and preparing for the group task. Group members are more trusting and respectful of each other as they begin to work together.

The fourth stage, **performing**, may also be referred to as the *task performance* or *production stage*. The focus of the group shifts to the performance of the task and effective occupational outcomes and goal attainment. There is positive interpersonal communication and a positive attitude for handling problems and disagreements. Not all groups may reach this stage completely, because some groups will struggle with the interpersonal interactions even while engaging in task performance. Some groups may engage well with others but have difficulty completing the task. There are varying degrees of effectiveness that may occur in this stage.

The fifth stage, **adjourning**, may also be referred to as the *dissolution* or *termination stage*. The group is over and no longer needs to meet. A group's entry into the dissolution stage can be either planned or spontaneous, but even planned dissolution can create problems for members as they reduce their dependence on the group. Group members may feel upset to be ending the group or may feel relieved that the group is over. It is helpful to spend time discussing the group's accomplishments and how best to end the group.

ESTABLISHING RAPPORT

For a group to be successful, the group leader establishes rapport with the group members; they should feel a sense of unity with each other. The group provides support and reassurance to the individual members. Members should feel comfortable sharing experiences and providing feedback to others. There are many **therapeutic factors** related to establishing rapport that can be facilitated in the group process[9,10]. These factors include the following:

- Instilling hope
- Universality
- Cohesiveness
- Imparting information
- Altruism
- Corrective recapitulation of the primary family experience
- Development of socializing techniques
- Imitative behavior
- Catharsis
- Interpersonal learning
- Self-understanding
- Existential factors

CASE STUDY

Priscilla is an occupational therapist who works in an assisted-living facility. She has recently noticed that several of her clients are depressed and isolating themselves

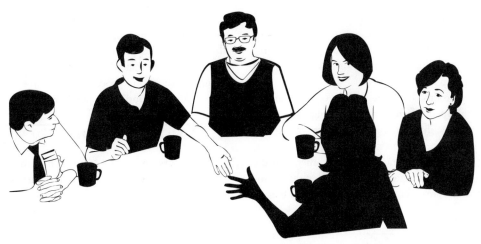

Figure 3-3 Small group of adults sharing similar life experiences.

from other residents. Priscilla plans a life experience group activity for four of her clients. Priscilla asks the clients to spend some time prior to the group writing down at least three and no more than five significant life experiences that occurred in their young-adult years. During a morning group session, Priscilla facilitates the sharing of similar life experiences (see Figure 3-3).

Instilling hope occurs in a group when a member is encouraged by another member who has dealt with a similar problem or issue. The occupational therapy practitioner as the leader can facilitate this process by asking group members to verbalize problems or issues that they are currently dealing with to see if other members have similar past experiences and are willing to share examples of how they dealt with the situation. This sharing of others' experiences can increase the hope that the individual has for dealing with the issue of concern. This relates to **universality** or the realization that other members have similar concerns and feelings and may have very similar experiences. The idea that one is not alone can be instrumental in improving one's emotional outlook. In realizing that a personal concern or feeling is a common human concern, the individual feels less isolated and more validated in his or her own experience. As members feel less isolated, a sense of **cohesiveness** develops. Members feel a sense of belonging, validation, and acceptance, which enhance the group experience.

Imparting information is often a key element of occupational therapy groups. The group leader generally facilitates this process by sharing information prepared for the group; however, the leader may also ask group members to share factual information that they may have learned based on their personal experiences. This information may be related to accessing services, obtaining products, or learning new skills. This relates to **altruism** through the experience of being able to help another person. The group process can encourage members to be supportive and give unselfishly to another group member through sharing experiences and knowledge for the sole purpose of helping a fellow group member.

Members of a group may unconsciously relate to the group leader and group members as if they were their own family members. If negative interactive patterns occurred in the past with significant others, these patterns may be present in current relationships and be expressed during the group process. A skilled group leader can assist the group member in identifying these patterns and in developing healthy interaction skills, resulting in **corrective recapitulation** of the primary family experience. The group setting can provide a safe and supportive environment for developing these healthy interaction skills or socializing techniques. The development of **socialization skills** is often a primary focus of occupational therapy groups through working with the other group members during the activity process and group discussion. The individual can improve and develop appropriate social skills through the process of modeling or practicing **imitative behavior**. This is achieved by observing the group leader and other group members interacting in an appropriate, socially acceptable manner. Behaviors such as showing empathy, using appropriate language, being polite and respectful, and sharing personal feelings appropriately are examples of behaviors that can be modeled and imitated.

For some individuals, the opportunity to tell their story to a group that is supportive and nonjudgmental is liberating. If the individual is able to talk freely and is able to express emotions in an uninhibited manner, then **catharsis**, the experience of relief from emotional distress, can occur. This can provide relief from chronic feelings of insecurity, shame, guilt, or fear. For many individuals, just the knowledge that others are listening to them and they are being heard is instrumental in their recovery.

An important aspect of occupational therapy groups is the learning that occurs through the group process. **Interpersonal learning** occurs when group members become more aware of their behavior and their interaction skills and how their behavior affects other people. It is closely related to **self-understanding**, the insight one has into one's problems and the understanding of how one's behavior positively or negatively influences the problems one is dealing with in life. A high level of self-understanding includes the understanding of unconscious motivations that affect one's behavior as well. In addition to interpersonal learning and self-understanding, the awareness of the **existential factors** of life such as the meaning of life, acceptance of mortality, and recognition of personal responsibility in one's life can be addressed in the group process. Difficulty coming to terms with these factors is a source of anxiety for many individuals and may not be accomplished by the majority of group members.

When facilitating groups, it is not feasible or necessary to include each of the therapeutic factors into each group. The therapeutic factors that emerge during the group process will depend on the purpose of the group, the functional levels of the members, the ability of the members to interact with each other, and the group leader's skill at guiding the group process so that the appropriate therapeutic factors are embraced by the group members.

◎ Clinical Pearl

An outpatient energy conservation group for individuals with chronic obstructive pulmonary disease (COPD) may be primarily designed for imparting information in the form of skills for conserving energy effectively; however, equally important elements may be instilling hope by increasing awareness of what one is able to do, recognizing the universality of concerns of others with COPD, and feeling less isolated as cohesiveness with other group members is established.

PLANNING THE GROUP

Effectively planning and leading groups requires a multitude of skills as well as experience in implementation. Occupational therapy practitioners lead groups in a variety of different settings. Many mental health programs use the group format to effectively provide treatment to individuals with similar diagnoses or skill deficits. Examples of other settings in which the group format works well include work simplification and energy conservation groups for clients in outpatient settings with diagnoses such as arthritis or chronic obstructive pulmonary disease. Occupational therapy practitioners in pediatric settings may use groups for improving gross motor and fine motor skills through interactive play. Groups focused on increasing strength and endurance for clients in skilled nursing facilities can also provide increased socialization opportunities for these clients. There are many other examples of settings appropriate for group interventions and the need for more cost-effective treatment may increase the demand for provision of services through this format in the future.

CASE STUDY

Henry is a certified occupational therapy assistant working in a skilled nursing facility. He has a daily group and uses light exercise to decrease generalized deconditioning. The perform upper-extremity movements to music (Figure 3-4).

The importance of careful planning cannot be underestimated in leading groups. In planning the group activity, an activity analysis of the group activity is essential so that an appropriate activity is chosen. The physical, psychosocial, sensory, cognitive, and developmental skill levels of the participants must be considered and matched so that interest is sustained

through appropriate task challenge. Tasks that are too easy or too difficult will not sustain interest and can lead to frustration. The ability to adapt activities or tasks should be considered ahead of time so that adaptations can be implemented without disrupting the group process. An example of a **group protocol** for planning a group is provided (Box 3-1).

LEADING THE GROUP

Cole[1] presents a model for learning how to lead groups that can be adapted to meeting the goals of a variety of different groups. This model can be used in conjunction with a group protocol to identify the leadership skills for the group activity. Seven steps are outlined in Box 3-2.

Using a format such as the one provided by Cole[1] ensures that the occupational therapy practitioner addresses the key elements for successful group implementation. The group leader is responsible for setting the mood and facilitating the progress of the group. The group leader's interpersonal skills and therapeutic use of self are extremely important. An awareness of one's leadership style is beneficial as well. Leadership styles can be considered on a continuum from a high level of control to a low level of control. Group leaders who lean more toward an **authoritarian style** are leaders who employ a high level of control in the decision making of the group. These leaders are more likely to control the progress of the group by dictating how the group activity progresses and what is discussed without allowing group members to have input or by not recognizing nonverbal cues of dissatisfaction provided by members. This can lead to frustration and lack of progress in achieving group goals.

On the other end of the continuum is the **laissez faire style** in which the leader allows the group to control all decision making and problem solving.[11] This is generally not a productive form of leadership for occupational therapy groups, because group members need some guidance for achieving the purpose of the group. Leadership styles that fall in the middle of the continuum include the **paternalistic style**, the **participative style**, and the **democratic style**.[11] A group leader using the paternalistic style closely regulates the behavior of group members to assist in achieving individual and group goals. The participative style of leadership is a more flexible approach in which the leader adapts the amount of direction and feedback to the specific needs and abilities of the group members. The democratic style allows for a higher level of involvement from group members in achieving the outcomes of the group; the group leader delegates responsibility for group tasks to group members as appropriate (Table 3-2).

The leadership style depends on the cognitive and psychosocial abilities of the group members. The three styles in the middle of the continuum are generally more effective when leading most groups. Allowing group members to have some control over the direction of the group results in greater group cohesiveness and increased satisfaction. The group leader provides the level of group guidance that is deemed most appropriate for the clients and the activity planned. This may vary

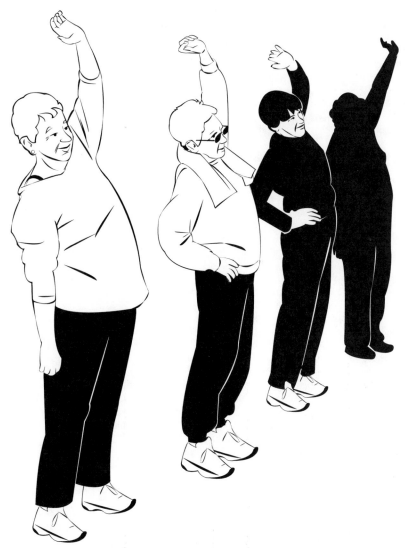

Figure 3-4 Group of older adult women exercising together.

BOX 3-1   Group Protocol

Group Protocol:

Topic: Teen Group: Finding your voice!

Purpose: Teens will be able to communicate to others verbally in a positive manner.

Members: Six adolescent girls.

Setting: Acute psychiatric hospital (adolescent unit)

Rationale: This group of teens will meet daily to develop positive coping strategies and communication skills. The teens will benefit from learning how to communicate effectively. During this group they will practice how to communicate to get their needs met to use as a positive coping skill.

Goals:

Long Term: Develop positive coping strategies to address life events.

Short Term: Communicate with others verbally in a positive manner.

Demonstrate positive communication with peers and adults.

State one's point of view in an effective manner.

Outcome Measures:

Express their needs in a positive and effective manner.

Identify resources that support them.

Listen to others' points of view.

Make their points to adults and peers verbally and in writing.

Meeting Schedule: 1 hour daily

Materials (for collage group):

List all materials needed—type, number, etc.

Assorted magazines and pictures, paper, scissors, glue, markers

Include cost of each item: magazines ($5-$8), paper—available in bulk on unit, assorted scissors ($5-$10), glue ($3-$5), markers ($5-$10)

Include method of acquiring each item: Available at local department stores.

Session Plan:

1. Introduction (10 minutes): This is the first session, so the practitioner will take more time for the introduction.

   ■ Introduce leaders and set the tone: Welcome to the teen group. We meet each day at this time. The goal of the group is to help you cope with the difficulties you face. Could you write down some things you find difficult? What are some things you find easy to do?

   ■ Introduce members (ice breaker): Please introduce yourself and tell the group a bit about yourself.

   ■ Review purpose and expectations: The purpose of the group is

Continued

BOX 3-1   Group Protocol—cont'd

to help everyone develop positive strategies for life. The focus will be on communication and helping everyone find his or her voice. Please do not discuss the group outside of group time. You are expected to participate in the activities and let me know if you can not attend the group. After today's session, the group will decide on the activities. It is meant to be fun and creative.

- Outline of the session: Today, because we are getting to know each other, we will complete collages. Once completed, you will briefly discuss your collage with others so that everyone can get to know each other.

2. Activity
- Describe the activity step by step in detail: Use these magazines, pictures, and markers to describe yourself to the group members. Include at least three healthy things you like to do.
- Identify the physical, cognitive, and psychosocial skills needed for participation:
  - **Physical:** Sitting endurance 30 minutes; bilateral hand use to reach and manipulate paper; fine motor skills to write on, tear, or cut paper; hand strength is minimal but required to press glue on paper.
  - **Cognitive:** Ability to follow simple two-step directions (find picture and glue to paper); processing to describe one's self in pictures; writing ability if plan on writing on collage; creativity for design of collage; spatial perception to place pictures; choosing and selecting pictures.
  - **Psychosocial:** Sharing supplies; asking for materials; identifying appropriate pictures to describe one's self; socially acceptable description; being able to limit information that is not acceptable; knowing when to speak up; using body language and mannerisms acceptably; supporting others; engaging in the process.
- Describe how the activity can be adapted if needed: The pictures could be precut (requiring that the teens select from limited pictures); more materials such as glitter, stickers, yarn,

could increase the demands. Less materials could change the emphasis. The instructions could be more emotionally demanding: "Show a collage of yourself currently and then show your future goals." Teens may be asked to share about their collage verbally or in writing. Sharing with a few teens or only one changes the activity.
- State the therapeutic goals:
  - Teens will identify healthy activities that promote a positive self-image.
  - Teens will communicate verbally with others in a positive manner.
  - Teens will identify three healthy activities in which they engage.
  - Teens will listen to others as they describe their collages.

3. Closure
- Review application to daily life: You did a nice job describing who you were and some activities that promote health. Did you learn about any activities that you would like to do not on your collage? What things did you like about the ways your peers presented? What did you learn that may help you in your daily life?
- Assess goal achievement: How did this group accomplish the goals:
  - Did you present yourself in a positive manner?
  - Did everyone listen to each other?
  - Did you learn anything about yourself?
  - What went well? What would you do differently?

4. End Group
- Based on this discussion, it seems you all really enjoy art. Would you like to do an art project tomorrow? Or we could. …
- See you tomorrow at the same time.
  Additional Information: Note: This group all picked art projects in their collages. Look into a trip to the art museum as the week progresses.

BOX 3-2   Model for Group Leadership

1. Introduction
- Warm-up and setting the mood: This includes lighting, room arrangement, materials, and position of the leader. Is the group formal or informal?
- Expectations of the group, explaining the purpose clearly: Describe the behavioral expectations and purpose of the group. For example, members are expected to remain in the group and participate. Everyone should support each other. If anyone is having difficulty remaining in the group or following the expectations, let the leader know.
- Brief outline of the session: Give an overview and show a completed project if applicable. Be sure to include time for clean up and remind group members to help.

2. Activity
- Timing and therapeutic goals: Carefully review the therapeutic goals and time each part of the activity. Being aware of time is essential.
- Physical and mental capacities of the members: Understanding the physical and mental capacities of members helps practitioners design group activities. Monitor the members' capacities as they work to be sure they can complete the activities. Guide members or adapt activities as needed so all can participate.
- Knowledge and skill of the leader: Be knowledgeable about the activity and skill level required prior to leading the group. Complete the activity and note the areas that may be difficult. Allow extra time for those areas and preplan how to adapt the activity if the group needs it.
- Adaptation of an activity: Examine each step and determine what changes can be made to the activity if needed. Have additional

materials that are already adapted available. For example, have directions in large print or precut materials.

3. Sharing
- Clients share experiences: Provide opportunities for each client to share his or her experience in the activity. Relate this experience to others.
- Leader acknowledges each member: Leaders should acknowledge each member positively, using the person's name and emphasizing improvement.

4. Processing
- Members express feelings about experience and others: Allow members to express their feelings about the experience and how the group performed. The leader must ask questions and be open to the feedback.

5. Generalizing
- Address cognitive learning aspects of the group: Reflect on the cognitive aspects of the group and determine how the group went.

6. Application
- How does this apply to everyday life: Ask members how they might use skills from the group in other settings and in their daily lives. Discuss different scenarios with the group.

7. Summary
- Review goals, content, process: Emphasize to members how the group addressed their goals. Did they feel challenged? Would they be able to use skills learned in other settings? Are there any areas on which they need to continue to work? What did they like or dislike about the process or content?

Data from Cole MB: *Group dynamics in occupational therapy,* ed 3, Thorofare, NJ, 2005, Slack.

TABLE 3-2 Leadership Styles

	Level of Control
Authoritarian style	High
Paternalistic style	Medium-high
Participative style	Medium
Democratic style	Medium-low
Laissez faire style	Low

greatly and requires the skill of the practitioner to determine what level will result in the best outcomes.

The sharing, processing, generalizing, and application steps can be the hardest for the group leader to facilitate. These steps should be carefully planned by determining the types of questions to ask and the best methods for encouraging the clients to participate. Again, this can vary greatly depending on the types of clients present in the group. Being aware of the roles or behaviors that participants engage in during the group process is important, too. Behaviors that may interfere with the group process include monopolizing the activity or discussion, criticizing others, or refusing to participate. Group leaders need to have excellent communication skills to positively facilitate the group process.

SUMMARY

Understanding interpersonal relationships and developing effective communication skills are essential for leading therapeutic groups. The development of group leadership skills requires experience over time. Learning what works best and understanding personal strengths and weaknesses evolves through the process of doing. Groups offer clients a rewarding and satisfying treatment approach through the opportunity to learn from other clients and to experience a sense of camaraderie and support.

REVIEW QUESTIONS

1. What are the components of communication?
2. How are groups defined?
3. What are the different types of group models?
4. What are the stages of group development?
5. How can you establish rapport within a group?
6. How do you plan and lead an effective occupational therapy group?

REFERENCES

1. Cole MB: *Group dynamics in occupational therapy*, ed 3, Thorofare, NJ, 2005, Slack.
2. Howe MC, Schwartzberg SL: *A functional approach to group work in occupational therapy*, ed 1, Philadelphia, 1986, Lippincott Williams & Wilkins.
3. Howe MC, Schwartzberg SL: *A functional approach to group work in occupational therapy*, ed 3, Philadelphia, 2001, Lippincott Williams & Wilkins.
4. Mosey AC: *Activities therapy*, New York, 1973, Raven Press.
5. Mosey AC: *Occupational therapy: configuration of a profession*, New York, 1981, Raven Press.
6. Schwartzberg SL, Howe MC, Barnes MA: *Groups: Applying the functional group model*, Philadelphia, 2008, FA Davis.
7. Tuckman B, Jensen M: Stages of small-group development revisited, *Group Org Manage* 2(4):419-427, 1977.
8. Tuckman BW: Developmental sequence in small groups, *Psych Bull* 63:384-399, 1965.
9. Yalom I: *The theory and practice of group psychotherapy*, ed 4, New York, 1995, Basic Books.
10. Yalom I, Leszcz M: *The theory and practice of group psychotherapy*, ed 5, New York, 2005, Basic Books.
11. Robbins SP, Judge TA: *Organizational Behavior*, ed 13, Upper Saddle River, New Jersey, 2008, Pearson Prentice Hall.

Therapeutic Use of Self: Applying the Intentional Relationship Model in Group Therapy

Renée R. Taylor, Laura VanPuymbrouck

KEY TERMS

dynamic	interpersonal style
interpersonal event	mode shift
interpersonal focus	multimodal
interpersonal reasoning	therapeutic mode

CHAPTER OBJECTIVES

1. Define therapeutic use of self in occupational therapy.
2. Understand how the intentional relationship model may guide use of self in occupational therapy.
3. Understand the application of the intentional relationship model in group therapy approaches.
4. Define the interpersonal skills necessary for successful group therapy outcomes.
5. Understand the difference between activity focusing and interpersonal focusing according to the intentional relationship model.
6. Understand the role of group dynamics (adaptive and maladaptive) in therapy outcomes.
7. Apply the intentional relationship model to a group therapy case example.

AN INTRODUCTION TO THERAPEUTIC USE OF SELF IN OCCUPATIONAL THERAPY

Occupational therapy (OT) lays claim to an ample literature base supporting a holistic understanding that includes the psychosocial and interpersonal characteristics of a client, in addition to his or her actual physical, sensory, or cognitive impairments.[32] In individual and group therapy applications, terms such as *client-centered care, empathy,* and *narrative* are referenced as talismans reflecting this emphasis. In recent history, there have been three central movements with which the client-therapist relationship has been associated:

- collaborative and client-centered approaches
- emphasis on caring and empathy
- use of narrative and clinical reasoning

Collaborative and client-centered approaches emphasize the readjustment of power within the therapeutic relationship and support client control over decision-making and problem-solving.[17,34] Generally, these approaches emphasize open communication, orientation toward the client's perspective, recognition of the client's strengths, shared goals and priorities, and a collaborative partnership. Group therapy leaders that emphasize collaboration derive wisdom from group and encourage mutual sharing and exchange during the process. Within this perspective, there has also been an emphasis on therapist self-awareness. Therapists are encouraged to recognize and control negative reactions toward difficult clients, incorporate their own life experiences into an understanding of their clients' perspectives, and draw on their personal reactions to clients to guide their clinical reasoning.

In conjunction with collaborative and client-centered approaches, the contemporary era has also been characterized by an emphasis on empathy and caring within the therapeutic relationship. This can be summarized as an emphasis on the emotional exchange that occurs between client and therapist, on goal-directed activity, and on activities that promote personal growth).[3,4,6,8,12,18,19-22,24,25,35]

Empathy has been written about extensively within the OT literature. Peloquin[19-21,23] emphasized the roles of art, literature, imagination, and self-reflection. She further argued that the fundamental characteristics required to develop one's therapeutic use of self are well conveyed through reading literature and viewing and doing art 18, 19. She believed that providing therapists with both fictional and nonfictional poems and stories that illustrate empathy and the depersonalizing consequences of neglectful attitudes and failed communication could be a powerful motivator for the development of caring.[20-22]

Clinical reasoning and narrative approaches compose the final general category of contemporary scholarship that includes the client-therapist relationship as a focal point.[9,10,13-16,27-31] These approaches emphasize the role of the therapist in understanding and reflecting about the unique way in which clients think about and summarize key events in their lives.[11] Clinical reasoning approaches incorporate thinking about the relationship as a component of one's overall approach to making sense of assessment findings and developing a treatment plan.[16] This element has been referred to as *interactive reasoning*[16] and it has been described as an "underground practice" in OT[7] because relatively little is known about the mechanisms that underlie it.

Narrative approaches (e.g., narrative reasoning) were developed in tandem with clinical reasoning approaches.[10,15] Narrative approaches seek to organize and make sense of information from clients by encouraging them to present information about themselves through storytelling, poetry, or metaphor. Thinking in story form is thought to allow both the client and the therapist to discover the meaning of the impairment experience according to the client's unique perspective. Therapeutic approaches are then focused toward reconstructing more hopeful narratives to reshape one's life story.

These concepts and values have been upheld in academic research as well as in clinical settings. For example, a growing number of studies indicate that the client-therapist relationship is a key determinant of whether OT has been successful.[1,3,5] However, there has been a lack of cohesiveness between evidence and discussion about the importance of these values and literature describing the concrete skills and competencies that are necessary to enact them within a clinical setting. According to the American Occupational Therapy Association's 2008 Practice Framework 1, therapeutic use of self is the "therapist's planned use of his or her personality, insights, perceptions, and judgment as part of the therapeutic process"[26] (p. 626). Although some believe that use of self is intuitive, a recent survey study found that most practicing occupational therapists within the United States agree that the field lacks sufficient knowledge about therapeutic use of self.[33] For example, only 4.3% of respondents reported taking a class that focused only and specifically on this topic in OT school.[33] In this chapter, we provide a rationale for the introduction of a new conceptual model of use of self, describe the model, and describe its application in group therapy. A case example is presented that illustrates a clinician's use of this model in a group therapy situation.

THE INTENTIONAL RELATIONSHIP MODEL IN OCCUPATIONAL THERAPY

Contemporary OT practice requires a therapist to understand how to manage the relationship with a client to optimize occupational engagement.[32] A conceptual practice model that provides a set of concrete tools and suggestions for development of interpersonal skills is a necessary guide in assisting occupational therapists in developing an understanding of use of self. The intentional relationship model (IRM) explains therapeutic use of self and its relationship with occupational engagement. It defines the most critical components of the client-therapist relationship as they are enacted in practice. According to IRM, "The client is the focal point. It is the therapist's responsibility to work to develop a positive relationship with the client and to respond appropriately"[32] (p. 48).

The IRM focuses on four main components of the therapist-client relationship. These are (1) the client, (2) the interpersonal events that occur during therapy, (3) the therapist, and (4) the occupation. The IRM asks therapists to observe and understand their clients from an interpersonal perspective, to be prepared to respond therapeutically to rifts and other significant interpersonal events that occur during therapy, and to communicate within a mode that matches the client's interpersonal needs of the moment.[32] This model, which is illustrated in Figure 4-1, provides a theoretical framework for understanding the significance that all interactions have and guidance in how to therapeutically respond in a manner that best serves the client. Each of the central components of the model is described in the following pages, and more extensive information is presented in Taylor.[32]

CLIENT INTERPERSONAL CHARACTERISTICS

At first appraisal, the relevant aspects that the client brings into a therapeutic relationship may appear to be obvious. For example, a client's heightened need for control becomes salient the moment he or she asks what seems to be an unnecessary question for the third time. A client's reluctance to engage in an activity may become apparent when he or she appears not to have heard a given instruction. One quickly learns of a client's limited capacity to assert his or her needs when the client

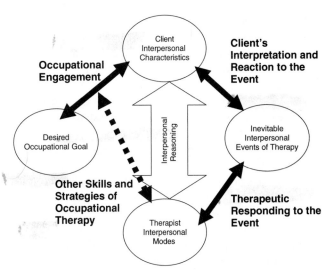

Figure 4-1 A model of intentional relationship in occupational therapy.

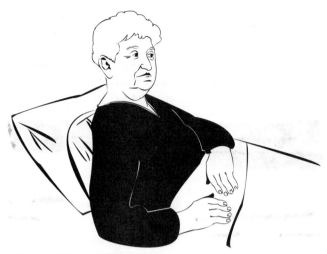

Figure 4-2 Client interpersonal characteristics may make it difficult for a person to get out of bed for therapy.

is found lying on a mat without a means to right himself or herself, not having asked anyone for help.

Although these are common characteristics of clients in everyday practice, they are not traditionally discussed as fundamental aspects of OT care plans or documented in a client's chart notes. Understanding the more challenging aspects of a client's interpersonal characteristics from an objective but empathic perspective assists a therapist to act in a way that is intentional and facilitating of occupational engagement (Figure 4-2).

IRM defines the essential interpersonal characteristics of a client in terms of 12 categories, presented in Table 4-1.

Communication style refers to a client's ability to communicate in a clear, well-paced, and detailed yet succinct manner that is appropriate to his or her developmental level and cognitive ability. Reticence to communicate or, by contrast, excessive loquaciousness will undoubtedly affect the therapeutic dynamic and the quality of occupational engagement that might otherwise be possible to achieve. Therefore, the IRM calls for therapists to consider communication difficulties such as these in building the therapeutic alliance, selecting an approach to communication, and ultimately in establishing the OT care plan. The same approach applies to the remaining categories of client characteristics. *Capacity for trust* refers to a client's ability to trust that the therapist has his or her best interests in mind and that every effort will be made to ensure his or her physical safety and emotional well being.

Need for control is defined as the degree to which a client takes an active versus passive role within the relationship and in determining the course of therapy. *Capacity to assert needs* defines a client's approach to expressing his or her wishes and needs for support, information, resources, or other requests within the therapeutic relationship, if they are expressed at all. *Response to change and challenge* refers to a client's ability to adapt to changes in the therapy plan or environment and his or her approach to OT tasks and situations that are new or challenging. *Affect* is defined as a client's general emotional expression during therapy, ranging from appropriately buoyant for the situation (flexible) to flat (absence of expression) to heightened (intensely emotional)

to labile (fluctuating anywhere between elation, anger, angst, and despair). *Predisposition to giving feedback* involves a client's ability to provide the therapist with appropriate negative or positive comments about his or her reactions to the therapist and experience of therapy as either helpful or unhelpful. *Capacity to receive feedback* describes a client's ability to maintain perspective when receiving praise from the therapist or when receiving correction during performance, limits on behavior, or information about his or her strengths and weaknesses.

Response to human diversity is defined by a client's reaction to ways in which he or she may be the same or different from the therapist in terms of observable sociodemographic characteristics (i.e., race, ethnicity, gender, age) and other interpretations of outward appearance or perceived worldview. Some clients have more difficulty than others relating to a therapist whom they perceive as differing from them in fundamental ways. *Orientation toward relating* defines a client's need for interpersonal closeness versus professional distance within the therapeutic relationship. Difficulties may occur when the client's expectations about the relationship differ from those of the therapist. *Preference for touch* involves a client's observed comfort with or expressed reaction to any type of physical touch, whether it be a necessary part of treatment or an expression of caring. Capacity for reciprocity refers to a client's ability to engage fully in the therapy process or show appreciation toward the therapist as a separate but connected partner within the therapy process. Some clients may be so focused on their own situations that they may lack this capacity, whereas others may function in an active and mutual way within the relationship. Regardless of the outcome, a client's capacity for reciprocity is always felt by the therapist and must be managed accordingly.

In summary, understanding client interpersonal characteristics is fundamental to planning how to respond during therapeutic interactions. Familiarizing oneself with the interpersonal characteristics of each of one's clients becomes particularly important in group therapy situations, in which it is important to consider the effects of one client's behavior on another, in addition to the effects of the therapist's behavior on each and every one of the clients and on the group as a whole. An extensive discussion of client characteristics may be found in Taylor.[32]

THE INEVITABLE INTERPERSONAL EVENTS OF THERAPY

Similar to client characteristics, difficult or emotional circumstances that occur during therapy are a normal part of everyday practice for the experienced therapist. However, knowing how to anticipate and respond to them in a deliberate and planned therapeutic way is not necessarily an assumed, universal skill. According to IRM,[32] an **interpersonal event** is a naturally occurring communication, reaction, process, task, or general circumstance that occurs during therapy and that has the potential to detract from or strengthen the therapeutic relationship. In therapy, these events may be precipitated by the following kinds of circumstances:

- Client resistance (e.g., a client refuses, either actively or passively, to communicate or participate in some activity)

TABLE 4-1 Client Interpersonal Characteristics

Interpersonal Characteristic	Group Therapy Example
Communication style	Elizabeth's group communication style appears to be a reluctance caused by a lack of confidence when asked her opinion on what activities the group should work on in a session. In one-on-one environments she is quick to provide her opinion.
Capacity for trust	During a session in which the therapist incorporated an overhead swing, all of the girls demonstrated hesitancy in attempting the activity despite encouragement. Alex has had multiple interactions both one on one and in the group with the therapist and displayed increased trust for this activity. Observing Alex enjoy the task encouraged the two other girls to engage in it.
Need for control	Iris' high need for control is evident during a parallel play activity of coloring because she frequently chooses and distributes crayon colors for the other girls to use, hoarding the most popular colors for herself.
Capacity to assert needs	In the coloring scenario, Elizabeth is unable to ask for a crayon color to be returned that has been taken from her despite her desire for it. Despite the therapist offering support for Iris to return the crayon, Elizabeth instead quickly picks up a crayon offered to her as a replacement by Iris.
Response to change and challenge	Unable to locate a commonly used CD for music during the group, Alex is quick to look for alternatives; however, Iris appears distraught by this inconsistency and withdraws from the group activity.
Affect	Because of Iris' high need to control the group and her dynamic affect, the therapist is careful to be sensitive to how her emotional vacillations effect the entire group and minimizes how these behaviors could be used by Iris as a tool for control.
Predisposition to giving feedback	During decision making for activity choice, Elizabeth infrequently provides input. When encouraged to provide a very basic choice, she displays prolonged hesitation; ultimately, she is dominated by others in the group and is unable to verbalize her opinion. Later, when alone with the therapist she acknowledges that she knew what she wanted to choose but was afraid the other girls would not like it.
Capacity to receive feedback	When Iris is encouraged to be more sensitive to turn taking when making choices, she is unable to receive this feedback without obvious disengagement and irritability for a brief time in response to the therapist.
Response to human diversity	In this particular playgroup, the girls all have historical difficulties with a male in their immediate family dynamic. Because of this, when attempts have been made for a male therapist to lead the group, each girl displays increased withdrawal behaviors and disengagement from activity.
Orientation toward relating	Each of the girls displays varying levels of relating to one another. Alex and Elizabeth have a nurturing and mutually helping relationship (e.g., they frequently hold hands together while walking); however, Iris has the need to remain safely distant with limited displays of intimacy to the other girls.
Preference for touch	Each child in the playgroup has different preferences for touch, most notable during times of distress. Iris prefers limited physical touch, withdrawing when it is attempted, whereas Alex prefers prolonged hugs to comfort her.
Capacity for reciprocity	During one session, the therapist gets a paper cut. Differences are noted with each child in her reciprocity toward the therapist's pain. Elizabeth is quick to ask her if the therapist is okay; Alex appears distressed by this occurrence, with decreased eye contact and verbalizations; and Iris begins telling a story about how many times she has had paper cuts and the effect they had on her.

- Therapist behavior (e.g., the therapist provides feedback that a client finds difficult to hear)
- Client display of strong emotions in therapy (e.g., a client becomes tearful when reflecting on the extent of his or her impairment before beginning therapy, as compared with the progress made recently)
- A difficult circumstance of therapy (e.g., a client is uncomfortable practicing toileting hygiene with the therapist)
- A rift or conflict between the client and therapist (e.g., a client disagrees with a treatment recommendation and confronts the therapist in a way that the therapist perceives is personal)
- Differences concerning the aim of therapy (e.g., a client insists on a goal that the therapist believes is not attainable, or the therapist recommends a goal that the client rejects)
- Client requests that test the boundaries or limits of the therapeutic relationship (e.g., the client invites the therapist to attend his or her wedding)

These are only a few of the myriad possible interpersonal events that occur during the course of OT. A more extensive list is presented in Table 4-2 and in Taylor.[32] When interpersonal events occur, their interpretation by the client is a product of the client's unique set of interpersonal characteristics. Sometimes the event may have a significant effect on the client and other times a client will be unaffected or minimally affected. When such events occur, it is important that the therapist be aware that the event has occurred and take responsibility for responding appropriately.

Interpersonal events are:
- Inevitable during the course of therapy
- Rife with both threat and opportunity

TABLE 4-2   The Inevitable Interpersonal Events of Occupational Therapy

Interpersonal Event	Definition	Group Therapy Example
Expression of strong emotion	External displays of internal feelings are shown with a high level of intensity beyond usual cultural norms for interaction. Can be positive or negative expressions.	During the end of playgroup and immediately following a power dilemma that was resolved with successful use of Empathizing Mode, Iris gives a hug to the therapist and exclaims she loves the therapist more than anybody else in the world.
Intimate self-disclosures	Statements or stories reveal something unobservable, private, or sensitive about the person making a disclosure. These can be stories about oneself or about close others.	Alex discloses during imagination time and story development that her mother and father are getting divorced. While casually brought up during the group conversation, this disclosure reveals an area of stress for Alex.
Power dilemmas	Tensions arise in the therapeutic relationship because of clients' innate feelings about issues of power, the inherent situation of therapy, the therapist's behavior, or other circumstances that underscore clients' lack or loss of power over aspects of their lives.	During clean up time at the conclusion of playgroup, Iris' refusal to put her toys away is coupled with her sitting in the middle of the floor with her arms folded. It is important that the therapist does not attempt to force her to participate here, because a power dilemma is a common end result.
Nonverbal cues	Communications do not involve the use of formal language. Some examples of these are facial expressions, movement patterns, body posture, and eye contact.	Elizabeth has a tendency to limit eye contact and engage in idle fiddling with a toy during discussion of client choices for activities at the beginning of playtime.
Crisis points	Unanticipated, stressful events cause clients to become distracted or temporarily interfere with clients' ability for occupational engagement.	During an outing to a playground, Alex becomes frightened by a passing dog, causing tearfulness and requiring the therapist to decrease attention to the group as a whole to console Alex. Careful attention had to be given to return to the group's needs as soon as Alex was consoled to avoid escalation of the crisis to others in the group.
Resistance and reluctance	Resistance is a client's passive or active refusal to participate in some or all aspects of therapy for reasons linked to the therapeutic relationship. Reluctance is disinclination toward some aspect of therapy for reasons outside the therapeutic relationship.	Elizabeth's refusal to follow the other children in rolling somersaults in the grass is reluctance based on her long-standing sensory processing difficulties.
Boundary testing	A client behavior violates or asks the therapist to act in ways outside the defined therapeutic relationship.	When asked to participate in an activity, Iris states she will only participate if the therapist will take her to the candy store after therapy.
Empathic breaks	The therapist fails to notice or understand a communication from a client, or communication or behavior initiated by the therapist is perceived by the client as hurtful or insensitive.	During the group's parallel play time Alex proudly displays her completed coloring project, which is below her age appropriateness. The therapist congratulates her but states that it must have been easy because it was from a baby's coloring book. Alex immediately responds with a deflated affect.
Emotionally charged therapy tasks and situations	Activities or circumstances can lead clients to become overwhelmed or experience uncomfortable emotional reactions such as embarrassment, humiliation, or shame.	During a physically challenging activity, Elizabeth suffers from increased oral secretions that she is unable to perceive. Iris points this out to the other group members, which embarrasses Elizabeth and makes her withdraw from the activity.
Limitations of therapy	There are restrictions on the available or possible services, time, resources, or therapist actions.	During playtime decision making, a promise was made that, at the conclusion of the hour, the group would be allowed to play with a favorite toy. At the appropriate time for this reward to occur, the toy has been misplaced and is unable to be found for follow through of the promised reward.
Contextual inconsistencies	Any aspect of a client's interpersonal or physical environment changes during the course of therapy.	This playgroup has three therapists who typically treat them; however, when a new therapist must assume the group session, the group requires some time to adjust to this new individual.

Interpersonal events are part of the constant give and take that occurs in a therapy process. They are distinguished from other events or processes in that they are charged with the potential for an emotional response either when they occur or later after reflection. Consequently, if they are ignored or responded to less than optimally, these events can threaten both the therapeutic relationship and the client's occupational engagement. When optimally responded to, these events can provide opportunities for positive client learning or change and for solidifying the therapeutic relationship. Because they are unavoidable in any therapeutic interaction, one of the primary tasks of a therapist practicing according to the IRM is to respond to these inevitable events in a way that leads to repair and strengthening of the therapeutic relationship.[32]

THE SIX INTERPERSONAL MODES

According to the IRM, effective use of self requires therapists to know and responsibly accept interpersonal blind spots,

recognize and cultivate strengths within their personalities, and develop less-used aspects of their personalities through honest appraisal of the effects of their behavior on clients.[32] The first step in accomplishing this is through an understanding of the six therapist interpersonal modes. **A therapeutic mode is a specific way of relating to a client.** The IRM identifies six therapeutic modes:

- Advocating
- Collaborating
- Empathizing
- Encouraging
- Instructing
- Problem solving

A brief definition of each mode and an example of its use in a group therapy situation are provided in Table 4-3.

Therapists naturally use therapeutic modes that are consistent with their fundamental personality characteristics. For example, a therapist who tends to be more of a listener than a

TABLE 4-3 The Six Therapeutic Modes		
Mode	**Definition**	**Group Therapy Example**
Advocating	The therapist ensures that the client's rights are enforced and resources are secured. May require the therapist to serve as a mediator, facilitator, negotiator, enforcer, or other type of advocate with external persons and agencies.	Speech therapy services will soon be discontinued for the client. However, following several playgroup sessions in which oral secretion management difficulties occurred, the occupational therapist discusses with the family the possibilities of working on this goal area and advocates for pushing back discontinuation of speech to allow for treatment focusing on this issue.
Collaborating	The therapist expects the client to be an active and equal participant in therapy, and ensures choice, freedom, and autonomy to the greatest extent possible.	A goal area for this playgroup is to facilitate equal decision making and turn taking by all members of the group. During activity selection the therapist structures a routine that requires each child to be responsible for different choices of the day. This routine is a constant, and the therapist uses collaboration mode to ensure all voices are heard during activity decision making.
Empathizing	The therapist continually strives to understand the client's thoughts, feelings, and behaviors while suspending any judgment. The therapist ensures that the client verifies and experiences the therapist's understanding as truthful and validating.	Following a failed attempt to manipulate the group, the client withdraws and becomes passive-aggressive during attempts to engage her. The therapist uses empathizing mode to allow the client to discuss her feelings. The use of empathizing mode demonstrates to the client that the therapist understands her behavior and is not critical of it.
Encouraging	The therapist seizes the opportunity to instill hope in a client and celebrate a client's thinking or behavior through positive reinforcement. The therapist conveys an attitude of joyfulness, playfulness, and confidence.	During a 10-minute span in which the three girls participated in a task that required a group effort from all to succeed, the therapist used appropriate reinforcement through the encouraging mode to identify positive behaviors from each child as they worked together successfully. At the successful conclusion of the task, encouraging mode was again used to celebrate their achievement.
Instructing	The therapist carefully structures therapy activities and is explicit with clients about the plan, sequence, and events of therapy. The therapist provides clear instruction and feedback about performance and sets limits on a client's requests or behavior.	At the onset of each playgroup session, the therapist initiates the activity with clearly established rules and goals of the group. Using instructing mode and a consistent approach with each session reminds the girls (and assists the client with her recall of the group's agenda) of what their tasks and expectations are.
Problem solving	The therapist facilitates pragmatic thinking and solving dilemmas by outlining choices, posing strategic questions, and providing opportunities for comparative or analytic thinking.	One activity that occurs during each playgroup is imagination play or story telling that will be acted out. In one session, the group is asked to create a journey through an imaginative land that has many physical challenges. The group works together with assistance from the therapist using problem-solving mode, facilitating input from each girl, to create a story of three princesses walking along a path with various challenges to save three puppies that must be carried home to safety.

talker and believes in the importance of understanding another person's perspective before making a suggestion would likely use empathizing as a primary therapeutic mode in therapy. Therapists vary widely in terms of the range and flexibility with which they use modes in relating to clients. Some therapists relate to clients in one or two primary ways, whereas others draw on multiple therapeutic modes, depending on the interpersonal characteristics of the client and the situation, or inevitable interpersonal events, at hand. One of the goals in using IRM is to become increasingly comfortable using any of the six modes flexibly and interchangeably, depending on the client's needs. A therapeutic mode or set of modes define therapist's general **interpersonal style** when interacting with a client. Therapists able to use all six of the modes flexibly and comfortably and to match those modes to the client and the situation are described as having a **multimodal** interpersonal style.

According to the IRM, a therapist's choice and application of a particular therapeutic mode or set of modes should depend largely on the interpersonal characteristics of the client and his or her reaction to any interpersonal events that may be occurring. Although a client may prefer that the therapist use one or two central modes, certain interpersonal events in therapy may call for a mode shift. A **mode shift** is a conscious change in one's way of relating to a client. For example, if a client perceives a therapist's attempts at problem solving to be insensitive or off the mark, a therapist would be wise to switch from the problem-solving mode to an empathizing mode so that she can get a better understanding of the client's reaction and the root of the dilemma. An interpersonal reasoning process, described in the following paragraph, can be used to guide the therapist in deciding when a mode shift might be required and determining which alternative mode to select. Because the interpersonal aspects of OT practice are complex and require a therapist to possess a highly adaptive therapeutic personality,

the IRM recommends that therapists learn to draw on all six of the therapeutic modes in a flexible manner according to the different interpersonal needs of each client and the unique demands of each clinical situation.

THE THERAPEUTIC REASONING PROCESS

The third therapist interpersonal competency involves the capacity to engage in an **interpersonal reasoning** process when an interpersonal dilemma presents itself in therapy. Interpersonal reasoning is a step-wise process by which a therapist decides what to say, do, or express in reaction to the occurrence of an interpersonal dilemma in therapy. It includes developing a mental vigilance toward the interpersonal aspects of therapy in anticipation that a dilemma might occur, and a means of reviewing and evaluating options for responding. The six steps of interpersonal reasoning and their definitions are presented in Table 4-4. An extensive description and discussion of these steps can be found in Taylor.[32]

APPLYING THE INTENTIONAL RELATIONSHIP MODEL IN GROUP THERAPY SITUATIONS

With the exception of educational and planning groups, most OT groups involve engaging clients in some level of activity. The demands associated with selecting, grading, and engaging all members in the activity can sometimes be so great that they may cloud a therapist's vision of important interpersonal dynamics within the group. The IRM principle that activity focusing must be balanced with **interpersonal focusing**[32] is particularly relevant in group therapy situations. This principle holds that therapists should not over rely on aspects of an activity to replace or compensate for the need to attend to

TABLE 4-4 The Six Steps of the Interpersonal Reasoning Process	
Step of Interpersonal Reasoning	Definition
Anticipate	Use observational skills, information from others who have interacted with the client, and your direct experience interacting with the client to anticipate the likely interpersonal events that may occur during therapy, given your knowledge of the client's interpersonal characteristics.
Identify and cope	Use IRM language to label a difficult client characteristic or interpersonal event when it occurs. Do what it takes to collect yourself and get emotional perspective on the situation. Remind yourself not to take it personally.
Determine if a mode shift is required	Ask yourself the following questions to determine whether a mode shift is required: What mode am I currently using with this client, if any? What are the effects of the mode on the client? Would another mode better serve the interpersonal needs of this client at this moment?
Choose a response mode or mode sequence	Interact within the mode or modes that you think the client prefers or needs at this moment. Think about a sequence of modes that you might use to accommodate changes in what the client might need from moment to moment.
Draw on any relevant interpersonal skills associated with the modes	Think about other communication, rapport-building, and conflict resolution skills that you might draw on in association with your mode use.
Gather feedback	Gather nonverbal or verbal feedback from the client as to whether he or she feels comfortable with the way you approached the event or difficulty.

IRM, Intentional relationship model.

the interpersonal aspects of the therapy practice. Dimming the lights or downgrading an activity in response to a toddler's emotionally laden refusal to participate in therapy are examples of activity focusing. By contrast, changing one's mode from instructing to collaborating (allowing the client to take the lead in therapy) or empathizing (observing and listening for a client's needs) is an example of interpersonal focusing. When focusing on the interpersonal aspects of a group therapy situation, therapists must consider a number of questions that will help them understand the group and decide how to interact with it in a way that serves the best interests of as many members as possible (if not all members). According to IRM, a *social systems perspective* calls for

therapists to understand the interpersonal aspects of their interactions with each client in the group as well as the interpersonal aspects of the mutual interactions between members (Figure 4-3).[32] Questions that characterize a *social systems perspective* include:

- What are the client characteristics of each member of the group? How are they similar and how are they different? What modes work best for group members individually and collectively (Figure 4-4)?
- Is there a member of the group that appears to present a greater number of difficult interpersonal characteristics as compared with others? How does this member's behavior affect others in the group? What modes are most effective in managing this person's behavior?
- Who are the most engaged members of the group? Who are the most disengaged? What modes work best to increase occupational engagement within the group?
- Who are the most prominent or influential members? How do they exert their power? Do they affect the group in a positive, negative, or mixed way? What modes work best to increase the likelihood of a positive outcome?
- What topics, general themes, or content of conversation dominate the group?
- What is the general emotional tone or mood of the group?
- Is communication within the group shared, open, and direct or are there certain alliances and indirect routes of communication?

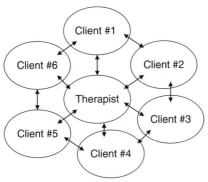

Figure 4-3 Viewing relationships from a social systems perspective.

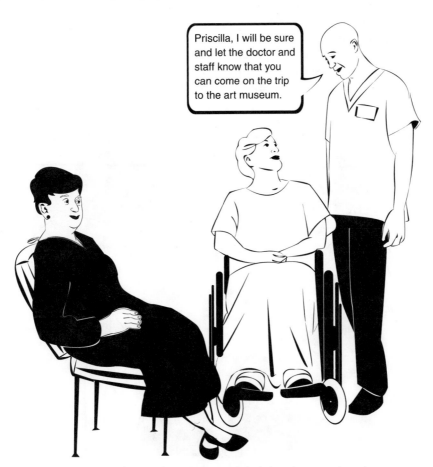

Figure 4-4 Advocating for one's clients includes helping them assert themselves

- What productive dynamics exist that support the group's best interests?
- What maladaptive dynamics exist? What modes are most successful in managing the maladaptive dynamics?
- How are disagreements or conflicts of interest managed?
- What other interpersonal events are likely to occur within the group or are emerging as potential patterns? What modes are most effective when responding to these events?

One of the most effective ways to begin to understand interactions from a social systems perspective is to observe a group of people interacting while keeping these questions in mind.

ADAPTIVE VERSUS MALADAPTIVE GROUP DYNAMICS

When one attempts to interact with a social system such as a group, the entire system becomes a kind of client in itself. As the therapist, you may take on one or more roles within the system and use modes to move into and out of the system in an intentional way to serve an individual client's or the group's best interests. To do this, one must be able to objectively identify and work within any number of dynamics that may emerge.

A **dynamic** defines the distinctive quality, emotional tone and specific interpersonal events that compose an interaction between individuals. For example, a dynamic involving competition for approval from the group leader may be observed between latency age girls participating in a dance group. Although it may not always be a productive dynamic, it is observed frequently in practice. If a dynamic serves a specific purpose within the system, it may become repetitive or entrenched over time. For example, a competitive dynamic between the girls may increase the likelihood that at least one of the girls will receive approval from a therapist who is otherwise weak in the encouraging mode (i.e., less likely to give open praise).

Dynamics can be productive or maladaptive. One example of a productive dynamic is a trusting dynamic. A trusting dynamic is characterized by evidence of trust between a client and therapist. For example, if a client feels confident about a therapist's ability to teach and demonstrate a sewing skill, his or her trust in the therapist will manifest in his or her earnest attempts to learn the skill. When a therapist returns the trust by showing a genuine investment in teaching, it constitutes further evidence that the therapist trusts that the client has a sincere desire to learn. If a client seeks input to check if the skill is being performed correctly, it constitutes behavioral evidence of this trusting dynamic. Similarly, if a therapist shows pleasure with the client's accomplishment, it is evidence of increased investment and emotional involvement in the trusting dynamic. Another example of a productive dynamic includes a collaborative dynamic in which members of the group work together to achieve a desired outcome (Figure 4-5). Similarly, a problem-solving dynamic in which different members brainstorm solutions and consider potential consequences of different actions typically leads to a productive outcome, and the end result is that important decisions are made and clients feel an increased sense of ownership and control.

If leaders are interpersonally self-disciplined about their mode use and strive to restrain their personal desires for control, approval, and success from influencing their behaviors, it is likely that most groups will be characterized by dynamics that are predominantly productive. However, even when therapists make all the best efforts to sustain productive dynamics, no one is invulnerable to being invited or drawn into a maladaptive dynamic. This is particularly likely in longstanding social systems in which maladaptive ways of relating can become entrenched over time. For this reason, it is critical that you be able to recognize maladaptive dynamics and differentiate them from dynamics that are productive.

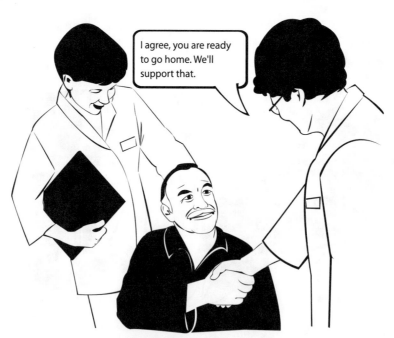

Figure 4-5 Many clients respond well to a practitioner who engages in collaborating.

All dynamics serve a specific interpersonal need or purpose. Maladaptive dynamics are similar to productive dynamics in that they serve the needs of at least one individual within the system. Distinct from productive dynamics, however, maladaptive dynamics are usually inefficient and involve negative feelings or outcomes for at least one of the involved individuals. An example of a maladaptive dynamic is one that commonly faces parents of adolescents who are struggling to differentiate themselves as individuals and take responsibility for the consequences of their actions. In this dynamic, the adolescent continually seeks guidance from the parents only to protest and explain why the guidance offered is unhelpful or would not work. This is commonly referred to as a *help-seeking and help-rejecting dynamic*. As a result, all individuals in the system end up feeling frustrated and ungratified. Some examples of maladaptive dynamics that have the potential to affect the process or outcomes of therapy are presented in Table 4-5.

In complex and longstanding relationships, multiple dynamics may emerge, some of which may be productive and others of which may be maladaptive. At times, it may be unclear whether a dynamic is ultimately productive or maladaptive. It is common for families, couples, or other social systems to assume that a maladaptive dynamic is productive because it feels familiar and defines the way people have always interacted within the system. Although it may be uncomfortable or painful at times, members participating in the dynamic may be unaware of any need for change. Also possible is that dynamics that were once thought to be positive may become negative over time (and vice versa). The nature and number of potential dynamics that can occur within a given social system are endless.

If a dynamic is prominent within a system, whether one is aware of it or not, it is inevitable that one will be invited or drawn into it when interacting with the system. The difference between being invited to join a maladaptive dynamic or simply drawn into it involves the issue of intentionality. An intentional therapist will recognize the dynamic before becoming involved with it. After identifying the dynamic, the therapist would then use interpersonal reasoning to decide how to interact within the dynamic. An unintentional therapist may not realize that he or she has become involved in the dynamic until his or her involvement has resulted in an interruption or disruption of the client-therapist relationship.

MANAGING MALADAPTIVE DYNAMICS OF SYSTEMS

At one time or another and to varying degrees of intensity, certain maladaptive dynamics are bound to emerge within almost any social system one encounters. The goal of learning about these dynamics is to:

- Understand their implications for the group and for occupational engagement.
- Anticipate their effects on relationships within the group.
- Remain an objective observer of the dynamic.
- Make an intentional decision about whether and how to manage the dynamic.

Even though maladaptive dynamics inevitably involve negative feelings for one or more members, they are very difficult to change. No matter how uncomfortable or unhappy they are, members of the system will habitually act together to sustain the dynamic because this is how they are most accustomed to interacting with one another. This is often the case even if members of the system recognize that sustaining the dynamic results in negative outcomes for the client or group. Because systems are, by nature, highly resistant to change, it is important to continually strive toward an empathic understanding of any social system with which you are working. In striving to understand maladaptive dynamics within a social system, you should:

- Look to the system for the problem (e.g., all persons involved in the interaction), rather than to the client alone.
- Try to understand why members are invested in sustaining the maladaptive dynamic.

What makes sense about the dynamic? What interpersonal needs are served by the members of the system who are enacting the dynamic? How does the dynamic serve the client's needs? What might each of the members lose if they were to stop interacting in this way?

- Try to assume a historic or multigenerational understanding of the dynamic. When did it begin? Do members of the system have a history of interacting in this way? What is known about the childhood family relationships of those most invested in sustaining the maladaptive dynamic? How do their unique histories make them prime candidates to function in their current roles within the system?

After you have achieved an empathic understanding of the system, the next step is to decide whether to remain an objective observer of the maladaptive dynamics or whether to try to manage or eradicate them. The decision whether to intervene in the dynamic is best made by asking yourself the following questions:

- Is the dynamic interfering with the course of therapy?
- Does the group perceive that this dynamic is negatively affecting outcomes?
- Are certain members of the group attempting to replicate the dynamic within the therapeutic relationship? If so, what are the potential long-term outcomes of this behavior?

If the answer to any of these initial questions is *yes,* then the IRM recommends that therapists use their interpersonal reasoning to select and change modes while working to attenuate or eradicate a rigid way of interacting. If, through the use of modes, therapists are interpersonally in tune with all of the members of the system, the system will be more amenable to additional systems-focused interventions that might be attempted in the future. The empathizing mode is reliable and effective regardless of the dynamic being addressed. In many cases, it is considered a prerequisite for the use of any other mode because of its powerful ability to allow therapists to create an alliance with any member of the system that is problematic or otherwise in need of empathy. Maladaptive dynamics create an emotional environment that is often characterized by tension and feelings of vulnerability in various members of the system. The empathizing mode is often effective in reducing

TABLE 4-5   Examples of Dynamics that Have the Potential to Interfere with the Process or Desired Outcome of Therapy

Dynamic	Description
Help Seeking– Help Rejecting	When an individual establishes a pattern of asking for assistance, guidance, or advice and then explaining why it would not work, a help seeking–help rejecting dynamic has been established. Potential negative outcomes include frustration or decreased performance in the help seeker. This dynamic is most frequently observed in parent-child relationships or in other relationships involving a power differential. If it is entrenched, it may be replicated within the therapeutic relationship.
Competitive	Individuals often compete to obtain an interpersonal need or a valued resource, particularly if it is perceived to be in short supply. If this competition is sustained, potential negative outcomes include conflict between the competitors or feelings of decreased self-esteem in the loser. Although they may occur in any system, competitive dynamics are often observed between siblings, friends, or client peers within a given milieu.
Enabling Negative Behavior	When individuals permit, facilitate, or support the behavior of another individual even though it is negative or potentially harmful, they further enable the negative behavior. The outcome is a continuation or worsening of the behavior. This behavior is frequently observed in couple's relationships or in families in which people are not able to show disapproval or take steps to limit the behavior for fear of disappointing the other individual, making the individual angry, or losing the relationship altogether.
Dominance- Submission	A dominance-submission relationship is a nondemocratic system that is characterized by a clear power differential that involves the consistent oppression of some individuals by others. Individuals may attempt to dominate others to increase their perceived control over their life circumstances or to compensate for feelings of insecurity or inferiority. Individuals may assume a submissive role because they have limited resources or options for independence; they are accustomed to being mistreated; they have low self-esteem; they perceive themselves as less powerful; they perceive themselves as physically, emotionally, or intellectually inferior; or they wish to avoid confrontation. Potential outcomes include passivity, vulnerability, learned helplessness, or feelings of low self-worth in the submissive individuals. In worst cases, this dynamic evolves into a pattern of emotional, sexual, or physical abuse. These dynamics are most likely to occur in relationships that involve one individual assuming a caregiving role for a more vulnerable individual. Dominant or abusive behaviors suggest that the caregiver is not emotionally capable of functioning in that role and should either seek mental health services immediately or discontinue his or her relationship with the vulnerable individual entirely.
Enmeshment	In an enmeshment dynamic, individuals have close ongoing contact. It is expected that individuals share information readily, even if it is highly intimate or personal. There is an expectation that all individuals conform and share similar worldviews and other behaviors and attitudes. Decision making is shared and the concept of individuality is downplayed. Members of enmeshed systems are fiercely loyal to each other despite conflicts or major transgressions. Caregivers in this dynamic often become over involved or controlling in reference to a client's treatment. The potential negative outcomes of an enmeshment dynamic include a closed or secretive system that is difficult for health care professionals to enter; psychological dependency between members; a lack of individuality between members; and occasionally feelings of angst or resentment related to the perception that one's efforts are being controlled, stifled, or smothered by the system. Enmeshment dynamics are most often observed in families and couples.
Disengagement	Disengagement dynamic occurs when individuals have little contact and do not share personal information readily. Individuals in the system view themselves as independent of one another in terms of worldview, attitudes, behavior, and decision making. The potential negative outcome is a lack of closeness, loyalty, communication, and connection between members. Caregivers in this dynamic are typically under involved in the client's care. Potential negative consequences of this dynamic include feelings of isolation and disappointment in others' lack of presence and investment. In worst cases, disengagement within systems can result in the physical or medical neglect of a client. Although they may occur in any system, disengagement dynamics are most often observed in families and couples.
Approach- Avoidance	When an individual enters a relationship with an expectation that the other will fulfill certain (often unrealistic) needs, there is often a period of intense contact and, in some cases, feelings of closeness. When people are ambivalent about this closeness or when their intentions for the relationships are limited to seeking need fulfillment, they promptly retreat into avoidance. This avoidance may be explained by the fact that they perceived that their needs were not met or by the fact that the relationship became so intense in their minds that it evoked uncomfortable or contradictory feelings (e.g., feeling smothered, fears of abandonment or rejection, feelings of rage, an intense and unfulfilled desire to be admired or unconditionally accepted). When approach-avoidance dynamics occur in couples' relationships, they often involve the same partner repeatedly approaching the other partner to obtain need fulfillment and the other partner repeatedly finding ways to withdraw. Because the approaching partner's needs are not gratified, the approach behaviors become increasingly intense (and sometimes demanding) over time. In return, the avoiding partner continues to find ways to increase withdrawal (e.g., falls asleep, leaves the environment, becomes emotionally unresponsive, is at a loss for words, remains at work later, spends more time with others, focuses more on the children, or turns to substances or other addictions) to counterbalance the approach behavior. The outcome is a relationship characterized by unpredictability, a lack of trust, feeling smothered or abandoned, and a lack of mutuality. Clients who suddenly appear intensely connected and divulge a tremendous amount of personal details during one session only to appear distant or fail to show up for the next session may be enacting this dynamic in therapy.

TABLE 4-5	**Examples of Dynamics that Have the Potential to Interfere with the Process or Desired Outcome of Therapy—cont'd**
Dynamic	**Description**
Idealizing-Devaluing	Individuals can be consistently idealizing of one another, consistently devaluing, or they can change between the two states. An idealizing dynamic is one in which individuals filter their perceptions of others in such a way that the positive characteristics of the others are exaggerated and any negative characteristics are downplayed or denied entirely. A devaluing dynamic is the opposite in which the negative characteristics are exaggerated. Some individuals have a tendency to relate to and know others only in terms of these two categories. Either state is characterized by an unrealistic and superficial knowledge of others. When others unwittingly allow themselves to become a part of this dynamic, they eventually find it uncomfortable, terrifying, or infuriating. At one moment they may be placed unrealistically on a pedestal only to find that they will be rejected or even vilified in a subsequent interaction. This dynamic is often observed in relationships with health care providers (including occupational therapists), particularly when clients, parents, or partners have unrealistic expectations of the provider and do not want to assume sufficient responsibility for the problem or for the solution.
Reluctance-Reassurance	When an individual (couple, family, or group) is consistently anxious, skeptical, or self-doubting about engaging in occupation and others reliably attempt to bolster, entice, and reassure them, a dynamic of reluctance and reassurance is occurring. Potential negative outcomes of this dynamic include psychological dependency, low intrinsic motivation, and limited opportunities for independence and progress.
Demonstrative-Voyeuristic	When individuals become involved in elaborating on, embellishing, or dramatizing their reactions or hardships, they often have a need for their hardship to be recognized and validated. When others are entertained by this behavior or do nothing but watch or listen, a demonstrative-voyeuristic dynamic is occurring. Negative outcomes include lack of progress and the eventual realization that the voyeuristic party is taking pleasure in the behavior. Although this realization may only serve to increase the demonstrative behavior, it is neither a therapeutic or a humane way of relating. If committed by the therapist, this kind of voyeuristic behavior is unethical because it does not represent an attempt to provide best practice.
Helpless-Rescuing	A helpless-rescuing dynamic occurs when individuals fall into a pattern of recruiting assistance when it is not necessary. Often the helpless behavior is a maladaptive expression of an entrenched need to be loved, attended to, or cared for. For some individuals, this need is strong and it exists no matter how much love, care, and attention is provided. The other part of the system enables the helpless behavior by rushing in to assist without recognizing that the behavior is maladaptive. The outcomes include increased dependency on the part of the helpless individual and eventual anxiety or resentment on the part of the rescuers. This dynamic can be culturally contexted and may not always result in maladaptive outcomes for the client. Although it may occur in any system, it is most often observed in parents of disabled children who feel guilty or responsible for the impairment and are unaware of the consequences of enabling the child's helpless behavior.
Chaotic-Organizing	A chaotic-organizing dynamic is one in which one aspect of a system is irresponsible, disorganized, slovenly, undisciplined, or lacking in emotional self-control. The other part of the system continually seeks to compensate by replacing lost items, reminding the individual of scheduled appointments or necessary tasks, cleaning up and organizing the person's physical environment, or providing required emotional and logistic support so that the person can function. One maladaptive outcome of this dynamic is an ongoing power struggle between the chaotic and organizing aspects of the system. Another consequence is the intensification of the chaotic behavior. Although it may occur in any system, this dynamic is most frequently witnessed in systems in which one member has an impairment that affects cognition, such as attention deficit hyperactivity disorder, bipolar disorder, a psychotic disorder, or another neurologic condition.
Manipulating-Conceding	Some individuals may be accustomed to getting their needs met through manipulation, particularly when they perceive that there may be an obstacle to getting what they want. This involves a pattern of knowing what the other likes or needs, and then giving it out in small doses with the expectation that the other will reciprocate by gratifying the manipulator's needs. When the other party concedes out of feelings of obligation or guilt, the conceding party is fuelling the dynamic. Negative outcomes include eventual feelings of resentment and anger in the person enabling the dynamic and a failure to learn to ask for needs in a more direct manner and a failure to accept limits imposed by others in the manipulator. In occupational therapy, this dynamic is often observed when working with parents who struggle to feel confident about disciplinary approaches and often feel guilty about setting limits consistently. It may also be witnessed in couples, friendships, or in student-teacher relationships. If it exists, it is also likely to play out in the therapeutic relationship.
Scapegoating	When two or more individuals collude to influence, criticize, reprimand, subjugate, shame, punish, or otherwise control another individual, a scapegoating dynamic has emerged. These dynamics may involve entire families or groups that decide to ally against a single individual. Individuals are most likely to engage in this dynamic when they are allied around a common ideology or when they perceive the scapegoated individual has threatened the status quo or equilibrium of the system or if they feel that the individual is otherwise problematic. Often triangulation reflects a need to displace anger within the system and the most vulnerable, powerless, or emotionally safe individual is usually selected as the convenient target. Although this dynamic is most likely to occur within families or groups, it may also occur when a therapist forms an alliance with one of two parents against the other, with one or more clients against another, or with one partner of a couple against the other.

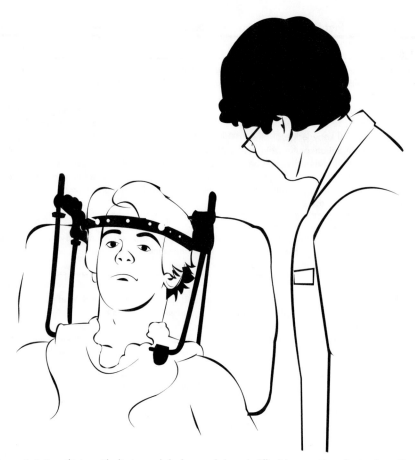

Figure 4-6 Empathizing with clients may help them work through difficult issues with professionals and family.

tension and bolstering peoples' self-confidence. If therapists explain the importance of hearing all voices upfront and then take the time and effort to hear and validate the perspectives of each member, a precedent for such behavior will be set within the system. The end result of beginning with an empathic approach toward the system is that members are ultimately primed to accept other modes and work to more receptively toward systems change (Figure 4-6).

APPLYING IRM TO CO-LEADERSHIP SITUATIONS

The interpersonal dynamics within a group become more complex when there is more than one leader present. When co-leading a group with another occupational therapist (or other professional), each therapist should be aware of the primary modes he or she is using and the effect of these modes on group dynamics. According to IRM, therapists should know what their strong and weak modes are[32] so that they may use each other's strengths to compensate for their own limitations while leading the group. The use of different modes and their effects on the different members and on the group dynamic as a whole should be discussed openly between co-leaders before and after each session. Adjustments in mode use should be made if it is determined that a certain mode or dynamic between the co-leaders is enabling counter-productive dynamics to occur within the group. Intentional use of modes by each co-leader

will increase the likelihood of occupational engagement for all group members and improve the overall dynamics and mood of exchange between members.

CASE STUDY: APPLYING IRM TO A CHILD'S PLAYGROUP

Three young girls, Alex, 11 years old; Iris, 9 years old; and Elizabeth, 11 years old, have routinely been placed into a group dynamic to focus on individual goals that address the ability to successfully function within group settings for return to a school environment. The group goals are for interactive imaginative play, rule following, and turn taking. In addition to group goals, each child has goals addressing deficits found that limit her ability for successful participation in school-based groups.

Alex is recovering from a head injury with deficits most significantly observed in short-term memory, initiation, abstraction, and other executive functions. Although her processing of speech is slow, she is open and social in her communication style and demonstrates a high level of comfort and trust with all therapists in the clinic. She presents with a mothering personality toward the younger children in the clinic; however, at times she is overly controlling within a group setting, offering uninvited assistance that overwhelms others in the group. She frequently demonstrates looks for approval from the therapist when she is assisting the other children. When confronted with challenges or change, she opts for tasks that are easy for her to perform and below her capacity cognitively and socially.

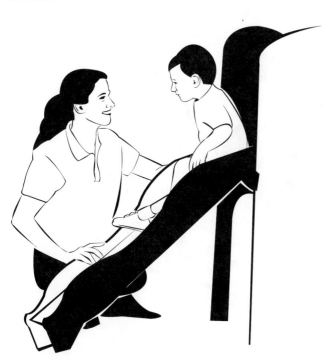

Figure 4-7 Encouraging clients to challenge themselves may be necessary.

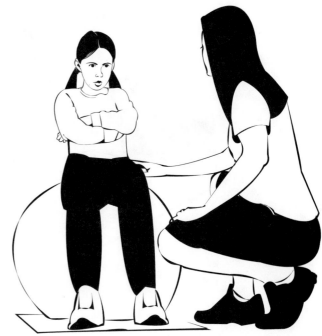

Figure 4-8 Practitioners using the instructing mode must be clear with directions.

Her affect is bright and positive in conditions she is familiar with but she has difficulty receiving feedback in her areas of deficits. She is open to touch and responds well to all levels of diversity, although she is withdrawn when in a room with an unfamiliar man. She frequently seeks out the therapist for affirmation of a job well done. An area of significant difficulty is her limited ability to provide feedback during group planning and decision making. She also has endurance and mild standing balance deficits. Individually and within the group setting encouraging mode and empathizing mode work best with Alex (Figure 4-7).

Iris is a 9-year-old girl recovering from removal of a malignant brain tumor followed by chemotherapy. She is in remission at this point. Her rehabilitation goals focus specifically on behavioral issues, emotional regulation, and cognitive deficits of attention to detail, divided attention, and impulsivity. Her interpersonal characteristics are representative of her behavioral and cognitive deficits. She is verbose and intrusive in her communication. She frequently interrupts the other children in the group and is tangential in her thoughts. Her need for control is very high. She frequently attempts to dominate the sessions and others and is manipulative in interactions with the other girls and therapists. She displays decreased capacity for trust, requesting frequent feedback from the therapist or others confirming their intentions. In conjunction with this, her intrusiveness occurs during group and individual tasks, frequently attempting to control the activity, conversation, or less outgoing group participants. She is overly assertive of her needs; however, her impulsivity predisposes her to spontaneously report her internal feelings on every subject. She is resistant to participate in tasks and activities that she has not identified as her own and attempts to bargain with the therapist to "get her way." She also frequently refuses to perform tasks that may challenge her cognitively or physically. Her emotional regulation displays itself most frequently when she is challenged or feels she has not

been allowed to do what she wants. Tantrums and physical threats toward the therapist occur when she senses she has lost control. She also appears to have a decreased capacity for touch because this frequently results in an aggressive response. This also occurs when limits are set or feedback is provided to her regarding her behavior or performance. Her verbosity includes providing unsolicited feedback to others in a group. The interpersonal characteristics of relating toward others, response to diversity, and capacity for reciprocity are immaturely developed in her at this time. Physical deficits include mild visual neglect and advanced balance deficits. Mode selection is much different with Iris in an individual setting than in a group setting. Individually, she at times works well in instructing and problem-solving mode; however, use of these modes in a group setting consistently creates power dilemmas (Figures 4-8 and 4-9). Within a group setting, empathizing mode is most effective at this time.

Elizabeth is an 11-year-old child with cerebral palsy from birth. She has no cognitive deficits; however, she is socially withdrawn and tactilely defensive. Her communication style is much better in one-on-one sessions than in group settings. She appears reluctant to offer her opinion or choices for activities and withdraws when encouraged. Her initial decreased capacity for trust of other children and therapists is evident in nonverbal cues such as standing in the background, making limited eye contact, and responses during group discussions or activity selection. Elizabeth has a problematically low need for control. She appears passive during most tasks and is dominated by the others in the group. She is indirect in her assertion of her needs and appears to lack confidence in her abilities through statements such as "I'm not good at that" or "I'm slow at everything I do." Because of this decreased self-confidence she is reluctant during tasks or activities that are new to her or perceived to

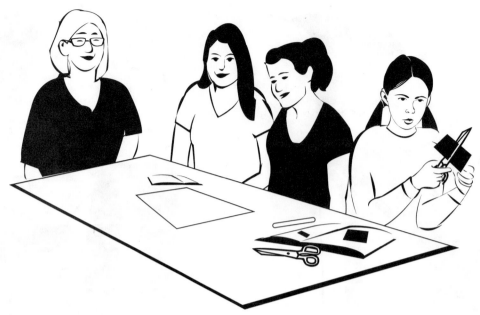

Figure 4-9 Using the problem-solving mode with clients allows them to figure things out.

be beyond her capacity. She does well with encouragement when in one-on-one sessions, often surprising herself when she achieves something new; however, this has not transitioned to behavior noted in group settings. Despite appearing anxious and shy, her affect and emotional regulation is good. She receives feedback and incorporates it; however, she rarely provides feedback and when solicited she is hesitant. Her sensitivity to others is significant. She demonstrates a high level of empathy toward other children and when given an opportunity to assist another, her affect brightens and her engagement increases. She responds well to diversity and relates well with her therapists. She prefers limited touch and does best with deep pressure, and this has created difficulty in group settings. Her capacity for reciprocity between herself and other children is high. She demonstrates the ability for increased tolerance and patience in all scenarios and often expresses gratitude to others when she has received outside help. She presents physically with decreased functional use of her right upper extremity for fine motor and gross motor tasks, decreased standing balance, and ability for transitional movements into and out of positions. During one-on-one sessions Elizabeth functions very well when the therapist uses collaborating and problem-solving modes. In a group setting she also functions well with these; however, encouraging mode and empathizing mode are used more successfully.

The group sessions with these three clients at times will focus on engaging in a form of parallel play; however, the majority of the time the main goal is for the clients to work together to create or achieve some end result as a unified group. The various interpersonal characteristics of the clients have created both productive and maladaptive dynamics. Because of her interpersonal characteristics, Iris presents both as the most prominent influence in the group and the most engaged. This creates difficulties for the therapist, because Iris exerts her power at times to the extent that it affects the group in a negative way. When Iris is allowed to manipulate and control the group activities and

individuals, the emotional tone of the group becomes less goal focused as a team, and often the end result is failure to successfully complete the group project. The other negative result is continuation of interpersonal characteristics that are reinforcing the inability of each of the girls to be a successful participant in group environments. Another dynamic that exists within the group is the dynamic between Alex and Elizabeth. This dynamic has mixed results in that it can be productive in facilitating a helping emotion within the group environment, but, when allowed to dominate, it is maladaptive for Elizabeth's independence and creates a conflict in Iris, because she feels left out of the group dynamic.

The intentional choice made by the occupational therapist is to use empathizing mode with advancement to collaboration mode during group activities. Other mode use is observed; however, these two facilitate the most productive dynamic scenarios during group play. The following is an example of the group in a recent treatment session:

The three girls quickly engage with each other in the kid's playroom. Alex and Elizabeth hold hands as they are walking into the room and Iris runs in front of them. Once the group has settled, discussion on the activity selection for the day begins. Alex and Elizabeth agree that they should do coloring and Iris shouts out that coloring is boring and they should do puzzles. Using empathizing mode, the therapist agrees that each of those activities sounds like a good idea but reminds the group that the goal is to do a big project together. The therapist suggests that the girls work together on a big activity and at the end of the session they can have 10 minutes of free-choice time. All the group members agree to this with positive affect. Sitting together in a circle on the floor, the group begins to think and imagine what fun story they can make up. The therapist asks each girl to provide input, taking turns creating a narrative of an imaginary journey of three girls traveling to a far-off land. Iris begins to dominate the story; however, the therapist, using empathizing mode, suggests that, although all her ideas are good, they will start with only one of the good ideas. Iris does *not feel deflated by this and instead chooses one aspect of her story to incorporate. The therapist then asks either Alex or Elizabeth to go next. Both girls hesitate, but, using empathizing mode again, the therapist, hoping to work on some memory areas, suggests to Alex that she might have good ideas from a story she has read or heard recently. She struggles to come up with an idea, but with some cueing is able to. The therapist used encouraging mode to reinforce to the group what good turn-taking they are doing and how good the story is sounding. Next it is Elizabeth's turn to add to the narrative. Despite having the strongest cognitive skills and ability to abstract, her withdrawn behavior makes this activity challenging. Alex appears to sense this and begins to provide suggestions, which is most interesting because she was unable to come up with ideas while it was her turn. Iris also begins to verbalize her ideas, which creates a dynamic furthering Elizabeth's decreased ability to provide feedback. Using empathizing mode, the therapist reinforces that each girl's ideas are good ones; however, the goal of the story making is that everyone has a chance to add an original idea. The therapist, using empathizing mode, moves very slightly in front of Elizabeth between her and the other girls to give her a sense of separation while she thinks. Elizabeth suggests two ideas and, using collaboration mode, the therapist asks the group to decide which of the two good ideas Elizabeth came up with they should put into their story. Elizabeth's affect is obviously more engaged by this. The group discusses how the story would sound with each idea and together make a decision. The group goal is to act out the narrative to a successful completion. Using IRM, this therapist's intentional incorporation of mode use allowed the group to successfully complete the creation of a narrative with each individual participating as an equal component of a productive dynamic.*

SUMMARY

As noted in the beginning of this chapter, OT is rich in literature supporting the effectiveness of a successful client-therapist relationship. Despite this, there has been an absence of a model for therapists to use as a source for developing concrete skills and competencies that are necessary to enact them within a clinical setting. This chapter introduced the IRM, and offers it as that source for skill development and competencies in group and individual OT settings. IRM provides a theoretical framework for understanding the significance that all interactions have and guidance in how to therapeutically respond in a manner that best serves the client. The defined suggestions for therapeutically responding to client interpersonal characteristics and inevitable interpersonal events are invaluable tools for any therapist. Introduction and instruction in six therapist interpersonal modes for relating to clients were provided both for individual treatment and group dynamics. The case example allowed the reader the opportunity to evaluate the significant effect of understanding clients' interpersonal characteristics and planned therapeutic mode use has on successful therapist-client interactions and productive versus maladaptive dynamics within the group. The combined elements of the IRM are established guides for better understanding the client, the interpersonal events that occur in therapy, and what the therapist brings to the situation and the occupation. IRM offers a tool for occupational therapists to learn how to understand the theoretical framework of therapeutic use of self and guidance in effectively positioning the client as the focal point of each therapy session, individual or group, for successful engagement in occupational tasks.

REVIEW QUESTIONS

1. The IRM focuses on four main components of the therapist-client relationship. These are: _____ _____ _____

2. When a therapist is planning a treatment session with a given client, the choice and application of a particular therapeutic mode or set of modes depend on two major qualities that the client brings to the therapy session. Describe these. _____ _____

3. A *dynamic* defines the distinctive quality, emotional tone, and specific interpersonal events that compose an interaction between individuals. Dynamics can be defined as *productive* or *maladaptive*. Provide one example for each. _____ _____ _____

4. In the case example that was provided, identified modes were empathizing, encouraging, and collaborative. As you read through the descriptions of the events of the group,

   another mode was used but not identified in the description. Based on reviews of the events, what other mode may have been used? _____ _____

5. In the group case example, describe how the dynamic between Alex and Elizabeth is a productive dynamic for the group. _____ _____

6. In the group case example, describe how the dynamic between Alex and Elizabeth is maladaptive. _____ _____ _____

7. Failure of a therapist to notice or understand a communication from a client or communication or behavior initiated by the therapist that is perceived by the client as hurtful or insensitive is what form of inevitable interpersonal event? _____ _____

REFERENCES

1. American Occupational Therapy Association: Occupational therapy practice framework: domain and process, *Am J Occup Ther* 62:625-683, 2008.

2. American Psychiatric Association: *2000 Diagnostic and statistical manual of mental disorders—text revision. IV*, Arlington, VA, 2000, American Psychiatric Association.

3. Ayres-Rosa S, Hasselkus BR: Connecting with patients: the personal experience of professional helping, *Occup Ther J Res* 16:245-260, 1996.

4. Baum CM: Occupational therapists put care in the health system, *Am J Occup Ther* 34:505-516, 1980.

5. Cole B, McLean V: Therapeutic relationships re-defined, *Occup Ther Mental Health* 19(2):33-56, 2003.

6. Devereaux EB: Occupational therapy's challenge: the caring relationship, *Am J Occup Ther* 38:791-798, 1984.

7. Fleming MH: The therapist with the three-track mind, *Am J Occup Ther* 45:1007-1014, 1991.

8. Gilfoyle EM: Caring: a philosophy for practice, *Am J Occup Ther* 34:517-521, 1980.

9. Jonsson H, Josephsson S, Kielhofner G: Narratives and experience in an occupational transition: a longitudinal study of the retirement process, *Am J Occup Ther* 55:424-432, 2001.

10. Kielhofner G: *Conceptual foundations of occupational therapy*, ed 2, Philadelphia, 1997, FA Davis.

11. Kielhofner G: *Conceptual foundations of occupational therapy*, ed 3, Philadelphia, 2004, FA Davis.

12. King LJ: Creative caring, *Am J Occup Ther* 34:522-528, 1980.

13. Lyons KD, Crepeau EB: The clinical reasoning of an occupational therapy assistant, *Am J Occup Ther* 55:577-581, 2001.

14. Mattingly C: The narrative nature of clinical reasoning, *Am J Occup Ther* 45:998-1005, 1991.

15. Mattingly C: The narrative nature of clinical reasoning. In Mattingly C, Flemming MH, editors: *Clinical reasoning: forms of inquiry in a therapeutic practice*, Philadelphia, 1994, FA Davis, pp 239-269.

16. Mattingly C, Fleming MH: *Clinical reasoning: forms of inquiry in a therapeutic practice*, Philadelphia, 1994, FA Davis. pp 178-196.

17. Mosey AC: *Three frames of reference for mental health*, Thorofare, NJ, 1970, Slack.

18. Peloquin SM: Moral treatment: contexts considered, *Am J Occup Ther* 43:537-544, 1989a.

19. Peloquin SM: Sustaining the art of practice in occupational therapy, *Am J Occup Ther* 43:219-226, 1989b.

20. Peloquin SM: The patient-therapist relationship in occupational therapy: understanding visions and images, *Am J Occup Ther* 44:13-21, 1990.

21. Peloquin SM: The depersonalization of patients: a profile gleaned from narratives, *Am J Occup Ther* 47:830-837, 1993.

22. Peloquin SM: The fullness of empathy: reflections and illustrations, *Am J Occup Ther* 49:24-31, 1995.

23. Peloquin SM: Art: an occupation with promise for developing empathy, *Am J Occup Ther* 50(8):655-661, 1996.

24. Peloquin SM: Reclaiming the vision of reaching for heart as well as hands, *Am J Occup Ther* 56:517-526, 2002.

25. Peloquin SM: The therapeutic relationship: manifestations and challenges in occupational therapy. In Crepeau EB, Cohn ES, Boyt Schell BA, editors: *Willard and Spackman's occupational therapy*, ed 10, Philadelphia, 2003, Lippincott, Williams & Wilkins, pp 157-170.

26. Punwar J, Peloquin M: *Occupational therapy: principles and practice*, Philadelphia, 2000, Lippincott, pp 42-98.

27. Rogers JC: Clinical reasoning: the ethics, science, and art (1983 Eleanor Clarke Slagle lecture), *Am J Occup Ther* 37:601-616, 1983.

28. Schell BA: Clinical reasoning: the basis of practice. In Crepeau EB, Cohn ES, Boyt Schell BA, editors: *Willard and Spackman's occupational therapy*, ed 10, Philadelphia, 2003, Lippincott, Williams & Wilkins, pp 131-152.

29. Schell BA, Cervero RM: Clinical reasoning in occupational therapy: an integrative review, *Am J Occup Ther* 47:605-610, 1993.

30. Schwartz KB: The history of occupational therapy. In Crepeau EB, Cohn ES, Boyt Schell BA, editors: *Willard and Spackman's occupational therapy*, ed 10, Philadelphia, 2003, Lippincott, Williams & Wilkins, pp 5-13.

31. Schwartzberg SL: *Interactive reasoning in the process of occupational therapy*, Upper Saddle River, NJ, 2002, Pearson Education.

32. Taylor R: *The intentional relationship: occupational therapy and use of self*, Philadelphia, 2008, FA Davis.

33. Taylor R, Lee S, Kielhofner G, Ketkar M: Therapeutic use of self: a nationwide survey of practitioners' attitudes and experience, *Am J Occup Ther* 63:198-207, 2009.

34. Townsend E: Reflections on power and justice in enabling occupation, *Revue Canadienne D'Erotherapie* 70:74-87, 2003.

35. Yerxa EJ: Occupational therapy's role in creating a future climate of caring, *Am J Occup Ther* 34, 1980. 509-679.

Teaching and Learning

Jean W. Solomon

KEY TERMS

aural perceptual mode	olfactory perceptual mode
case method of instruction	perceptual learning styles
direct teaching	print perceptual mode
haptic perceptual mode	teaching
indirect teaching	universal design for learning
interactive perceptual mode	(UDL)
kinesthetic perceptual mode	visual perceptual mode
learning	

CHAPTER OBJECTIVES

1. Discuss the relevance of teaching and learning from an occupational therapy perspective.
2. List and describe methods of teaching.
3. List the principles of universal design and apply these principles to learning.
4. List and discuss perceptual pathways or styles of learning.
5. Discuss teaching and learning concepts during occupational analysis.
6. Discuss teaching and learning concepts during group processes.

Occupational therapy (OT) practitioners teach clients how to reengage in occupations after trauma, disease, or developmental disability. Understanding the teaching and learning process is essential to OT practice. In this chapter, the author describe specific methods of teaching, teaching tools, and the application of teaching to OT practice. A description of universal design, perceptual pathways, and motor learning principles provides readers with specific techniques for practice.

Teaching and learning are reciprocal and lifelong processes. A reciprocal process is one in which the roles of the teacher and learner alternate during the interactions. It is human nature to continue to learn throughout one's life. From a pediatric perspective, infants gain skills in performance components to become actively engaged in the areas of occupation (e.g., an infant's ability to sit supported promotes independence in self-feeding). From an aging perspective, as one's strength, balance, and endurance lessen, alternate ways of performing occupations may be learned (e.g., sitting while dressing). **Learning** is gaining awareness and understanding by active participation in activities that lead to skills. **Teaching** refers to imparting knowledge or skill.

The teacher facilitates learning by designing appropriate lesson or activity plans and sharing information. OT practitioners teach clients through doing. Helping clients engage in the problem-solving process engages them for learning. OT practitioners use a variety of methods when teaching clients to reengage.

METHODS OF TEACHING

The two major categories of method of instruction are **direct** and **indirect**.[10] The combination of direct and indirect instruction is known as an *eclectic approach.* The practitioner using a direct method teaches in a formal style. The environment is not a free-choice for instruction. The learner is expected to pay attention. The practitioner uses an autocratic leadership style.[1,7] Box 5-1 lists the characteristics of a teacher who uses the direct method of instruction.

Using an indirect method involves an informal style of teaching. The environment allows the learner to make choices.[1,7] For example, reading, writing, and math centers in a preschool setting allow children to learn on their own. This method encourages self-initiation and expression. The teacher uses a laissez faire leadership style.[1,7] Box 5-2 describes the characteristics of a teacher who uses an indirect method of instruction.

OT practitioners frequently set up the environment and allow the client to problem solve through the activity with little instruction. This indirect method may help clients gain ability and feel empowered. They may develop unique ways of doing things. Their problem-solving abilities allow them to work through a variety of situations and are helpful for the future. Practitioners also use a direct method of teaching that involves instructing or demonstrating each step of an activity. Often a combination of approaches serves clients best, allowing clients some direct instruction to learn basics before allowing them to problem solve and figure out solutions on their own. See Box 5-3 for examples of each method.

LEARNING ENVIRONMENT

Instruction occurs both in **formal** and **informal environments**.[7] A formal instructional environment is characterized by individual work, emphasis on assessment, and use of external motivators. The result of formal instruction is typically academic achievement. For example, the OT practitioner uses

formal instruction during prewriting and handwriting groups. The OT practititoner teaches the steps, strokes, and patterns sequentially. Children complete work independently and are assessed to determine how well they have achieved the needed skills.

An informal instructional environment is characterized by freedom in choosing activities and minimal emphasis on assessment or the use of external motivators. This type of environment fosters thoughtful and creative learners. Learners must decide how to do things and develop solutions. Informal environments are helpful for clients who must learn to problem solve. Therefore, this type of learning requires some basic skills and is often used after periods of direct instruction.[1,10] The occupational therapy practitioner uses informal instruction during sensory processing groups. Throughout the occupational therapy process a combination of formal and informal teaching styles is applied.

TOOLS FOR TEACHING

The choice and use of teaching tools depend on the content and context of the subject matter (Box 5-4). The **objects and materials** used in the activity may serve to teach clients. For example, providing an adult who has experienced a stroke with a shirt to put on may remind the client of the technique. The adult may be able to recall putting on a shirt and now needs to figure out how to do this with limited arm use. In this way, the object serves as a reminder to facilitate the learning. **Media** and **methods** are terms that an occupational therapy practitioner uses when planning interventions on an individual or group basis. *Media* is the plural form of the word *medium*. A medium is the materials used during the intervention process.[2] For example, a child engaged in making paper bag puppets uses media that include the paper bag, glue, and other materials and supplies, and the *method* refers to the set-up, steps of the process, and cleaning up. A method is a means of accomplishing a task.[2] OT practitioners use an eclectic approach combining the direct and indirect methods while providing interventions. Examples of therapeutic media are playdough, arts and crafts supplies, and scented markers.

Visual aids may be useful to remind clients of key points, sequences, and directions. Visual aids used for teaching can be based in low or high technology. Visual aids provide cues to remind clients of the steps. Examples of low-technology visual aids are picture boards, handouts for sequencing the steps of an activity, and handwritten transparencies projected from an overhead (Figure 5-1).

BOX 5-1	**Direct Teaching: Characteristics of the Teacher**

1. Analyzes student's behavior.
2. Responds to observable behavior.
3. Directs decisions and activities.
4. Keeps records.
5. Uses external motivations such as grades.

BOX 5-2	**Indirect Teaching: Characteristics of the Teacher**

1. Cares for and respects students.
2. Encourages student-initiated behaviors.
3. Solicits ideas for students.
4. Focuses on nonobservable behaviors such as thoughts and feelings.
5. Encourages learner's inner potential.

BOX 5-3	**Examples of Direct and Indirect Methods**

Direct Method

The OT practitioner uses direct instruction when teaching a group of children the proper mechanics of letter and number formation. The children are seated at a table with writing materials available. The OT practitioner instructs the children to start their letters at the top and to stay on and between the lines on the paper.

The OT practitioner may use a direct instructional approach while teaching a client to perform a transfer. The steps of the specific transfer are taught. The client is tested for accuracy and safety prior to performing the transfer.

Indirect Method

The practitioner uses indirect instruction during a sensory processing intervention session. The environment is structured to meet the sensory needs of the members of the group. The children choose which activities to engage in with facilitation from the OT practitioner.

An informal instructional approach may be used when planning what clothes to wear during activities of daily living interventions. The session may first begin with a discussion of the weather and clothes available. The client may want to have a conversation about the colors and types of clothes to wear.

BOX 5-4	**Tools for Teaching**

- Objects that stimulate learning
- Visual aids (e.g., colorful handouts)
- Meaningful repetition
- Plain language
- "Just-right" challenge
- Active engagement
- Activity analysis

High-technology visual aids include things such as PowerPoint shows or DVDs for teaching. Auditory aids may also be used to facilitate learning. Recorded music incorporated into the learning environment or auditory feedback systems are examples of auditory aids. Many learners benefit from a kinesthetic approach to teaching. This means learning through moving and doing. A multisensory approach using several sensory pathways simultaneously with teaching is often the most successful (Figure 5-2). For example, while working with a preschool child who has autism spectrum disorder, the OT practitioner may incorporate music to help the child focus while engaging the child in movement experiences.

Clients learn by doing and OT practitioners help facilitate clients' engagement in activity. This involves providing clients with **plain language** (sixth-grade level). Using clear and concise directions to highlight key aspects of the activity helps clients learn. **Meaningful repetition** provides clients with the practice needed to fully integrate the movements or sequence of steps.[6] Learning how to divide the parts of the activity into basic actions is an essential part of practice. Practitioners teach clients by providing the **"just-right" challenge**, a challenge that is not so easy as to make clients bored nor a challenge that is so difficult as to make clients frustrated. Often, the key to successful intervention is understanding the activity and how to change the demands for specific clients.

Active engagement in a variety of activities helps clients learn. Using visual, auditory, and movement methods reinforces learning. OT practitioners rely heavily on learning by doing. In this way, much time is spent in OT teaching clients through "doing." As clients become actively involved in activities, they learn.[6]

Frequently, practitioners use home programs, handouts, or visual cues to help clients remember, learn, and follow through. Colorful and attractive handouts written in plain language are most effective. Handouts should not be overwhelming or include extraneous language.

Table 5-1 provides a completed chart to help students examine the tools they are using in practice. This example shows how a meal preparation activity making pasta can be organized to address each suggested guideline when providing direct or indirect instruction.

TEACHING TECHNIQUES

Although one-on-one direct instruction may be the primary mode of teaching, OT practitioners also use indirect methods as described earlier in this chapter. Other techniques may be beneficial. For example, role playing, case methods, and group projects are effective techniques to facilitate learning.

Role playing helps clients see things from a different perspective. This technique can be effective in helping clients try out new skills and abilities in a safe environment. Clients must understand that they are engaging in a "pretend scenario" and

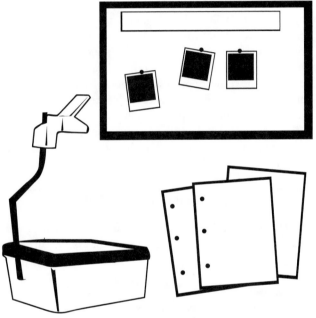

Figure 5-1 Low technology instructional tool: overhead projector.

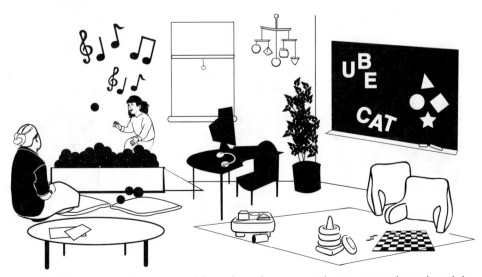

Figure 5-2 Students being directly instructed during dance class using a multisensory approach: visual, vestibular, and somatosensory pathways.

be able to verbalize. Role playing may help clients prepare for new activities. For example, a client may role play the expectations that are required to participate in a community outing. The practitioner may add obstacles to the role play, such as asking the client how he or she might react if someone gets too close on the bus. Role playing may provide clients with some insights into others' feelings or may allow the client to express feelings. The OT practitioner must carefully design role playing sessions. These sessions are best performed with a few clients.

TABLE 5-1   Using Tools for Teaching: Meal Preparation

ACTIVITY: PASTA

Tool	Example Related to This Activity
Meaningful repetition	Repeat pouring, measuring, stirring. Clients will make a variety of pastas (e.g., spaghetti, bowties, ziti).
Plain language	Recipe is written in plain language in large print on one sheet of paper.
"Just-right" challenge	Some members will be able to work independently from written directions; others will be guided with one-on-one directions.
Objects to stimulate learning	Familiar foods will help clients associate cooking tasks and remember familiar tasks (that they may have lost).
Colorful handout	Handouts and directions will be colorful, attractive, and professional. A picture of the completed dish will be included.
Active engagement	Clients will each make a dish of pasta and eat the meal together. They will participate in all steps of the activity.

The **case method** of instruction offers the learner the opportunity for brainstorming and application of the knowledge being learned. A brief case study is reviewed by the learners. The teacher serves as the facilitator, asking guiding questions. The teacher records the ideas from the learners (Figure 5-3). At the end of the session, the learners come to a consensus as to the best practices and approaches for the particular case. Using the case method of instruction gives the learner more opportunities to explore a variety of options for interventional strategies.

The case method is useful in brainstorming social behaviors. Clients are provided with social scenarios and asked to discuss possible responses. Clients read social stories and consider how they would respond or act in the scenarios. This type of learning may help clients reintegrate into social settings or prepare for new situations.

Group projects are frequently used in occupational therapy practice to facilitate learning. Group projects allow members to assist others. Members may contribute to the final project without having the burden of completing all aspects of the project. The sense of teamwork and camaraderie is often helpful in the recovery process. Members learn that they can contribute and make a difference despite their areas of weakness. Together, the group celebrates the outcome. The OT practitioner ensures that all members are contributing and may group certain members together so that they can help each other.

UNIVERSAL DESIGN FOR LEARNING

The Higher Education Opportunity Act (2008) defined **universal design for learning (UDL)** mandates as the curricular

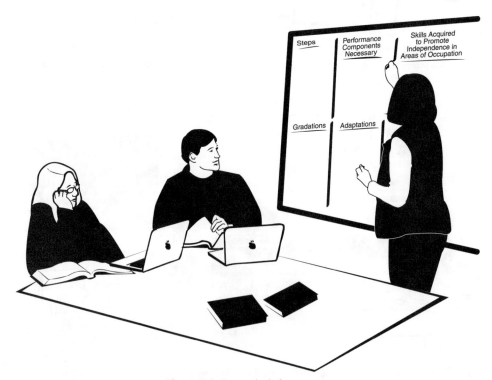

Figure 5-3 Case method of instruction.

flexibility to reduce barriers to provide appropriate supports and challenges, and to maintain high academic achievement standards for all students enrolled in primary and secondary public education programs. UDL applies equal access, flexibility, simplicity, perceptibility, and efficiency principles to the educational environment and to the process of teaching and learning. OT practitioners use activity and task analysis to determine if the environment and the teaching and learning processes are designed universally.[5,7] By analyzing the tasks required to complete activities, the practitioner can determine how best to adapt or change the steps so clients can be successful in completing the activity.

The principles of universal design for learning are derived from architecture. Products and environments following universal design are usable for all people without the need for adaptation or specialization.[3,5,7,9] Seven principles are considered for determining if a product or environment meets the criteria for universal design:

1. Equitable use or same means for all users
2. Flexible use or choice in methods
3. Simple and intuitive use or complexity eliminated
4. Perceptible information or different modes of use (perceptual pathways for learning)
5. Tolerance for error or removal of hazards
6. Low physical effort or minimal sustained or repetitive actions required for use
7. Size and space for use or adequate space for use[5,7]

UDL examines learning using multiple and flexible ways of representing, expressing, and engaging in the learning process. This approach allows students with different strengths, weaknesses, and preferences to actively engage in the learning process. OT practitioners use UDL principles and guidelines when designing and implementing occupation-based intervention.[7]

PERCEPTUAL PATHWAYS FOR LEARNING

Three neuronal networks interact during the process of learning: recognition, strategic, and affective.[4,9] The *recognition* network identifies patterns of sensory information and what is being learned. The *strategic* network assists in determining how learning is planned, executed, and monitored. The *affective* network determines the importance of what is learned and the emotions associated with learning. These three neuronal networks interact to make sense of the sensory information and result in an action. **Perception** refers to making sense of the information.[8,11] For example, visual perception is the ability to interpret what one sees. Visual perception is required to make sense of letters for reading (Worksheet 5-1).

Perception requires interactions between the central nervous system (CNS) and peripheral nervous system (PNS). The CNS and PNS have afferent (sensory) and efferent (motor) nerves.[8] The *afferent nerves* bring sensory information from our internal and external environments to the CNS for processing. The sensory information is processed in the CNS, which makes sense of the information received. The CNS uses this perception to determine the *efferent messages* to be sent to body structures or body functions to be effected. The nervous systems function primarily by a feedback mechanism. Sensory information is received (afferent), processed (cerebral cortex) and a command message is sent from the CNS to the effector[8] (Figure 5-4).

Perceptual modes of learning are the pathways for processing sensory information from the environment for use. These include **print**, **aural**, **interactive**, **visual**, **haptic**, **kinesthetic**, and **olfactory** learning styles[11] (Table 5-2). Individuals have preferred perceptual pathways for learning. For example, some college students enjoy learning through reading texts (print) whereas others enjoy listening to lectures (aural). Many students prefer interactive (discussion, small group) learning. OT students often prefer learning by doing (kinesthesia). Practitioners identify the style of learning best suited to the client.

Often the activity highlights a particular learning mode. For example, while one is engaged in cooking, the olfactory sensory system processes the odors to monitor the cooking status without looking. While one is learning a new dance routine, the visual and kinesthetic sensory systems are the preferred pathways. Table 5-3 provides examples to describe seven perceptual pathways as identified by Perceptual Styles Theory.[3,11]

WORKSHEET 5-1	Understanding Pathways of Learning

Use the following worksheet to identify how an activity can help clients learn.

ACTIVITY:

Process	Questions	Examples
Recognition	What is required for this activity? What must the client process? What is the sensory input?	Client must see clothing, feel buttons, sense where muscles and joints are for movement.
Strategic	What must the client "figure out?" What steps in the activity require problem solving? Must the client arrange things in relationship to others?	Client must place mixing bowl close and stir for a certain amount of time, sequence steps, monitor force, time events, and arrange materials.
Affective	What does the learner feel about the activity? What is the importance of the activity? Was the activity pleasurable? How did the learner assess his or her performance? What did the learner gain from the activity?	Client enjoyed making a familiar meal. The client is the primary caregiver of the family so making this dish was important to regaining some identity. The learner felt good about his or her performance.

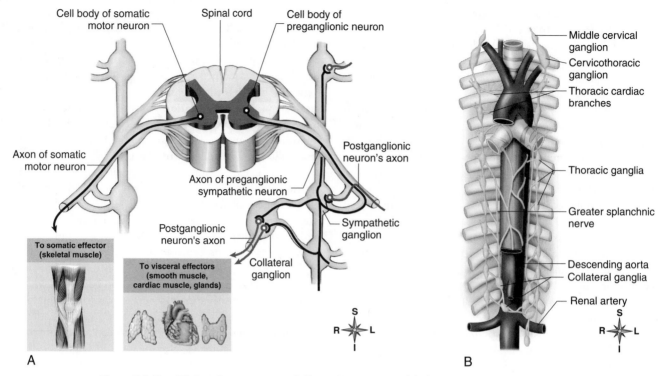

Figure 5-4 (A and B) Central nervous system and effectors. (From Patton KT, Thibodeau GA: *Anatomy and Physiology,* ed 7, St Louis, 2012, Elsevier.

TABLE 5-2	Perceptual Learning Styles and Characteristics[11]
Perceptual Learning Style	**Characteristics**
Print	Takes notes. Learns best by seeing. Reads often.
Aural	Remembers and repeats ideas. Excellent listener. Enjoys drama, music, dialogues.
Interactive	Enjoys small-group discussions. Prefers to discuss things. Learns best through verbalization.
Visual	Learns through watching demonstrations. Drifts when extensive listening is required. Likes picture graphs and other visual aids.
Haptic	Learns through touching. Likes to trace words and pictures. Likes tasks that require manipulating objects.
Kinesthetic	Learns by doing and moving. Gestures while speaking. Finds reasons to move, which increases concentration.
Olfactory	Learns best by smelling and tasting. Associates smell with past experiences. Scents increases learning.

TABLE 5-3	Perceptual Pathways
Pathway	**Example**
Print: reading	Providing a written recipe for a cooking group
Aural: listening	Providing clients with verbal instructions of the steps of an activity
Interactive: discussing	Facilitating a discussion as to the possible sequence of an activity
Visual: watching demonstrations	Providing a motor model, such as drawing a circle and then asking the child to draw a circle
Haptic: manipulating	Encouraging an adult to assemble a puzzle
Kinesthetic: moving	Engaging clients in sensory motor activities, such as imitating postures
Olfactory: smelling	Incorporating scents (e.g., peppermint or cinnamon) into an activity

BOX 5-5   Characteristics of an Effective Teacher

1. Knowledgeable and enthusiastic
2. Effective communicator who provides feedback
3. Positive attitude toward students and teaching
4. Fair in offering learning opportunities and grading
5. Flexible in instructional approaches
6. Cognizant of individual and group needs

APPLICATION OF TEACHING AND LEARNING CONCEPTS TO OCCUPATIONAL ANALYSIS

Occupational analysis is a systematic and thoughtful process that guides an OT practitioner's clinical reasoning for planning and implementing interventions. The OT practitioner uses the knowledge of his or her teaching characteristics to design interventions. See Box 5-5 for a list of the characteristics of an effective teacher.

The OT practitioner uses activity analysis and synthesis in designing and planning individual or group interventions (see Chapter 2). The OT practitioner also considers the **perceptual learning styles** of the client. Optimal learning occurs when the "just-right challenge" is presented. For example, once a child can independently finger feed, the next challenge is to introduce spoon feeding.

Backward Chaining

In backward chaining, the last step is taught first (e.g., the child first learns to return the spoon to the bowl). When teaching a child to spoon feed independently, backward chaining is more effective and successful than forward chaining. Using backward chaining the practitioner physically assists the child in scooping the food and taking the spoon to the mouth. The child independently takes the spoon back to the plate. In this case, the child is successful early on and therefore the behavior is reinforced.

Forward Chaining

Forward chaining teaches the first step of the process and proceeds to the next. For example, in forward chaining, a client would learn first to pick up the spoon. The practitioner completes the activity by providing hand-over-hand assistance.

APPLICATION OF TEACHING AND LEARNING CONCEPTS TO GROUP PROCESS

A group is two or more people who have come together because of one or more common interests or needs. In an effective group the roles of teacher and learner are shared by all of the group members. The group leader or facilitator learns and adjusts as the group process evolves.

The OT group leader is concerned that each member achieve his or her individual goals. Working with a group of clients presents different challenges when compared with providing one-on-one intervention. Planning the interventions is critical to the success of the group process. The sequence of the activities is carefully considered. A successful sequence includes **warm-up (preparatory)** activities, practicing **purposeful activities**, engaging in **occupations**, and then **wind-down activities**. For example, the OT practitioner applies moist heat to the client's left elbow prior to gentle stretching, followed by active assisted exercises (preparatory, warm-up activities). Next, the client practices reaching into kitchen cabinets to retrieve food items (purposeful activity). The client opens the packages and prepares the casserole (occupation). While the casserole is cooking, the practitioner applies moist heat to the involved

TABLE 5-4	Checklist for Teaching Process	
Activity:		
Preparation		
	Space	
	Supplies and materials	
	Completed project	
	Handouts	
	Time needed	
	Costs	
	Travel	
	Precautions (allergies, sunscreen)	
	Activity plan (introduction, activity, conclusion)	
Activity	Group members needs	
	Special considerations	
	Directions	
	Wrap-up—reminders	
	Clean up	
Follow up		
Suggestions for next time		

elbow followed by gentle stretching and active-assisted exercises (wind-down).

Teaching and Learning Process

Teaching requires that the leader be prepared, provide structure, follow rules, and follow-up. Table 5-4 provides a checklist for preparing to lead a group activity. The OT practitioner is careful to consider that all materials and supplies are available and in working order. Importantly, the practitioner ensures that there are enough materials for everyone. The space requirements are also factored into the preparation, as is consideration of the time to get to the space and prepare it for the activity. The leader is responsible for time management, which includes providing enough time to prepare the space, complete the activity, and clean up the space.

The leader monitors each member's performance and skillfully adjust steps so that each member is addressing his or her goals as well as group goals. The group process is essential to effective teaching. It requires that the teacher be aware of members' strengths and weaknesses and artfully figure out how to challenge members without overwhelming them. This may require special seating arrangements or advance preparation. Leaders prepare by considering who the group members are and how they may perform. Discussing group management strategies prior to the activity helps leaders act in therapeutic ways to the benefit of the group members. Spending time preparing for all possible situations is perhaps the best way for a group to succeed.

This preparation involves having sample end products available. Some groups may need a few samples, whereas other groups may become overwhelmed by choices and need only one sample. The leader can foresee any steps that may cause difficulty by doing the activity beforehand. Identifying steps that may be difficult allows the leader to adapt or change the techniques to allow for success.

Group leaders will introduce the group (or choose a member to do this), provide the supplies, and set the ground rules for the activity. As the activity progresses, the group leader adapts and modifies steps to help all members achieve their goals. Keeping track of time, the leader gauges how to help members succeed. The leader is aware of the group dynamics and may need to intervene to allow for positive interactions. Once the group is complete, the leader facilitates the wrap up or conclusion and clean up.

Follow up may be necessary. This is an integral part of the therapeutic relationship. For example, in one group a member left her completed picture in the OT clinic while it dried. The member asked if the OT group leader could return it to her at the end of the day. The OT group leader said yes and was sure to return the picture to the client at the end of the day. The client beamed with pride as the leader returned the picture and showed it to all of her peers. Following up with requests is part of the OT practitioner's professional responsibility.

MOTOR LEARNING PRINCIPLES APPLIED TO OCCUPATIONAL THERAPY PRACTICE

OT practitioners use principles of motor learning to provide effective strategies for the teaching-learning process to help people regain motor skills. *Motor learning principles* refer to those principles found to assist people in gaining motor skills[6] (Box 5-6).

Feedback refers to the messages the person receives from the movement.[6] For example, when a person kicks a ball, he or she feels the ball, how the leg moves, and the extension at the knee. These sensory experiences provide feedback to the person known as *internal feedback*. The person interprets the sensations. *External feedback* is provided by someone else, such as the practitioner.

Feedback may also refer to the person's assessment of the performance, also known as **knowledge of performance**. **Knowledge of results** includes information on the end product of the performance.[6] For example, knowledge of results may be relayed by responding, "You made a goal!"

The general rules of feedback suggest that feedback be specific, clear, concise, and consist of a few key words. Internal feedback is best for learning. Knowledge of performance is best for fine-tuning one's motor performance. For example, "You extended your knee fully" is better than "Good job!" Asking the client to reflect on his or her performance helps a person become aware of the motor requirements.

Practice is used to help clients remember the steps, motor requirements, or details of activity. Practice is therefore an essential part of learning and requires repetition. When teaching someone a new skill, the practitioner may decide to practice separate steps or even actions repeatedly with limited rest breaks. This type of practice is called **blocked** or **massed practice**. Blocked or massed practice may help a person fine-tune a skill or action.[6] For example, basketball players repeatedly practice the same shot to become proficient. **Distributive** or **random practice** provides for better carryover and allows the person to fine-tune skills and use the skill in a variety of situations. Distributive practice involves repeating a variety of movement or activity with varied rest breaks. For example, distributive practice may involve the basketball player taking five shots, running down the court, taking three more steps, and resting.

Meaningfulness of an activity helps the client engage more fully and produce a better result. Studies have shown that people will complete more repetitions when they find the activity meaningful. OT practitioners help clients return to meaningful activity and seek to find out the person's interests before engaging them in activity.[6] Practitioners may help clients see activity as meaningful by providing an end product.

Directions are key to teaching and learning. Practitioners frequently provide verbal or demonstrative directions. Verbal directions should be clear, concise, and emphasize the key parts to the movement. The practitioner should avoid speaking while the person is performing. The practitioner often provides a demonstration prior to the movement. The demonstration should be short, clear, and slow enough for the person to grasp the key components. It may be necessary to demonstrate small steps of the activity. Some clients may benefit from written or pictorial directions for activity.

Variability refers to the multiple ways in which an activity or movement can be performed. Typical movements are variable, which makes it possible for people to perform movements in a variety of **contexts** (situations and environments).[6] Research shows that helping clients practice movements in variable conditions in a variety of contexts produces better learning and results. Furthermore, allowing clients to perform the whole movement versus only a part of the movement is most effective. These principles support occupation-based movements that suggest that performing the movement within the natural context and in a real-life situation is the best for motor learning. OT practitioners may work on parts of movement until the person is able to perform, but the goal of intervention is for the person to preform the occupation in the natural environment. This requires practice in a variety of sitatuions.

SUMMARY

This chapter discusses the relevance of teaching and learning as a part of the occupational therapy process. Teaching and learning are defined. Methods of teaching are presented. The principles of universal design are presented and applied to the learning process. The perceptual pathways or styles of learning are discussed and examples are given for each mode of perceptual learning. The relevance of teaching and learning during occupational analysis and group processes is presented and exemplified with clinical examples.

| BOX 5-6 | Williams Motor Learning Principles[6] |

Transfer of Learning
- Skill experiences need to be presented in logical progression.
- Simple, foundational skills should be practiced before more complex skills.
- Skill practice should include "real-life" and simulated settings.
- Skills with similar components are more likely to show transfer effect.

Feedback

Modeling or Demonstration
- Demonstration is best if it is given to the individual prior to practicing the skill and the early stages of skill acquisition.
- Demonstration should be given throughout practice and as frequently as deemed helpful.
- Demonstrations should not be accompanied by verbal commentary because this can reduce attention paid to important aspects of the skill being demonstrated.
- It is important to direct the individual's attention to the critical cues immediately before the skill is demonstrated.

Verbal Instructions
- Verbal cues should be brief, to the point, and involve one to three words.
- Verbal cues should be limited in terms of numbers of cues given during or after performance.
- Only the major aspect of the skill that is being concentrated on should be cued.
- Verbal cues should be carefully timed so they do not interfere with performance.
- Verbal cues can and should be initially repeated by the performer.

Knowledge of Results and Knowledge of Performance
- A variety of different combinations of both knowledge of results (KR) and knowledge of performance (KP) typically helps to facilitate learning.
- KP error information may help the performer change important performance characteristics and thus may help facilitate skill acquisition.
- Information about "appropriate" or "correct" aspects of performance helps to motivate the person to continue practicing.
- It is important to balance between feedback that is error based and that based on appropriate or correct characteristics of the performance.
- KP feedback can also be descriptive or prescriptive; prescriptive KP is more helpful than just descriptive KP in early or beginning stages of learning.
- KP and KR should be given close in time to but after completion of the task.
- KP and KR typically should not necessarily be given 100% of the time.
- Learning is enhanced if KP and KR are given at least 50% of the time.

- A frequently used procedure for KR and KP is to practice a skill several times and then provide the appropriate feedback.

Distribution and Variability of Skill Practice
- Shorter, more frequent practice sessions are preferable to longer, less frequent practice.
- If a skill or task is complex, requires a relatively long time to perform, or requires repetitive movements, relatively short practice trials or sessions with frequent rest periods are preferable.
- If the skill is relatively simple and takes only a brief time to complete, longer practice trials or sessions with less frequent rest periods are preferable.
- It can enhance skill acquisition to practice several tasks in the same session.
- If several tasks are to be practiced, divide the time spent on each and either randomly repeat practice on each or use a sequence that aids the overall practice.
- Providing a number of different environmental contexts in which the skill is practiced appears to facilitate learning.
- With regard to the amount of practice, more is not necessarily always better.
- Clinical judgment should be used to recognize when practice is no longer producing changes; at this time, a new or different task could and probably should be introduced.

Whole Versus Part Practice
- Whole practice is better when the skill or task to be performed is simple.
- Part practice may be preferable when the skill is more complex.
- If part practice is used, be sure that the parts practiced are "natural units" or "go together," so to speak.
- To simplify a task, reduce the nature and complexity of the objects to be manipulated (e.g., use a balloon for catching instead of a ball, etc.).
- To simplify a task, provide assistance to the learner that helps to reduce attention demands (e.g., provide trunk support during practice of different eye-hand coordination tasks).
- To simplify a task, provide auditory or rhythmic accompaniment; this may help facilitate learning through assisting the learner in getting the appropriate "rhythm" of the movement.

Mental Practice
- Mental practice can facilitate acquisition of new skills as well as the relearning of old skills.
- Mental practice can help the person prepare to perform a task.
- Mental practice combined with physical practice work best.
- For mental practice to be effective, the individual should have some basic imagery ability.
- Mental practice should be relatively short, not prolonged.

REVIEW QUESTIONS

1. Define and describe the interrelatedness of teaching and learning.
2. List and describe the two major instructional approaches.
3. Describe two tools to teach.
4. List and describe the principles of universal design and apply to learning.
5. List and describe the seven perceptual pathways for learning.
6. What is the relevance of teaching and learning during the OT process?

REFERENCES

1. Flanders, NA: *Analyzing teaching behaviors*, Reading, MA, 1980, Addison Wesley.

2. Hanner N, Marsh A, Neideffer R: Therapeutic media: activity with purpose. In Solomon J, O'Brien J, editors: *Pediatric skills for the occupational therapy assistant*, ed 3, St Louis, 2011, Mosby.

3. Kratzig G, Arbuthnott K: Perceptual learning style and learning proficiency: a test of the hypothesis, *J Educ Psych* 98:238-246, 2006.

4. Meyer A, Rose DH: The future is in the margins: the role of technology and disability in educational reform. In Rose DH, Meyer A, Hitchcock C, editors: *The universally designed classroom: accessible curriculum and digital technologies*, Cambridge, MA, 2005, Harvard Education Press.

5. North Carolina Center for Universal Design. Retrieved 04/08/2012 from http://www.ncsu.edu/project/design-projects/udi/.

6. OBrien J, Williams H: Motor control and motor learning. In Case-Smith J, O'Brien J, editors: *Occupational therapy for children*, ed 6, St Louis, 2010, Mosby.

7. Park K: Universal design for learning. Retrieved 04/08/2012 from http://www.aota.org/Consumers/Professionals/WhatIsOT/CY/Fact-Sheets/UDL.aspx?FT=.pdf.

8. Patton KT, Thibodeau G: *Anatomy and physiology*, ed 7, St Louis, 2012, Elsevier.

9. Rose DH, Meyer A: *Teaching every student in the digital age: universal design for learning*, Alexandria, VA, 2002, ASCD.

10. Teaching strategies and learning styles. Retrieved 07/25/2011 from http://www.garysturt.free-online.co.uk/teachin.htm.

11. Unknown: Overview of the seven perceptual styles. Retrieved 04/08/2012 from http://miworks.org/VirtualCareerLab/Assessment%20to%20Successful%20Employment/7%20perceptual%20styles.pdf.

Managing and Facilitating Groups

Kerryellen Vroman

KEY TERMS

authoritarian	open groups
blocking	personal disclosure
client-centeredness	productive
feedback	questioning
forming	reflecting and paraphrasing
group climate	short-term goals
laissez-faire leadership	structure
linking	summarizing
long-term goals	time-limited groups

CHAPTER OBJECTIVES

1. Develop group programs.
2. Describe strategies to manage and facilitate group process.
3. Write long-term and short-term goals for groups.
4. Identify the key components of goals.
5. Describe the group climate.

In an effective group, managing the group process appears effortless. This is an illusion, because facilitating a group requires competent communication skills and proficient knowledge of group process and is the result of careful preparation and planning. This process begins with selecting a frame of reference (i.e., group model or an approach). The frame of reference provides the conceptual and practical format on which group interventions then are planned and implemented. It also determines what evaluations, group activities, and interventions the practitioner uses. Leading groups also involves facilitation skills, which the practitioner employs to manage group dynamics and foster group members' communication and interaction. This chapter describes the steps in developing a group program. It outlines the process of writing therapeutic group goals, instructs about how to plan a group program and individual sessions, and describes the strategies that practitioners use to manage and facilitate group process.

THE FUNDAMENTALS OF GROUP DEVELOPMENT AND MANAGEMENT

The group frame of reference and the leadership style are determined by the clients' needs and characteristics. As previously discussed, there are different types of group structures: open, closed, continuous, and time-limited groups. In **open groups** members may be heterogeneous, change frequently, and have diverse abilities; therefore, cohesiveness among the members is low. The open group sessions focus on autonomous short-term goals associated with general outcomes in a particular area such as the acquisition of skills. For example, open groups are offered in acute inpatient psychiatric units where there is a high turnover of patients. In this setting, the changing membership creates challenges such as the level of trust among members and practitioners' lack of opportunity to meet and assess members before they attend a group. In contrast, a **time-limited group**, such as a psychoeducational group, usually has closed membership once the program has started, and new members are admitted when a new psychoeducation program is started. These groups have members who are homogeneous (similar characteristics—e.g., diagnosis, problem, or age) and the length of the program is a predetermined number of structured sessions. The long-term goals are clearly delineated and sessions are sequentially organized to facilitate change in behavior or acquisition of knowledge and skills. An example is a community-based psychoeducational stress management group based on a cognitive-behavioral therapy frame of reference, with 10 weekly sessions, in which there are explicit criteria for members, such as diagnosis or gender (e.g., women with children diagnosed with anxiety disorder). However, irrespective of the group type, core principles apply to the development of a group program, the planning of a group session, and the facilitation of a group session. This process starts with assessing the needs of the target client population and selecting the type of group intervention based on the evidence of best practice.

DEVELOPMENT OF A GROUP PROGRAM

In this section, the process of developing a group program is outlined in three stages. These are the preplanning needs assessment and proposal stage, the development of a group program, and finally designing individual sessions. The initial stage of determining whether a group-based intervention is the optimal occupational therapy service to meet the clients' and organizational needs begins with a practitioner asking and answering critical programmatic questions. These questions are designed to identify the research evidence to support the proposed group program as the most effective intervention to meet the targeted clients' needs and to determine if the proposed program is feasible within the organizational infrastructure in which he or she is employed. The *Preplanning a Group Program* template (Box 6-1) provides a list

---

BOX 6-1   Development of a Group Intervention

Preplanning a Group Program
List the characteristics of the target population (age; diagnosis; status such as inpatient, outpatient, or community-based; socioeconomic status; health insurance; etc.).

_____

List the occupational therapy needs of the target population.

_____

Are the needs of the target population most effectively met by a group intervention? Justify the answer with empiric evidence that supports a group intervention as the optimal mode of therapy.

_____

Identify the type of group intervention (frame of reference) that is supported by the empiric evidence for these clients' needs (e.g., psychoeducation, cognitive-behavioral therapy, motor-relearning theory, sensory integration theory, social learning theory, gestalt therapy, illness management and recovery).

_____

Identify the type of group structure (open, closed, time limited, directive, problem-diagnosis, or population specific).

_____

Identify the schedule of group and time frame (number of sessions; whether they are daily, weekly, or biweekly; and duration, such as 8 weeks, permanent program, or as needed).

_____

Identify criteria for admission: define the gate-keeping process (e.g., all inpatients admitted to unit, all presurgical total hip patients, self or physician-referral, children currently enrolled in occupational therapy).

_____

List resources required to implement program and costs: Practitioner expertise to deliver program (does it require specialized skills such as cognitive-behavioral therapy training, or sensory integration certification to implement group), space, equipment, and materials. How will these resources be provided? Create a budget if necessary.

_____

Source of reimbursement

_____

Identify how the group intervention's effectiveness will be measured and reported to clients and payment providers. Measurement and communication of group outcomes are often overlooked in the planning phase. Pretesting is fundamental in demonstrating the effectiveness of occupational therapy services and the communication of outcomes is crucial to sustaining services.

_____

of questions a practitioner must address in the process of determining the group intervention to be offered. Working systematically through the template yields the necessary data for making a programmatic decision about providing a group intervention as part of occupational therapy services before moving forward and investing time and resources in stages two and three. It also is the basis of a proposal for a new service initiative that will be submitted to either a funding source or administration for resources or as a tool to review an existing program. Although this stage may seem time consuming, especially if the decision has been made to provide a group intervention, it should still be completed. It ensures that the type of group program developed will meet the clients' needs, be based on the best practice model, and have the necessary resources to deliver the service, and will therefore meet our ethical responsibility to "use, to the extent possible, evaluation, planning, intervention techniques, and therapeutic equipment that are evidence-based and within the recognized scope of occupational therapy practice."[1]

◎ Clinical Pearl: Don't Reinvent

Look at programs that already exist. There are many excellent examples and resources available in journal articles, books, and on websites. You can save time and learn from these successful programs and use the activities, strategies, or entire group interventions that have proved effective. These resources will be helpful in developing your own program.

PLANNING GROUP PROGRAM

The process and the core elements of planning a group intervention are generic in that they follow a common structure. Taking the time to create an overall program plan leads to a logical development of clients' skills or a successful process of change, coherent delivery of information, and therapeutic outcomes being met. Therefore, when the decision has been made to provide a group intervention based on the data gathered in the preplanning stage, the next step is to develop systematically a group program that involves outlining the purpose, writing the long-term goals, determining the sessions that will be offered, identifying materials and evaluation methods, and meeting the practicalities of offering the group program. An inexperienced practitioner may be tempted to jump straight in to planning the individual sessions. The results will be poorly articulated goals and a lack of coherence among the group sessions designed to meet the long-term goals. Box 6-2 provides a template for the practitioner to work through this planning process and an example is provided in Chapter 9, "Groups for Adolescents."

GROUP GOALS

A well-written goal is elegant; it is concise, easily understood, and clearly articulates what will be achieved, when, and by whom. The clarity of its intent means a colleague can read the goal, understand it, and therefore identify an appropriate intervention that could be provided to meet the goal.

A group program can vary in length from a few sessions (e.g., inpatient or education group) to an entire semester (e.g., hand writing group for elementary school children) or an indefinite length of time in which members come and go depending on their needs (e.g., an older adults caregivers' support group or social interaction group for adults with developmental delays). The overall intervention being delivered in this group format has **long-term goals** that delineate what group members will achieve over the life of the group program. These long-term goals operationalize the purpose of the program in explicit, measurable terms and are influenced by structure and frame of reference of the group program.

Based on the long-term goals, each individual group session will have measurable **short-term goals**. These short-term goals, which are often referred to in educational settings as *objectives,* are the specific outcomes to be achieved and the process by which the long-term goals will be attained. Hence, they are the stepping stones to the end point group members are working toward.

Short-term goals define the desired outcomes of a single session and do not always depend on all members having attended previous sessions. Time-limited groups are more likely to be interrelated and require a progression from one group to the next, whereas in open groups with a fluid membership it is important that the sessions are more discreet entities in which the short-term goals can be attained without previous group attendance. However, in all groups the purpose of the individual sessions is to move members forward to achieving the long-term goals while also presenting achievable immediate outcomes specifically related to the current group activity. Similarly, they need to accommodate clients' different rates of progress. In addition to the group goals, it is common for clients to have individualized goals that are integral to their occupational therapy intervention plan (see Chapter 7).

Writing Group Goals: Long-term and short-term goals are structurally the same.[9] The wording and the order of the components of a goal may differ from practitioner to practitioner or among settings, but goals *always* have four mandatory components and a component that is usually present, though not essential. The mandatory components are:

Subject or Actor—The *subject* or *actor* specifies who will do the behavior (e.g., *Group members* will. . .).

Behavior or Skill—Group members will develop, practice, or modify a behavior or skill through the group intervention to participate in their occupations successfully or to enhance their occupational performance in their natural context. A behavior is *not* a single action performed solely in the group session; it must be transferrable to the clients' occupational performance beyond the group.

This is an example of a poorly written goal that is *not behavioral,* but is instead an action or activity that will be completed within a single group session. Do not write:

Group members will make a list of six of their fears *by the end of the communications skills group session.*

Making a *list of fears during the group* is a task; it does not state the behavior or skill that members will develop through engaging in the task. If we examine this short-term goal we can

BOX 6-2 Planning a Group Program

WHEN PROGRAM WILL BE IMPLEMENTED: DATE_____
WHERE PROGRAM WILL BE IMPLEMENTED: ROOM_____
NUMBER OF SESSIONS_____
STAFF_____
NUMBER OF GROUP MEMBERS TO BE ENROLLED_____

Purpose of Group
The practitioner outlines the overall purposes of the group in a language that can be used to describe the program to team, clients, and reimbursement agency. The purpose will be occupation-based and have clearly delineated outcomes. Completing this step provides the practitioner with a description of the purpose of the group that can be used in a variety of ways such as on information brochures or to explain the group to new prospective clients.

Outline Frame of Reference and Core Assumptions of this Approach
It is beneficial to articulate the conceptual tenets of the group's frame of reference that underpins the group sessions. For example, in planning a social interaction skills group, a practitioner could decide to use a social learning theory (i.e., social cognitive theory) frame of reference. Some of the assumptions of this approach that influence the structure and activities in the group are the belief that people are self-determining and can make choices and self-regulate their behavior given the appropriate skills, and that by observing another person these skills can be learned. A person may also change his or her behavior because he or she sees others experiencing negative consequences. A frame of reference also outlines what evaluations and intervention techniques are used. For example, behavioral rehearsal such as role play, and role-modeling strategies such as mentoring are important strategies in the social learning theory frame of reference.

Write Long-Term Goals
Long-term goals are broad, observable outcomes that will be achieved at the end of the group program. The long-term goals are congruent with the frame of reference and use language that is consistent with it. For guidelines, see the goal writing section later in this box.

Screening and Pre- and Posttest Evaluations
Screening assesses clients' suitability for a group is important. For example, groups that are based on a psychoeducational frame of reference are designed for clients with similar needs and characteristics (i.e., clients who are homogeneous). As clients engage in preparing to attend the group, you are beginning to develop a therapeutic relationship that will ease their transition into the group and reduce their anxiety. The pre- and posttest evaluation measures serve important functions. The pretest measures may be completed prior to starting the group program as part of a screening process or incorporated into an initial group session as the first activity. Although in some situations a practitioner will have knowledge of clients' abilities, this information does not replace pretest measures as they measure group outcomes. This process also orients the clients to the group and its goals, and is important information for documenting intervention effectiveness.

Involving clients in the pre- and posttest process is therapeutic. A pre- and posttest assessment provides them with a tangible measure of their gains during therapy. This pre- and posttest assessment can also be individualized so that each client documents his or her tangible behavioral outcomes that will be representative of successfully achieving his or her personal goals.

Outline the Sessions
State the number of sessions and time frame (e.g., closed group with two sessions per week for 6 weeks or continuous daily sessions with floating membership). Outline the title and a brief description of the purpose or focus of each session

List All Materials, Personnel, and Resources Needed to Implement Program
In this step, the practitioner identifies and meets all the specific requirements of delivering the program.

---

recognize that the practitioner's goal for this group session is that members will identify their fears so that they can become aware of how their fears affect them and how these fears inhibit their participation or occupational performance in social situations. This "consciousness raising" activity in a behavioral change group for clients learning to manage their anxiety symptoms such as panic attacks is a short-term goal of a group session early in a program.[3,8] However, as the goal is written, it does not clearly demonstrate the intention (goal) of the session or the behavior (i.e., ability to recognize and articulate one's fears) to the group members. To make the previous short-term goal a behavioral goal the practitioner could revise the goal in the following way:

Group members will identify six fears *that interfere with their ability to talk in social settings demonstrated by verbally sharing these fears by the end of the stress management skills group session.*

In this version of the short-term goal the outcome is that members are learning to identify their fears, a behavior that is meaningful and transferrable to their everyday lives. One exercise to help them begin to recognize their fears might be "to make a list of their fears." This task could also be used as one measurement that members have achieved this goal because the

list is an observable indication that they can identify their fears. Other relevant short-term goals for this session are goals that specify recognizing either their cognitive or physiologic reactions to their fears. An example is:

By the end of the stress management group session, group members will be able to recognize the faulty thinking pattern that accompanies *at least two of their identified fears by listing five thoughts for each fear on the worksheet.*

The second two short-term goals clearly communicate to clients what behaviors they are working on and why they are relevant to their problematic area of occupational performance. Therefore, clients will see how they are developing adaptive behaviors that are prerequisites to modifying their thinking patterns that increase physiologic arousal in social situations. The level of understanding provided by these short-term goals results in a more therapeutic outcome than a goal that merely specifies making a list of fears without a context for the task or acquisition of transferrable behaviors. In the second of the two goals, the relationship to the long-term goal related to their occupational performance in social participation is explicitly and consistently articulated across the sessions. Those who are familiar with cognitive-behavioral therapy will recognize that these short-term goals are congruent with this frame of reference, which previous research indicates is an effective intervention approach for dysfunctional occupational performance associated with anxiety disorders.

Measurement—Some texts write about the *measurement*, whereas others use the term *criterion* to refer to the statement in the goal that identifies the observable outcome. This component defines the standard and evidence required to indicate the quality of the performance or the frequency of behavior required to deem that the goal has been successfully achieved. Two essential characteristics of the measurement are that it is relevant to the behavior or skill being measured, and that it is observable to others (practitioner, group members, and client). A common error of measurement for a novice goal writer is to use either time frame or frequency as the measurement of a behavior when the quality of the performance needs to be the outcome measurement. To identify the measurement, a practitioner asks what evidence would represent that a client has acquired the desire behavior or skill stated in the goal. The gold standard is always whether the skill or behavior can be demonstrated or used by the client in a naturalistic context.

Time Frame—A goal states a realistic time frame in which the behavior, component of a skill, or a complete skill will be acquired or demonstrated. A common mistake in writing group goals is overestimating what can be achieved in a given time frame. All learning, adaptation, or behavioral change is incremental and it takes time to integrate a new skill or behavior or eliminate a behavior from a person's occupational performance repertoire. Consider how difficult and challenging it was when you last tried to learn a new skill (e.g., skiing, body surfing, knitting, measuring range of motion) or to modify your behavior (e.g., go to the gym regularly; make a change in your eating patterns; give up a habit such as smoking; or recover and adjust to a change in your life such as a relationship ending, death of a family member, or moving to a new town).

Condition—The condition component of a goal is not essential, but goals frequently include them. Conditions provide useful parameters for the goal that will make it achievable and add clarity. The conditions are the contingencies of the goal. They can describe the characteristic of the behavior and the context in which the behavior will be demonstrated. Therefore, conditions are an important element for grading goals. Conditions make goals achievable within the time frame or context of therapy by outlining the circumstances under which the client is expected to exhibit the behavior. The conditions can make the goal more demanding or increase the support for the behavior. An example of how the condition component is used for grading is that a short-term goal may be that the group members will initially demonstrate the behavior in the supportive environment of the group. As members develop competence in the desired behavior in the group setting, the goal will be graded by changing the condition

---

BOX 6-3   Reviewing Goal Structure

Until you are proficient in writing goals, check off that you have included all the elements within each of your goals. This box identifies the components of the earlier example:

Group members will identify six fears that interfere with their ability to talk in social settings,
Actors   Behavior   Condition
demonstrated by verbally sharing these fears by the end of the communications skills group session.
Measurement or Criteria   Timeframe

---

such that the group members will demonstrate the behavior in a more natural context such as a classroom, within the family, in the community, or in a work setting. Each subsequent short-term goal might modify the conditions by changing or adding to the demands of the setting, the behavior or the frequency. In the earlier example of a short-term goal for members of a stress management group, the condition was that *Group members will identify six fears that* **interfere with their ability to talk in social settings,** *demonstrated by verbally sharing these fears by the end of the stress management skills group session.* The parameter (condition) was that members identify only the fears that *interfere with their ability to talk in social settings* (Box 6-3).

There are other important therapeutic dimensions in the use and construction of occupational therapy goals. These include:

- **Client-centeredness** means that goals are discussed with clients and that the language used is straightforward, appropriate to the client's educational level, and if possible his or her language of choice. The purpose of this is to is have clients actively involved in setting their therapy goals, fully understand what is expected of them in the intervention process, what it means to achieve their goals successfully, and how their goals are relevant to them. One way to do this is to have clients in the group discuss in their own words the purpose and goals of the group and describe how they will recognize that they have achieved them in the context of their own lives. This process can be revisited throughout a group program or built into each group session. In groups based on Mosey's cooperative or mature developmental activity group model, members are expected to develop the group goals with the practitioner and take responsibility to monitoring the progress toward the desired outcome.[5,7]

- *Goals are consistent* with the values, policies, and the mission of occupational therapy profession and in the practice setting. The goals emphasize occupation-based outcomes, reflect a top-down approach recommended in the American Occupational Therapy Association practice framework, and are client-centered.

- *Goals are reimbursable.* The crafting of the goals should meet the criteria set by the funding agencies covering the cost of occupational therapy intervention. Knowledge of reimbursement policies is a practitioner's moral and professional responsibility. It results in his or her ability to advocate clients' access to therapy and to write goals that will be reimbursed.

DESIGNING AND MANAGING INDIVIDUAL GROUP SESSIONS

Similar to a teacher developing a lesson plan, a practitioner uses a standard structure to design a group that includes goals and specific activities. Box 6-4 is a template for designing an individual session that includes descriptions of each explicit step in leading a group. Over time, templates of individual session outlines become valuable resources that the practitioner will review, revise as necessary based on the previous group and the needs of the new clients, and then use when repeating the group program with future groups of clients.

◎ Clinical Pearl: Acknowledging Group Participation

It is common practice to thank members for attending group sessions. Thanking members "for coming to group" is patronizing and not client-centered. It diminishes their autonomy, ownership of their achievements, self-agency, and accentuates the power differential between the group leader and the members. Individuals, irrespective of condition or age, choose to attend a group and do not attend "for" the practitioner. The practitioner's role is to provide an effective intervention and work *with* the clients to meet their goals. In the conclusion phase of group, the practitioner provides positive *behavioral* feedback that reinforces group cohesiveness and what has been achieved. For example, in a cognitive strategies group of individuals with head injuries who have been working in a group on using recall-memory strategies, a group leader might say, "*We* worked hard, and successfully concentrated for 20 minutes without a break today in group. This is better than last week." This statement could be used to then have group members individually state what aspect of their performance they felt pleased about and how they will incorporate this into their occupational performance in the following week. The practitioner might join in this activity to intentionally role model how to recognize one's behavior constructively by focusing on behaviors and not personal characteristics. For example, the practitioner might state, "I was pleased with myself today because I introduced the activity clearly because I used the checklist I made to organize my thinking and aid my recall. I know this worked because I did not have to clarify the steps of the activity as I did last week."

FUNDAMENTALS OF GROUP DYNAMICS: THE ART OF FACILITATION AND THE EFFECTIVE MANAGEMENT OF GROUP DYNAMICS

This section outlines practical strategies used to effectively manage the group process and facilitate group dynamics. These strategies are germane irrespective of the type of leadership or group frame of reference used because they pertain to managing the interactions among the group members, including the leaders and the group process that occurs when people come together in a group.

GROUP CLIMATE

Group climate is the emotional atmosphere that the group members experience. A collective level of comfort with each other and a sense of trust among members and with the leader are critical to the initial development of a group and the ongoing group process from session to session. Both the physical environment and the leader's ability to develop feelings of trust, acceptance, friendliness, and mutual supportiveness contribute to the climate. It is also influenced by and expressed in the rules that become the group norms, expectations, and level of mutuality that is developed and maintained by the group members and leader across sessions.

Developing, monitoring, and maintaining group climate are fundamental tasks of the group leader and the type of leadership will significantly influence group climate. A nonjudgmental, respectful, client-centered leadership style that is consistent fosters trust and client-group interactions. In contrast, a **laissez-faire leadership** style that is inconsistent and has unclear expectations can result in an unproductive, discordant group with poor outcomes. An **authoritarian** style of leadership makes the leader responsible for group climate. In some situations, this authoritarian style might reduce anxiety among members and maintain structure and task achievement, but it does not give members a collective sense of ownership for the group outcomes or interactions and therefore generalization to everyday occupational performance in social participation will be less likely. Therefore, different styles of leadership require different strategies to maintain and ensure an optimal group climate.

The physical environment, namely the characteristics of the space and how the space is organized also influences group climate. Under ideal circumstances, the practitioner chooses a space that is most conducive to the type of group, its activities, and goals. However, as the space is usually determined by the setting and space availability, leaders often pay minimal attention to this important aspect of group management. A group leader needs to evaluate whether the space is appropriate and how it will influence the group climate and productivity. Even if the space is predetermined, a practitioner may still have options in how the space is organized.

Aspects of the space to be assessed and modified to suit the group include how the seating is arranged, comfort, and flexibility (e.g., seats that can be moved to create small working groups or made into a circle for discussion); the availability of tables or work surfaces; and access to equipment such as data projectors or flip charts. Practitioners also evaluate the suitability of the lighting, the level of privacy, whether the setting is free of distractions (e.g., interruptions from staff and other clients). Lastly, the practitioners need to be sure that in this space the group members feel safe.

The use of physical space is about achieving a balance between comfort and group function. A discussion or brief interpersonal therapy group with 8 to 10 people who will be sharing personal issues is best held in a quiet private room where seating can be arranged in a circle to create a feeling of intimacy and members can see each other. In this arrangement the leader's physical position is equal with other group members. In an activities group, the space may require tables, access to a sink and running water, and an area where projects can be left until completed. A group for adolescents

BOX 6-4 Guidelines for an Individual Session

This template provides instructions for an individual session. Write this outline so another occupational therapy practitioner could follow it and run the session. Once these instructions are developed, they can be reused for future groups.

Purpose of Group Session:
Briefly state the purpose of the session. This will be used in the introduction of the session.

_____
_____
_____

Goals for Group Session:
Write the specific goals to be achieved in this group. The relationship to the long-term goals need to be clear because these short-term goals are the steps to achieving them.

1. _____
2. _____
3. _____

Materials Needed:

_____
_____
_____

Introduction:
Outline the key points for the introduction that state the purpose of the session and expectations of the session, including goals, and reiterate group norms as applicable to individual sessions. Describe what will happen in the session and the time frame.

_____
_____
_____

Warmup: Describe the Warmup (Icebreaker):
A warmup is short (e.g., 5-10 minutes of a 1-hour session). It energizes and focuses on bringing group members together around a common purpose expressed by the short-term goals of the group. Therefore, the warm-up is not a random activity. It is carefully chosen to orient the members to the theme or topic of the group activity and its demands are consistent with the stage of group development. For example, when a group is new, warmup activities are likely to emphasize common themes or shared problems

to reinforce members' sense of belonging and similarities. At the productive stage of group development, the warmup may require disclosure of more personal information or be more emotionally demanding.

_____
_____
_____

Activity or Intervention:
Outline the steps of the activity. This might be a discussion group, in which case the talking points are outlined, or it might be a task group in which the directions for a specific activity are documented.

_____
_____
_____

Conclusion of the Group:
In the conclusion phase of the group a number of tasks need to be complete so it is important to make sure there is adequate time to address them. These are (1) summation of the group by either members or group leader, (2) application and generalization to occupational performance in everyday life, and (3) homework to reinforce transfer of learning and generalization of skills or behaviors.

_____
_____
_____

Postgroup Evaluation:
Document immediately following a group session. Critique the group and write comments and recommendations for the next time this group session is run. In a busy schedule, it is difficult to recall the details of a specific group. Taking 5 minutes to document an evaluation of the group will significantly reduce time planning this session in the future and continue to improve occupational therapy services. This feedback could include changes to the activity, points about structuring the activity, time management, or points for facilitating this group.

_____
_____
_____

might be more suited to a gym where there is space for physical activities and games, but will also need smaller more intimate space for discussions and instructions. The use of space involves creating a sense of comfort that will reduce the anxiety of being in a clinic or hospital. However, this process does not mean creating informality that undermines purpose. On a sunny day, it might seem a good idea to hold the group session outside, but before changing the setting, the practitioner needs to consider what effect this change will have on the group dynamics. If you want to increase member-to-member interaction and playfulness, the informality and social atmosphere outside might facilitate these goals. Conversely, the distractions of being outdoors might reduce the members' attention to the task and lower productivity. All decisions about space are based on the answers to the questions: *How does this space support a therapeutic climate and enhance the group members' ability to meet group and individual goals?*

GROUP FACILITATION TECHNIQUES

A practitioner uses numerous techniques when facilitating a group. Monitoring and observing members' behaviors, the interactions among members, and relations among the members and the leader are critical to this process. As a facilitator, the group leader works with members to participate in the group successfully by encouraging them to interact, by creating a supportive, safe, nonjudgmental setting for learning and taking risks to gain skills and practice alternative ways of interacting and behaving. Sometimes it means challenging or confronting members. Some of the techniques used in leading a group are discussed in the following paragraphs.

Listening and *observing* include hearing what members say verbally, but also recognizing the message conveyed in their nonverbal body language and actions. These also involve observing changes in posture, voice tone or pace, facial expressions, and gestures. An extension of listening is being aware of members' behaviors and what this *may* mean, such as where people sit in the group, tardiness or absences, who speaks, who does not speak, and how and when members respond to each other.

The process of listening and observing group members' verbal and nonverbal language, behaviors, and the interaction among group members are critical and occur on two levels. The first is the listening and observing that serves as a subtext to the group. The practitioner is constantly noting, processing, and using this information to facilitate the group session. The second is the broader and cumulative observations made following an individual group session. These reflective observations are the basis for group and individual client documentation and are used to plan the next group.

◎ Clinical Pearl: Mindfulness is Being Present in the Group

A barrier to a group leader listening and observing effectively occurs when the leader is preoccupied with his or her role as group leader or other work demands. It is difficult for group leaders to attend to the group members and the group process when they are overly concerned or anxious about their performance because they are evaluating themselves. Group facilitation means being able to listen, to step into another person's experience empathetically, and to be aware of both the needs of the group member who is speaking and the group, so the response made is therapeutic and advances the work of the group.

The group leader is often in the role of *giving feedback* and modeling how to give constructive feedback to others. In groups this may be giving group feedback about how the group is functioning or feedback to individual members. Feedback, whether positive or aiming to address a problem behavior, is *always* focused on behaviors and not personal characteristics. It should be presented using an "I" statement. An example of productive feedback is, "It is difficult for me, Mary, when you arrive late because I need to repeat the instructions and I am thinking that the group is not important to you."

Different group models use less or more **structure** to organize the group. By introducing structure, the leader gains more control over aspects of the group such as the activity and how it is done, and members' interactions and communication with each other. Structure may also increase the role of the leader. By reducing the level of structure the leader increases members' control of the group process, giving them greater autonomy in determining their roles and actions in the group.

A leader uses the level of structure to lower or raise the demands of an activity, increase participation, and achieve the group goals. Structure is introduced to a group by the type of group model used, the level of instructions provided to members, the leadership style (i.e., authoritarian and directive leaders provide the most structure), and by modifying the environment. In some groups, especially with clients who have behavioral problems, are acutely psychotic, or have significant cognitive deficits such as older adults with dementia disorders, structure is often required to achieve group goals, ensure that members are safe (real and perceived safety), and to create the

"just-right" challenge for members to participate fully at their current level of occupational performance.

A leader's goal is to facilitate member-to-member interactions rather than have a question-and-answer session with the members; therefore, **questioning** directed collectively to the members is more effective. Open questions start with what, how, when, where, and who. These questions encourage members to provide narrative or descriptive responses. "Why" questions should be used judiciously, because they require members to consider their reasons for an action, feelings, or beliefs and in responding they disclose personal information. "Why" questions used early in the group discussion or group's development can feel intrusive or make clients feel defensive because it may seem group members are being asked to explain themselves or to justify how they are feeling.

Questioning assists members to expand on issues and develop skills and knowledge. However, a leader needs to be respectful of members and provide a group climate that can work at a pace that is therapeutic. Practitioners new to group leadership may be reluctant to ask probing questions for fear of distressing a client. If clients are aware that they do not need to talk about topics until they are ready and have the right to pass on a question, probing is an essential aspect of questioning. An astute open-style question asked with genuine interest or concern can be the strategy that assists a member to take the next step in his or her therapy. For example, a leader asking a key question about the effect of a behavior on the individual's relationship allows him or her to examine the consequences of an unhealthy behavior as an initial step in changing it.

The communication techniques of **reflecting and paraphrasing** used in one-on-one interactions (i.e., interviewing) are extensively used in facilitating groups. They are not distinctly different techniques, but rather a pattern of responses. The most straightforward are repeating and paraphrasing. The leader repeats briefly key words of the speaker or puts into his or her own words what the speaker has said. This technique serves to indicate the leader is hearing the speaker accurately. It can prompt the speaker to continue and to elaborate, or the speaker can be cued about the direction to take the conversation.[10]

The outcome of paraphrasing is accuracy of communication within the group. Paraphrasing is often presented in the form of a question because it serves to help the leader clarify what the speaker means. It can also highlight for the speaker what the leader thinks is his or her main message to the group. The speaker is encouraged to respond with agreement or disagreement as to the accuracy of the paraphrasing.

Reflecting is a more skillful form of paraphrasing because the leader's response captures the core message that is being communicated. It can reflect the essential content of what the group members or a member has been saying (*reflecting content*). This is the simplest form of reflection because it pulls out the key facts or information. The other type of reflecting involves the reflecting of feelings. In this type of response the leader reflects back to the group the feelings that are being expressed verbally or less overtly within the content of what is being said.

Leader: So school starts next week?

Jason: I have so much to do before next week. I don't know what class I will be in and who my teacher is. I don't want the summer to end. I hope I am in Miss Brown's class, I have heard that she is nice.

Leader: "You are worried about going back to school?"

Sometimes the feelings are conveyed in the members' behavior and the leader gives these feelings a voice by reflecting. It is useful in reflecting to include why or how you have recognized the feelings being expressed.

Leader: "Chris, you are quieter than usual and seem restless, I sense that you are anxious about being discharged this afternoon. Do you want to talk about it?"

Reflecting uses interpretation and therefore is undertaken with care and sensitivity and it is important that members or a speaker respond to the accuracy of reflective statement.

Linking is a strategy used by a group leader to facilitate member-to-member interactions to enhance group productivity, and enhance members' sense of ownership for group outcomes (Figure 6-1). Linking is the technique of relating what one member of the group has said with another member's concerns, interests, experiences, or previous comments to the group.[2] When a group leader notes similarities, it reduces a person's feelings of isolation such as, "I am the only person with this problem" or "I am the only person who feels this way."

Linking is particularly useful in the group in the **forming** stage of group development or when new members have recently joined the group, because it highlights commonalities and increases members' sense of belonging. Later in the **productive** stage, linking moves the direction of communication from predominantly leader centered to member to member. For example, a leader identifies similarities among members' responses and facilitates a response directly among members. For example, a leader might state, "Molly, what you are saying about how your siblings are not recognizing the time it takes to take takes to care of your mother with Alzheimer's disease similar to what others have said about their family members who are not providing day-to-day care. Sam, I recall you mentioned something about a family conference when you were in this position. Could you tell Molly and us more about this?"

Summarizing is a strategy a leader uses to clarify that he or she understands what group members are thinking and feeling. It brings group members together and voices the common understanding of the group purpose, the task, or reviews what has occurred in the group up to this point. This organizing process helps group members gain insight and perspective by presenting relationships among events or topics that might otherwise have been overlooked.[10] Summarizing can be used as a transition strategy. A leader might review what has happened or has been decided in the group before moving on to a new activity. This review process gains everyone's attention and brings the group's focus back to the leader. At this point the leader highlights the key points of the previous group work and can indicate that the group is moving to a new stage or introduce the next activity. If a group is becoming fragmented or disorganized, a summary can clarify, provide **feedback**, or refocus the group. The following is an example of brief summation in a group working on assertiveness skills and how nonassertive behavior affects mood, emotions, and actions.

We were discussing examples of how saying yes to a request made us feel, when we really wanted to say no. Many of you mentioned how it made you feel frustrated, resentful, and used. But now it seems the group has become distracted and there are side conversations. Let's talk about how we deal with these feelings.

Summation has specific roles at the beginning and end of the group. At the beginning of a group a leader summarizes the work achieved in previous sessions if the group sessions are interrelated as part of a group program. This sets the context for the current group session and reinforces the relationship among the group goals and transfer of learning between sessions. The leader *always* uses summation at the end of the group. Sometimes a leader will provide a summary; at other

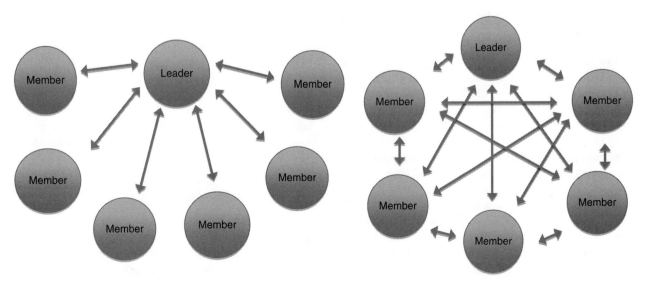

Figure 6-1 Patterns of communication in leader-centered and member-centered groups.

times he or she will facilitate the members to summarize the session and what they or the group have achieved. When members summarize the group, they are able to self-evaluate and put the group experience and their understanding into their own words, which reinforces their group experience.

Blocking is a technique used to manage group members' behaviors such as excessive talking, dominating, gossiping, and acting out disruptive behaviors. The group leader needs to maintain the group norms such as confidentiality, taking turns, and respect for all members. It is essential to block any interactions that personally attack a member's personhood.[2]

Blocking requires that the leader intervene directly and verbally to address the behavior that is interfering with the process and integrity of the group. This requires sensitivity and a tolerance for conflict. A leader must be directive and be able to give constructive behavioral feedback. The blocking strategy can be redirecting a member who gets off topic or who in recounting a story is long-winded. The leader might ask the storyteller to finish the story with one sentence that relates to purpose of the session; for example, the leader might state, "I can see this trip home was important to you, can you finish with it now with one sentence that states what this story tells us about your relationship with your brother? Then we will hear from Mary." In being specific and stating who will speak next, the leader has introduced structure that shifts control from the member speaking back to the leader and then to Mary, who will speak next. Another example of blocking is when the leader calls attention to a behavior, such as interrupting other people or speaking for them and describes the behavior's effect on the leader and the group. For example, the leader might state, "Tom have you noticed when the last two members were speaking, you interrupted them?" The leader may invite the members to say how they felt when they were interrupted. This feedback will need to be managed carefully so the person receives constructive comments on his or her behavior and does not feel attacked or scapegoated. The leader can role model and stress the importance of using "I" statements and own one's feelings. For example, the leader might state, "Tom when you interrupt me, I feel that you do not think what I have to say is important." Depending on the purpose of the group, the leader might also use this situation to teach interpersonal skills. For example, the person who is interrupted might use this opportunity to practice being assertive and reclaim the conversation. This will also enable Tom to become aware of how his behavior, which he mostly likely exhibits in other social situations, interferes with his ability to communicate effectively.

Last, the leader can use nonverbal body language and structure as blocking strategies. Nonverbal actions include avoiding making eye contact with an excessively verbal member and body posture that directs the group members' attention away from the person. Introducing turn taking, setting time limits on speaking, and having members address the person they are talking about are examples of the use of structure. Another strategy is to give a person a specific task in the group that will reduce the unwanted behavior. For example, the person who always has the answers in a game can become the person who asks the questions.

PERSONAL DISCLOSURE

Personal disclosure should be used judiciously and selectively. It means that when a leader contributes personal information, it is done with the intention to be therapeutic, enhance the group process, and contribute to a group member or members collectively meeting the group goals. When disclosing personal information, leaders should be mindful of the purpose of sharing the information; the value of the information; the effect on the group and themselves; and what, when, and how much to disclose.[2] Self-disclosure can occur on three levels: (1) the least intimate information is purely information about past or future feelings, beliefs, and thoughts; (2) moderately intimate information consists of sharing feelings and thoughts about present events; and (3) the most intimate information is shared when a person expresses feelings and thoughts about the person or persons with whom he or she is speaking.[6] A leader can use disclosure to role model what is expected in a group activity or session or to demonstrate risk-taking. It can enhance the level of trust and intimacy. It needs to be appropriate and beneficial and must not shift the attention from the group members to the group leader.

It can be challenging to navigate direct personal questions. Again, the key question a leader asks is, "How would my disclosure or nondisclosure influence the group dynamics and outcomes?" In some situations, declining to answer a question and redirecting the focus back to the group is an important step in clarifying boundaries or diffusing members' confrontational interaction with the leader. At other times, a thoughtful, therapeutically relevant answer can be valuable and will increase trust and members' confidence in sharing personal information. A good self-evaluative strategy helps a leader assess his or her motivation for sharing the information.

The guidelines for using self-disclosure apply to all groups, whether a practitioner is leading children in activities, coaching adults with developmental delays in work skills, or leading a brief interpersonal therapy group for clients with substance abuse disorders. However, the occupational therapy group in which the leader's interactions and interpersonal relations with the clients are integral in the intervention requires more advanced knowledge of self-disclosure as a therapeutic technique. Further information on disclosure in the psychotherapeutic process is available in Yalom's book,[11] *The Theory and Practice of Psychotherapy*, which discusses both the primary therapeutic factors of groups and the use of self-disclosure as a therapeutic technique. Similarly, McKay, Davis, and Fanning[6] include a chapter on self-disclosure that focuses on interpersonal self-disclosure in relationships in their book, *Messages: The Communication Skills Book*.

POSTGROUP ANALYSIS

In addition to the documentation required following the group session, the practitioner must assess the group and his or her leadership. What occurred in the group is not the result of a single person, the group leader, or any group member. Instead, what occurs is understood by examining the actions and

Clinical Pearl: Managing Complaints and Conflict in and Out of Group

Discontent will inevitably arise in a group. There can be tension among members, some may be isolated or scapegoated, collaboration can decrease among members, and subgroups may form. When this occurs members will often seek out the group leaders with complaints and concerns. An inexperienced leader will feel that he or she needs to "fix" the problem and meet with individual members. Avoid resolving these issues outside the group. The issues arise from and within the group and should be resolved by all group members of which the leader is but one member. In the process of resolving conflicts, members learn and acquire interpersonal skills. With the leader's support and facilitation, members address their concerns in the group. Alternatively, a leader might introduce a session that explores issues that underline the concerns and in doing so provides the context for the issues to addressed.

Conflicts among members or between members and the leader occur in all kinds of groups, from activity groups with children to cooking groups with clients with acquired brain injuries, and often reflect everyday life situations for the members. Working on resolving conflicts with others or making requests for changes when facilitated by the group leader has the potential to develop communication skills; offer positive experiences of conflict resolution; lead to interpersonal awareness, growth and agency; and build cohesiveness among members. In addition to dealing with issues in the group, the leader needs to consider how he or she might have recognized the issues among members earlier and how process and structure may have contributed to the conflicts, and identify strategies that might be employed to prevent similar issues in future groups.

reactions from the perspective of the individual members as influenced by their cognitive, social, and psychoemotional factors; the interactions and relationships of the group members with each other and the leader; as well as the characteristics of the group such as the activities used. Group observation and evaluation can be broken down into a number of areas, many of which have been discussed in this and other chapters. Box 6-5 provides areas a practitioner would observe and critique following the group. This information is used in preparing the next group session and the process helps the practitioner reflect on his or her practice.

SUMMARY

Because of the therapeutic value of groups, occupational therapy interventions are often provided in a group setting. The effectiveness of a group or group program is the result of planning, preparation, and skillful leadership that is a process of ongoing learning. This chapter provides information about the strategies, techniques, and procedures that novice and experienced practitioners could use and develop to facilitate occupational therapy groups in a variety of clinical and community settings. Groups are dynamic and each session can be both demanding and rewarding. Each group session will require the practitioner's full attention and repertoire of skills.

BOX 6-5 | **A Postgroup Observation Checklist**

Postgroup Evaluation
Area of Observation   **Comments and Actions**

Group Climate
☐ Space—room
☐ Lighting, heating, ventilation, seating suitability
☐ No interruptions or distractions
☐ Organization and materials supported group goals
☐ Openness and appropriate level of trust among members
☐ Sense of cohesiveness among members

Group Norms
☐ Therapeutic group norms maintained
☐ Lateness, absences
☐ Members listened to each other
☐ Members were respectful of others
☐ Decisions made collectively and accepted

Group Goals—Productivity
☐ Goals were clear and stated
☐ Goals understood by members
☐ Goals relevant to members
☐ Goals for group met

Group Activity
☐ Occupation-based
☐ Facilitated members' goal attainment
☐ Activities supported group goals
☐ Activities presented clearly and understood
☐ Activity demands appropriate and relevant

Continued

BOX 6-5	A Postgroup Observation Checklist—cont'd

Postgroup Evaluation—cont'd
Area of Observation

Comments and Actions

Participation —Interaction

☐ Cooperation encouraged participation
☐ Member-to-member interaction
☐ Members interested and involved
☐ Members restless and disengaged
☐ Balanced participation (no member dominant or withdrawn)
☐ Members listened and built on each other's ideas and actions

Leadership

☐ Directions and introduction clear
☐ Positively facilitated members' participation
☐ Encouraged group interaction
☐ Constructively set limits
☐ Elicited members' feelings and ideas
☐ Time management ensured completion of activities with full member participation
☐ Concluded group with summary
☐ Reinforced generalization of learning beyond group session

General Comments

Box developed using Dimock.[4]

REFERENCES

1. American Occupational Therapy Association: Occupational therapy code of ethics and ethics standards, 2010. Retrieved from http://www.aota.org/Practitioners/Ethics/Docs/Standards/38527.aspx.

2. Corey MS, Corey G, Corey C: *Groups: process and practice*, ed 8, Belmont, CA, 2010, Brooks/Cole.

3. DiClemente CC, Procaska JO, Fairhurst SK, Velicer WF, Velasquez MM, Rossi JS: The process of smoking cessation: an analysis of pre-contemplation, contemplation and preparation stages of change, *J Consult Clin Psych* 59:295-304, 1991.

4. Dimock HG: *How to observe your groups*, ed 3, North York, Ontario, 1993, Captus Press.

5. Donohue MV: Theoretical bases of Mosey's group interactive skills, *Occup Ther Int* 6: 35-51, 1999.

6. McKay M, Davis M, Fanning P: *Messages: the communication skills book*, Oakland, CA, 1995, New Harbinger Publications.

7. Mosey AC: *Psychosocial components of occupational therapy*, New York, 1986, Raven Press.

8. Procaska JO, DiClemente CC: Stage of change in the modification of behavioral problems. In Hensen M, Eisler RM, Miller PM, editors: *Progress in behavioral modification*, Sycamore, IL, 1992, Sycamore Press, pp 184-214.

9. Sames KM: *Documenting occupational therapy practice*, ed 2, Upper Saddle River, NJ, 2009, Prentice Hall.

10. Sampson EE, Marthas M: *Group process for the health professions*, ed 3, Albany, NY, 1990, Delmar.

11. Yalom ID: The theory and practice of group psychotherapy, ed 5, New York, 2005, Basic Books.

Group Process and Management: Attaining Individual Goals

Jane Clifford O'Brien

KEY TERMS

group dynamics   occupational profile
just-right challenge   preparation
long-term goals   short-term goals
objectives
occupational or activity
    analysis

CHAPTER OBJECTIVES:

1. Describe the process of developing individual goals and objectives for members in groups.
2. Discuss how to address individual goals within group settings.
3. Identify strategies for working on individual goals with in group settings.
4. Using occupational analysis, define the relationships between individual and group goals.

This chapter describes the process of developing individual goals for each participant involved in a group. A review of developing individual goals is presented. This chapter outlines the processes involved in addressing individual goals and effective strategies used to individualize interventions while managing group dynamics and meeting group goals. This is illustrated in a case example of a group in a rehabilitation center focusing on activities of daily living (ADLs) such as self-feeding.

SETTING INDIVIDUAL GOALS

Kielhofner[2] emphasized the need for practitioners to understand the client's motives, volition, interests, values, and personal causation (belief in self and perceived efficacy in one's occupational performance) as ways to develop occupation-based goals for intervention. Once a practitioner has determined the client's occupational desires, he or she is in a position to develop goals with the client. These goals serve as the road map for the course of therapy. Consequently, developing goals are key components of occupational therapy (OT) practice and as such demand careful consideration because they determine all that follows.

Engaging clients in developing goals helps ensure that clients are invested in therapy. An **occupational profile** is used to understand the client's history, roles, and motivations.[1] The occupational profile provides a brief picture of the client and serves as the foundation for developing meaningful intervention. The OT practitioner interviews and observes the client to obtain information on the client's story, including the client's identity, occupations, routines, and concerns. This information provides an understanding of the context in which the person performs. All this information is needed for individual goal setting. The following questions serve to explore goals:

- What would you like to do during therapy?
- What kinds of things would you like to be able to do again?
- What is your favorite activity?
- What is causing you the most trouble?
- What is the one thing you want to do within the next month?
- What bothers you the most right now?

Once the practitioner has the relevant information, the goals can be developed with the client. All clients can be involved in the process irrespective of age or disorder. Keep the goals as clear and concise as possible so that the client and his or her family understand the goals. Use plain language and state the outcomes in understandable terms. Avoid medical jargon and write the goal in terms that the client can relate to easily and can explain to family or friends.

Developing clear and meaningful goals that the client understands and hopes to achieve ensures that the client will be invested in reaching the goals. Clients who are positive and invested in goals do better than those who are unclear about the goals and not invested in reaching them. Writing down the goals and placing them close to the person (perhaps on an index card) or reviewing the goals each session helps the client stay focused on meeting the goal. It also serves to remind the practitioner and other health care professionals of the goals so that everyone is reinforcing goal attainment.

Practitioners (and students) may decide to write goals in the client's words and later edit the wording of the goal so it is measurable. This technique works very well for verbal clients. The practitioner can revise the questions as needed. For example, the practitioner might ask questions such as:

- What would you like to accomplish in therapy?
- What would tell you that therapy has been successful?
- What do you want to accomplish over the next month?
- What is bothering you the most right now that you could work on?

The practitioner records the response exactly as stated. The practitioner tries to get these answers from the client directly. Spending time collaborating with the client on the goal benefits the client and ensures that intervention is meaningful and purposeful to the client. Using information learned from the client, the practitioner may follow up with further questions, such as:

- How will you measure success?
- Can you describe what success would look like in everyday activities?
- How would you know the goal was accomplished?
- How long do you want to work on this goal?

After determining the client's long-term goal, standards, and expectations for success, the practitioner outlines the steps in the short-term goal. Using skills or activity analysis, the practitioner is able to divide the activity into even smaller steps to determine how to best address each member's goals.

DEVELOPING INDIVIDUAL GOALS

The foundation of OT intervention lies in the development of client-centered, meaningful, long-term, and short-term goals. **Long-term goals** are the broad targets of intervention. These goals provide a view of the outcome of the intervention over time. The length of time for a long-term goal varies with settings. **Short-term goals** are designed to measure the steps required to meet the long-term goals and thus require less time to accomplish. Some settings require even more immediate goals, often referred to as **objectives**. When developing goals and objectives, practitioners must carefully examine the progression and

consider how the objectives and short-term goals address the long-term goals. This sequence should be clear to the client.

CASE STUDY

Figure 7-1 illustrates the analysis of goals and objectives. Karli's long-term goal is measureable, yet very broad. Her goal is to feed herself again. The practitioner reasons that Karli may always need adapted equipment to be independent, but that this is an obtainable long-term goal. To reach the goal, the practitioner decides that Karli must be able to bring the spoon to her mouth and thus this becomes a short-term goal. The practitioner may have other short-term goals that address swallowing or positioning for feeding oneself. The practitioner develops the objectives as small steps that may be addressed in the intervention session to help Karli reach her short-term goals. Clients need to accomplish the objectives to meet the short-term goal. However, objectives should not be the intervention activity. Rather, objectives are measurements that inform the practitioner about how the intervention program is progressing. The entire process of goal setting is based on clinical reasoning and consideration of the client, diagnosis, context, and environmental factors.

WRITING INDIVIDUAL GOALS

Writing goals and objectives in concise, meaningful terms is beneficial. This helps clients, family, and other professionals understand the purpose and direction of therapy. Therefore, goals and objectives must be written in measurable clear terms and include:

Who: Who is the client?

Action: What will you see as the performance? What is the observable result of the intervention?

Condition: Under what circumstances will the client complete the action?

Criteria: What are the standards for success? How will you measure the success?

Practitioners use their skills in **occupational or activity analysis** when developing goals and objectives. The objectives are steps toward the short-term goal. Practitioners can change the goal requirements by altering the conditions. For example, asking a child to complete an obstacle course in a shorter amount of time or with more accuracy makes the goal more difficult. Requiring a client to complete less repetitions or take more rest breaks makes the goal easier to accomplish. See Table 7-1 for suggestions to change the activity demands.

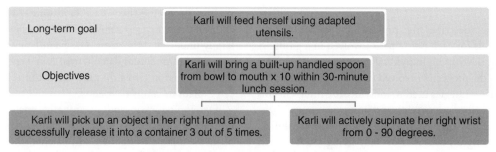

Figure 7-1 Sample progression of goals and objectives.

TABLE 7-1 Suggestions for Changing Activities

Activity Requirement	Easy	Difficult
Time	Shorten length of task	Add more time
Strength	Small objects Light objects Limit lifting	Large objects Heavy objects Add lifting, pulling, pushing
Repetitions	Few repetitions Frequent rests	Numerous repetitions Limit rests
Speed	No time limit	Limit time for steps
Accuracy	Gross movements Large target No goal	Fine movements Small target Goal is precise
Variety	Limit variety Few choices	Variety available Many options
Cognitive	Simple steps or directions Limited problem solving	Multiple steps or directions Advanced problem solving
Materials	Built-up handle Easy to grasp Larger Simple everyday materials	Small materials Precise manipulation needed Small and difficult to hold Unfamiliar materials
Attention	Simple and clear tasks Few distractions Limit sensory stimuli	Complex and demanding tasks Many distractions Multisensory stimuli

DEVELOPING GROUP GOALS

Writing goals for groups helps members understand the group purpose. Once the group purpose is established, members who will gain from the group experience can be invited to join. Working with clients who have similar goals makes it easier for the practitioner to develop activities. For example, addressing handwriting difficulties in preschool children with developmental delays requires preparation and planning, but all participants can benefit from the same activity. The practitioner sets up the activity and monitors each child's progress to be sure that the child is engaging to his or her fullest.

OT groups focus on the areas of occupational performance: ADLs, work, play and leisure, and social participation. Within these topics, the purpose of the group may vary and therefore it is important for practitioners to be clear about the goals. See Table 7-2 for examples of group goals.

Once the goals and purpose of the groups have been established, practitioners invite members to join. Decisions must be made on the size of the group and types of activities in which they will participate. The practitioner considers the location, equipment, and resources needed for the group. The practitioner establishes the group guidelines, which may include how long members can participate in groups and any rules (Box 7-1).

ADDRESSING INDIVIDUAL GOALS IN A GROUP SESSION

Once group members are selected, the OT practitioner reviews individual goals with each member and determines how to best facilitate the client's progress. The group may serve as the catalyst or reinforce a client's goals. For example, a peer may have more experience or knowledge of resources that benefits another client. Members may find support from others

TABLE 7-2 Goals for Selected Groups

Group Name	Member Characteristics	Goal	Purpose
Cooking	Group is a day treatment group for adults 25-50 who will be living independently.	Develop meal preparation skills for independent living.	Members will learn to shop for food; prepare simple, healthy meals; and stay on a budget.
About Town	Group consists of older adults who have poor social skills. Some adults have behavioral problems or cognitive delays, resulting in poor judgment regarding social participation.	Improve social participation skills to engage in healthy occupations in the community.	Members will explore and participate in community activities. Emphasis will be on establishing social behaviors required in community (e.g., eye contact, language, space).
Sports and Leisure Games	Group consists of young adults and adults with SCI.	Explore adapted sports and leisure activities in the community.	Members will explore a variety of sports and leisure activities that can be completed in a wheelchair. This group will help members integrate into the community after an SCI.
Fitness, yoU, and Nutrition (FUN program)	Group consists of elementary school children.	Develop healthy physical and nutritional activity patterns.	Members will participate in healthy physical and nutritional activities. Lessons will encourage healthy habits as a way to promote fitness and health.

SCI, Spinal cord injury.

BOX 7-1   Group Guidelines

Name of Group: Walk in the Park
Group Goal: Leisure exploration, community mobility, health and
    wellness
Leader (s): OTR and OTA
Members in Group 10
Length of sessions: 2 hours Number of sessions: weekly
Location: City park, local zoo, Audubon Society (all located close
    to the facility)
Cost per week: Zoo entrance fee; others free to public
Equipment: None (water needed)
Types of sessions: Prepare for walk in the woods; discuss weather,
    proper clothing, transportation, food and snacks. Members will
    describe their goals for the outing (explore leisure opportuni-
    ties in the community). Members will discuss proper behaviors.
Comments: Sunscreen; medications; water; physical abilities
    of membrs must be considered; weather and transportation
    needs

BOX 7-2   Considerations When Planning a Group Session

- Age: Will some members serve to mentor others? Will their pairings help facilitate progression toward goals?
- Gender: Are there members who will work better with the same or opposite gender?
- Personality characteristics: Consider the extrovert, introvert, passive, aggressive, manipulative, blocking, caring, empathetic characteristics of clients when requiring group members to interact.
- Goals: How do group members' goals relate?
- Physical: Are there certain members who need help with physical tasks? Consider how you will encourage success for all members in the group.
- Cognitive: Consider how each member can handle the cognitive tasks of the group.
- Social: What are the social requirements of the group? How can you facilitate social participation?
- Emotional level: What are the psychosocial characteristics of members? What is the purpose of the group and what type of intensity of emotions may be displayed? Are members able to support each other? Are group members safe to disclose personal information if needed?

---

to enable them to progress more quickly in therapy. There are many benefits of the group session if it is planned well and its members chosen accordingly.

The OT practitioner carefully designs the group session, considering the multitude of individual goals. The practitioner considers a variety of interpersonal issues as well. Asking two clients who are angry to complete a task together may not benefit the clients or the group. Rather, the practitioner may decide to pair an angry member with the practitioner for the first session. It may benefit a client who is new to his or her condition (e.g., spinal cord injury) to be paired with a client who has experience with the condition. Clients with experience may feel empowered in teaching a novice, and the novice may find hope in relating to the experienced client. Box 7-2 presents a list of considerations that may help facilitate the group process.

The OT practitioner carefully considers the group dynamics and individual goals throughout the group process. While leading the group, the practitioner facilitates the **just-right challenge** for all members by skillfully modifying the requirements. The *just-right challenge* refers to developing activities that are not too easy or too difficult for clients to help them reach their goals.

CASE STUDY

For example, Tom is working on improving his ability to ask for help when needed instead of becoming frustrated and giving up. In a group session, he is working well with Vicky who seems to be taking care of completing all the difficult parts of the project. The practitioner notices this and decides to ask Vicky if she could assist a new member in finding supplies for the project. This leaves Tom alone to problem solve and work on his ability to work through difficult tasks. This allows Vicky to "care for" a new member by showing her knowledge of the supply area. Later, the practitioner comments on how Tom worked through the project and reinforces Vicky's helpfulness during the session.

The practitioner is continually monitoring how each member is working toward his or her goal during the group session. With experience, practitioners become skilled at intervening in

subtle ways, redirecting members, and setting up opportunities that challenge and allow members to succeed. Practitioners reflect on each group session as a way to develop these abilities. Practitioners realize that they often learn when things do not go as well as expected and that reflection is key to developing new strategies.

CASE EXAMPLE APPLICATION: GROUP DYNAMICS

Leading group sessions requires that OT practitioners consider and respond to the dynamic nature of individuals and settings. **Group dynamics** refers to the many factors influencing group members during a session. Experienced OT practitioners are aware of the group dynamics and quickly develop strategies to reinforce positive behaviors in the group, while ignoring or intervening when negative behaviors arise. Reflecting on techniques that worked or did not work with particular individuals helps novice practitioners develop a therapeutic intervention style for a variety of groups. **Preparation** is the key to "thinking on one's feet" and working effectively with groups. Having materials, a well-developed plan, and ideas for adaptations and modifications is essential when working as the leader. OT practitioners also must be aware of each individual's goals, conditions, precautions, and daily status. Knowledge of safety issues related to the group session is required. Prior to leading a group, the practitioner determines the time, space, and location. The following example provides a description of some of the complex issues of addressing individual goals in a group session.

CASE STUDY

Steve, an OT student, has been asked to lead a group for adults who are currently in a rehabilitation center. He will have four members in the group. Participants have a variety of physical needs (Figure 7-2).

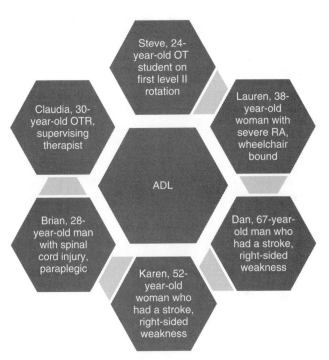

Figure 7-2 Group members.

The first step in the process involves setting individual goals with each client so that Steve understands the direction of the intervention. After meeting with each client, Steve determines they all hope to return to completing their ADLs (e.g., feeding, dressing, bathing, grooming, toileting). Steve decides to begin the group session working on feeding skills. All members will require adapted feeding equipment for independence. Lauren has rheumatoid arthritis so she is familiar with some equipment and may be of assistance to other group members. Furthermore, Steve notes that Lauren appears frustrated with her recent admission to the hospital. He does not want to challenge her in the first session, but rather hopes she will leave the session feeling positive about her future. Karen and Dan both have right-sided weakness, so the OT student asks his supervising therapist (Claudia) to work with them in the group. Finally, Brian is a paraplegic after a recent spinal cord injury. Brian has minimal involvement in his hands, so should be very successful in this group session. Because this is Brian's first OT session, the practitioner plans to instill confidence and establish a rapport while addressing ADL skills.

Steve addresses group session dynamics by providing an overview, introducing himself, and asking members to introduce themselves. He provides a variety of adaptive equipment that may be helpful and asks members to try out the equipment and discuss how they might use it. He has a variety of food available (tailored to each member's dietary needs) so that they can try the equipment. He encourages group members to help each other out. Claudia (the OT practitioner) explains the equipment and shows specific pieces that may be helpful as she observes members trying things out. Interestingly, Lauren has seen some of the equipment and she engages Brian in a discussion of pieces that were exceptionally helpful to her. Brian is not really interested in the equipment until Lauren says her best friend

and mother both have the adapted can opener. The group members discuss how much of the equipment would be helpful to the general public and that perhaps Brian should get that for his mother. He decides to try it out and decides that he will use it for a week. Lauren feels useful and she begins to explain to Karen, "You should try it. You don't have to use it once you get more use of your hand." Karen appreciates the sentiment that she will get more use of her hand and Steve reinforces this concept to the group. Dan is quiet, but he watches Karen carefully (because they both have right-sided weakness). Steve notices this and asks Karen to demonstrate how to use a piece of equipment for Dan. Karen fumbles with feeding herself and they laugh. Dan mumbles, "Well at least it's not just me."

The group session has gone well and each member identifies at least one piece of equipment he or she would like to try for the week. The OT practitioners have observed feeding abilities and documented areas in which members may need individual attention. For example, Dan is experiencing some swallowing and communication difficulties. Lauren reassures Dan that she was "as bad as you" when I came in last week. Dan seems relieved.

The small group intervention has allowed all members to receive attention from the OT practitioners and support from the members. Group members looked to each other for answers and empowered each other. Steve documents each member's progress. He also reflects on how he performed and discusses his performance with his supervisor. Steve acknowledges how difficult it was for him to see a man his age with a spinal cord injury. Claudia complements Steve's professionalism at being friendly yet therapeutic with Brian.

The group session allowed for members to work on ADL skills while finding support, reassurance, socialization, and resources from the members. The rich discussion among members benefited everyone. At the conclusion of the group, the members decided that they would continue to work on self-feeding at the next session (tomorrow), but they wanted to move quickly to dressing.

Understanding and being aware of the group dynamics help practitioners develop effective group intervention sessions. Practitioners and students must practice "thinking on your feet" in a variety of situations prior to leading group sessions in clinical practice. Asking students to role play a variety of conditions or behaviors provides leaders with practice in adapting and modifying activities quickly.

SUMMARY

Addressing individual goals in group sessions can be extremely effective. Practitioners must develop skills in observing group dynamics and multitasking to ensure that individual goals are being met. Preparation is key to the success of group interventions. The practitioner develops groups with knowledge of individual member's goals. Understanding all the elements of the activity and being prepared allow the practitioner to focus on the group dynamics and facilitate the just-right challenge for all clients.

REVIEW QUESTIONS

1. What are the parts to a goal?
2. How do practitioners develop individual goals?
3. How do practitioners address individual goals in a group setting?
4. What strategies are used in group sessions to facilitate individual goals?

REFERENCES

1. American Occupational Therapy Association: Occupational therapy practice framework: domain and process, ed 2, *Am J Occup Ther* 62:625-683, 2008.
2. Kielhofner G: *A model of human occupation: theory and application*, ed 4, Baltimore, MD, 2008, Lippincott, Williams & Wilkins.

Occupational and Group Analysis: Children

Jean W. Solomon

KEY TERMS

collaborative group	parallel group
cooperative group	prewriting group
dress-up group	process group
functional group	special occasion group
handwriting group	task-focused group
occupation-based group	

CHAPTER OBJECTIVES

1. Discuss and describe the classifications of the types of groups.
2. Discuss the differences and similarities of task-(performance component) and occupation-based groups.
3. Develop long-term goals and short-term objectives for task- and occupation-based groups.
4. List and describe target outcomes for task- and occupation-based groups.

Occupational therapy (OT) practitioners enable children to develop skills and abilities for play, education, and self-care. While engaging in small group activities, children interact with peers and develop abilities.

This chapter presents a variety of types of small groups effective in improving young children's motor, cognitive, and social-emotional developmental skills. The areas of occupations addressed in these groups are prewriting, handwriting, and activities of daily living (e.g., feeding, dressing, bathing). The chapter describes the process of developing groups for children with

special consideration and how to integrate groups in the educational system.

TYPES OF GROUPS

Children participate in groups at school, at home, and in the community. They enjoy interacting with other children and learning. Thus, OT practitioners may use groups to engage children in a variety of activities that promote development. **Functional groups** refer to groups that result in end products or help members achieve desired skills and abilities. In OT, functional groups can be used to help members develop motor, cognitive, or social skills. **Process groups** refer to groups that work on the members' interpersonal abilities. Process groups can be used to help children play with other children. These groups are interested in using the process of being involved in a group to address the member's goals.

Groups can be classified as *parallel, cooperative,* and *collaborative.* In a **parallel group** the members work in close proximity to each other, but do not share materials or interact with each other. The only thing that is shared is the physical space. Each group member interacts with separate materials and supplies and works for individual outcomes. For example, children exploring activities in a "sensory room" are engaged in a parallel group. Each child seeks out the sensory input he or she requires. The children do not need to interact with each other to have their needs met or to achieve the goals of the group.

◎ Clinical Pearl

Wiggle or sensory rooms can be designed to promote individual sensory experiences that help a child to be focused and on task in a school setting. Equipment, materials, and supplies are available to meet individual sensory needs or "diets." Sensory rooms typically have suspension systems with a variety of swing options. Trampolines or other bouncing options (e.g., balls or other inflatable items) are available to promote body awareness. Other materials and supplies to address sensory seeking and sensory avoidance behaviors in the tactile, visual, auditory, and olfactory sensory systems are also available based on the needs of the individual children in the group.

Cooperative group members share materials and supplies while striving for individual projects as the outcome. For example, children making bird seed pine cones share the peanut butter, spreading utensils, and other media, but each child completes an end product (i.e., a bird seed pine cone).

◎ Clinical Pearl

> The bird seed pine cones can be hung outside the classroom and used as unique educational tools to reinforce knowledge of colors, numbers, and other concepts when birds are eating.

During a **collaborative group** members share materials and supplies while working on a single project as the final group outcome. An example is a group of adolescents making a poster board collage sharing magazines, scissors, glue, and other materials and supplies to make one collage that represents the group's thoughts and feelings. A variety of types of groups for adolescents is discussed in Chapter 9.

◎ Clinical Pearl

> Cooperative and collaborative groups promote the development of socialization skills (e.g., taking turns, requesting items to be passed along to another child).

Groups are also classified by tasks, activity, or occupations being addressed. **Occupation-based groups** focus on an area of occupation, such as activities of daily living (e.g., feeding, dressing, bathing), instrumental activities of daily living (i.e., care of pets, meal preparation and cleanup), education, rest and sleep, work, and play. Occupation-based groups engage in activities that give children meaning in the natural context. Engaging children in a play group on the school playground with peers to promote playfulness and socialization skills is an example of an occupation-based group. The OT practitioner leads the group, paying attention to facilitating play and playfulness in a nonobtrusive manner with the children.

Activity groups engage children in meaningful activity but may not necessarily occur within the context of the actual occupation. For example, a practitioner may work on socialization skills in a small-group setting in the clinic instead of within the natural context of the playground. Helping children develop skills and abilities through activity groups is often a precursor to the occupation-based group.

Task-focused groups address specific client factors and performance skills such as sensory processing, fine motor skills, strength, endurance, and range of motion. The OT practitioner analyzes the activity at the very basic level and designs group activities to address the performance components.

PLANNING PEDIATRIC GROUPS

Although a pediatric group session can appear fun, spontaneous, and effortless, OT practitioners must consider a variety of issues to lead such a group. Those groups that appear effortless and spontaneous are actually well planned and organized. Effective planning and flexibility are critical when designing groups for children. Gaining experience in adapting and

BOX 8-1   Physical Environmental Considerations

> What is the best lighting for the intervention? Low, bright, or black lights?
> What equipment is available? Moving or stationary?
> What materials and supplies are available? Paper, pencils, crayons? Wipe board and markers?

modifying activities quickly is essential to effective intervention. Having materials and directions for alternative activities readily available helps the practitioner skillfully adjust the plan when needed. For example, the practitioner may need additional activities when he or she realizes that the planned activity is completed too quickly or that the children are not invested in continuing the group activity.

The OT practitioner leading groups for children must pre-plan all aspects of the group to ensure success by considering the following:

- Individual OT goals and objectives for group members
- The present functional levels of the group members
- Physical, social, and personality traits of group members
- Materials, supplies, equipment needs of the group
- The physical environment in which the group is held (e.g., lighting, equipment, materials, supplies; Box 8-1).

Understanding and defining the OT **goals and objectives** for each child help the practitioner design activities that meet the children's needs. One group activity may address multiple objectives. The practitioner must be aware of the individual objectives to arrange materials and steps to facilitate the requested performance. (See Chapter 7 for a description of how to address individual goals in group sessions).

OT practitioners identify the **present functional levels** of the group members to determine the fit of each member or to decide if additional personnel are needed for the group to convene. Groups may function more efficiently if members are of similar functional levels. However, practitioners may decide that having children at different functional levels can be effective, because members work to help each other. Peer role models may facilitate skills and abilities. This has been shown to be exceptionally true for social behavior. The practitioner considers the functional level of the group members and explores the activity requirements. For example, the practitioner may decide that a handwriting group is too advanced for the group members and change the activity to a prewriting group.

Factoring in the **physical, social, and personality traits** of group members is necessary when planning groups for children. The practitioner attempts to create a group that will support each member and allow each member to achieve his or her goals. Placing children together who can physically complete similar activities allows the practitioner to plan group activities that challenge children. Understanding the social skills of each member provides the practitioner with information on how to most successfully group children. For example, the practitioner may decide to position an outgoing and verbal child next to a shy and timid child as a way to encourage interactions, whereas positioning a child who is apt to misbehave next to a timid and shy child may result in disruptions to the group process. Understanding the personality traits of the children in the group helps the practitioner develop strategies prior to the implementation of the session.

While considering the children's functional levels and objectives, the practitioner also examines the **materials, supplies, and equipment** needs for the group activity. Determining how the children may respond to the materials helps the practitioner plan alternative ways of completing the activity. The practitioner secures the equipment and supplies prior to the group and becomes familiar with the variety of ways the activity can be accomplished. For example, in an obstacle course a trampoline activity may be overwhelming for some children. The practitioner may decide that those children bounce only once on their way to another activity. Some children may bounce longer and others may throw a ball to a peer who is bouncing. In this example, all children are engaged in the obstacle course, yet they are bouncing on the trampoline in a variety of ways that are appropriate for them.

The **physical environment** can have an influence on the success of group activity for children. Settings that are over-stimulating or unwelcoming may cause children to experience stress and anxiety, affecting the group process. Children may not want to participate in groups that are not viewed as fun. Therefore, practitioners set up playful environments that are structured and welcoming. Having a space that allows children to move and interact is important. Allowing children the opportunity for choice and time to explore may be beneficial.

LEADING GROUPS WITH CHILDREN

Structuring and planning groups for children are necessary for success. The OT practitioner must have all materials, supplies, and equipment organized and in good working order. Once a group starts, there is little time to look for needed supplies. Children require constant supervision, hand-over-hand assistance, and frequent redirection. Providing children with a list of rules enables everyone to understand the expectations. Practitioners lead groups with gentle but firm expectations. Care should be taken to be specific with feedback, to speak directly to the child, and to correct with gentle redirection. Understanding each child's behavior, personality traits, and functional abilities allows the practitioner to anticipate when a child requires a redirection or assistance. Stepping in before a child becomes frustrated and upset is always preferred. Allowing children to take breaks or start over may help them continue.[5]

Practitioners who display playfulness, positive up-beat attitudes, and compassion work well with children. (See Chapters 3 and 4 for insight into communication and the intentional relationship model). Children need structure and firm, gentle reminders about the expectations of the group. Using humor and imagination helps children engage in playful behaviors, but can be overused. Getting feedback from professionals and reflecting on groups once completed are effective techniques to improve one's therapeutic skills.

Being prepared and having a variety of alternative activities that allow the children to address their own goals is essential when leading pediatric groups. Being flexible and changing plans may be necessary if the group activity is not going well.

PREWRITING GROUPS

OT practitioners frequently design **prewriting groups**. Prewriting skills are the foundation for efficient and legible handwriting. A young child first learns to scribble. Early scribbling is large and not confined to a specific or designated area. Children enjoy scribbling in a variety of positions, on various surfaces, and using different media. Scribbling helps children develop hand strength and fine motor control, and explore movements required for prewriting and writing skills.

◎ Clinical Pearl

Drawing on a sidewalk with chalk or using a small stick to draw in sand offers a child a multisensory experience.

Young children sit, stand, or lie on their stomachs while coloring, painting, or manipulating playdough to develop strength, coordination, and motor planning for prewriting. **Prewriting strokes** are learned through imitation and copying. Imitation is the physical or motor modeling or demonstration of the desired stroke to be drawn.[4] For example, a child imitates by drawing the stroke at the same time as the practitioner. **Copying** refers to drawing the stroke from a picture. In this case, the child is shown the stroke and asked to draw the same thing. When copying a stroke, the child is not observing how the stroke is drawn. Children learn to imitate strokes before they can copy them. Last, they learn to draw a stroke from memory on verbal request. Table 8-1 provides the progression of the development of strokes.

These prewriting strokes are used to form the uppercase and lowercase letters and numbers. For example, the uppercase letter D consists of vertical and circular strokes. The early prewriting strokes are combined to draw simple and complex geometric shapes. Simple geometric shapes include a cross, square, and rectangle that are composed of vertical and horizontal lines. Complex geometric shapes such as triangles and diamonds require children to cross the midline of their body to draw diagonal lines. The following scenario describes the process of a preschool prewriting group.

PRESCHOOL PREWRITING GROUP

Carlos is an OT practitioner who visits a rural elementary school each week. His caseload includes six 3-year-old students who have fine motor and prewriting objectives as a part of their individualized educational plan (IEP). The IEP is a school-based plan that describes the intervention goals and objectives for the child who receives special education services in the school system. OT practitioners develop educationally relevant goals and objectives for children who are receiving therapy as part of their educational plan. Carlos consults with the preschool teacher as to her preference for the delivery of small-group services. They agree

TABLE 8-1   Prewriting Skills: Development of Visual-Motor Integration Skills

14 months	Scribbles vertically	
23-24 months	Imitates vertical stroke at least two inches	
27-28 months	Imitates horizontal stroke at least two inches	
33-34 months	Copies circle with end points within ½ inch of each other	
39-40 months	Copies cross with intersecting lines within 20 degrees of perpendicular	
41-42 months	Traces line with a maximum of two deviations by no more than ½ inch	
49-50 months	Copies square using straight lines and closed corners	
59-60 months	Colors between parallel lines, crossing lines no more than two times	

Based on the Peabody Developmental Motor Scales.[2]

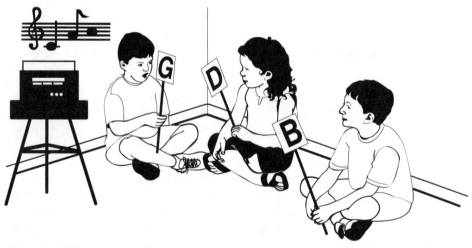

Figure 8-1 Children learn to identify uppercase letters using a multisensory approach (seeing, hearing, and feeling).

that the prewriting group will be scheduled in the fine motor area of the multipurpose sensory motor classroom. The fine motor area is partitioned from the gross motor area of classroom. There is a rug and low table in the center of the area. The table has several incline (slant) boards available for children to use during their prewriting activities. There are four easels on one side of the fine motor area. Because music is used during "warm-up" and "wind-down" activities, there is a CD player located in the fine motor area.

Each group is scheduled for 30 minutes per week. A classroom assistant helps facilitate each group. The warm-up activities help the children to learn basic concepts important to prewriting skills (e.g., directionality concepts such as up, down, across, and around, and imitation of body movements). The prewriting activities include coloring in a designated area, imitating prewriting strokes using various media (crayons, markers, finger paints), and forming shapes with wooden straight and curved sticks. The wind-down activities include cleaning the room and washing hands while listening to instrumental soothing songs (Figures 8-1 through 8-5).

Teachers make a majority of referrals for OT because of **handwriting**. According to Cermak, 30% of a child's day is spent on handwriting and this is the primary means for which

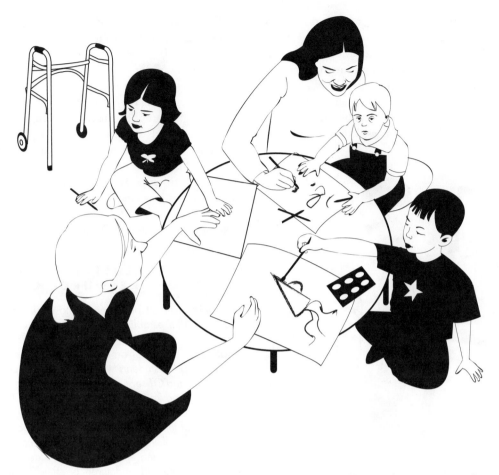

Figure 8-2 Children improve fine-motor and prewriting skills by seeing, feeling, and hearing (the practitioner provides verbal cues) regarding letter formation.

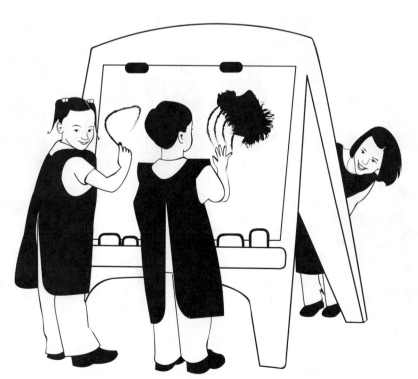

Figure 8-3 Children develop hand skills by manipulating objects and feeling textures.

they communicate learning.[1] In many states, handwriting is not a part of the general education curriculum. Therefore, young children do not learn the proper mechanics of handwriting. Consequently, OT practitioners who work in school systems are frequently asked to intervene in this area. The *Handwriting without Tears*[3] curriculum outlines seven elements of handwriting important for efficient and effective handwriting:

1. Memory: recall of upper and lower case letters and numbers

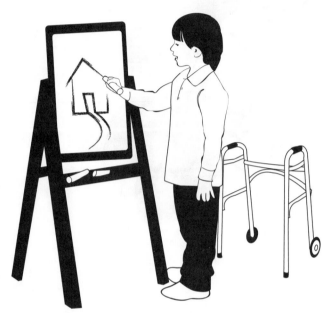

Figure 8-4 Using a paint brush for details requires fine-motor coordination.

2. Size: appropriate sizes of letters and words for age
3. Orientation: letter or number facing the correct direction (no reversal)
4. Placement: putting letters, words, and numbers on the line or above and below as appropriate, such as g, p, k
5. Start: beginning the letters at the top
6. Spacing: appropriate spaces between letters in words and between words and sentences
7. Control: grasp of writing tool, posture, use of helping hand to stabilize paper

OT practitioners working with young children in educational settings may effectively provide services in small groups to meet their caseload demands. Leading prewriting and handwriting groups lends itself to group instruction and can be integrated into the classroom.

INCLUSIVE HANDWRITING GROUP: RESOURCE CLASSROOM

Jeannie is an OT practitioner who works for a local school district. After establishing a relationship with Erica, the first grade resource teacher, they communicate and collaborate on the idea of an **inclusive ("push-in")** *handwriting group for students who receive both special education resource and OT services. Jeannie and Erica mutually decide that the handwriting group will occur at the table in the front of the resource room because it is partially partitioned from the rest of the classroom by a wall and bookshelves. There are four small chairs on either side of the table and an adult-sized chair at the end of the open side of the table. Four students (one girl and three boys) will participate in the handwriting group that is scheduled weekly for 45 minutes.*

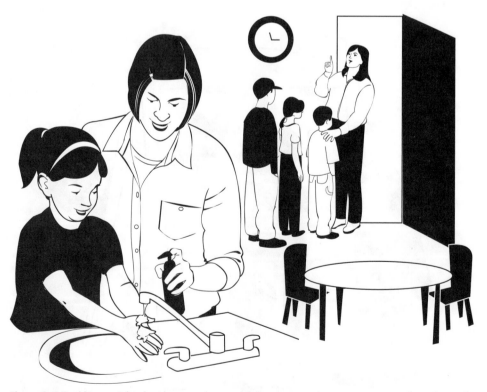

Figure 8-5 Scrubbing one's hands with soap and water while listening to soothing music serves to indicate the conclusion of the activity (wind down).

Each group session begins with warm-up activities to address posture, range of motion, and strength. Examples of therapeutic exercises incorporated include shoulder rolls forward and backward, imitation of movements of the arms against gravity, and waking up the finger muscles by popping bubble wrap. These warm up activities help prepare the child for writing tasks.

Following the warm up activities, the students complete worksheets that reinforce the proper mechanics of letter formation and spacing. They draw the letters in sand before completing the paper tasks. The OT practitioner provides instruction as needed and reinforces success. The practitioner ensures that the children are sitting upright and are holding the pencil appropriately.

The children are asked to print their names, or one letter from their names, on the top right-hand corner of a piece of paper so that they can use it in class today. This helps emphasize the occupation of handwriting and increases the meaning of the activity.

The end of the session consists of "wind-down" or "cool-down" activities. These wind-down activities may include shaking out stiffness in the arms and hands, stretching the arms and fingers, walking around the room with the hands clasped together, bending toward the floor with clasped hands and swinging the arms from side to side like an elephant swinging his trunk. These activities serve to relax

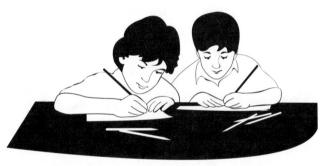

Figure 8-6 Students benefit from practicing handwriting.

the children and rest their muscles after activity so they can continue with school work (Figures 8-6 through 8-8).

There are two models for providing direct OT services in an educational setting: *inclusive* and *direct service (pull out)*. The inclusive model may also be termed *push in*, and requires the OT practitioner to provide direct services in the special education classroom. In the **direct service (pull-out)** model, the OT practitioner provides services in the school environment outside of the special education classroom. The OT practitioner carefully assesses the most effective model to use based on the child's and group's needs.

ACTIVITIES OF DAILY LIVING

Activities of daily living relevant in daily routines in a classroom include personal hygiene such as washing hands and dressing skills (e.g., donning and doffing coat and manipulating clothing during toileting routines). Incorporating washing hands at the end of a small group promotes turn taking and independence in self-care. Playing dress up in a preschool classroom helps the child gain gross and fine-motor coordination. There are many commercially available materials, (e.g., dressing capes, doll clothes, buttoning boards) that can be used to increase a child's ability to manipulate fasteners or clothing. However, children enjoy playing dress up and this allows the OT practitioner to engage children in play while addressing dressing skills.

PRESCHOOL DRESS UP GROUP

At the beginning of the school year, the preschool teacher asked Shawntionya, the OT practitioner, how to best work on increasing his students' ability to dress and undress and manipulate fasteners. Together, the practitioner and teacher decided that in addition to working on these skills during naturally occurring opportunities (e.g., toileting, arriving, leaving),

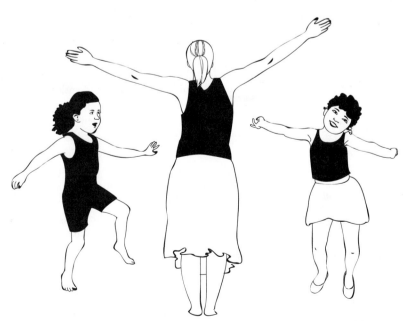

Figure 8-7 Stretching and "shaking out any stiffness in arms and hands" can serve as wind-down activities.

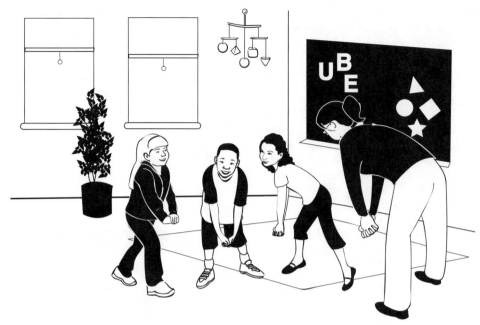

Figure 8-8 Swinging one's arms "like an elephant" is a fun way to wind down.

playing **dress up** two to three times per week would provide opportunities for teaching and learning basic self-care.

Shawntionya gathered a box of dress-up clothes, which consisted of brightly colored, oversized dresses, shirts, pants, hats, skirts, and other accessories. She included clothing and accessories with a variety of fasteners. Four to six 3- to 5-year-old children participated in each session, which lasted 30 minutes (including clean up) two times a week. The preschool teacher and a classroom assistant helped the OT in leading the group.

The preschool children gathered around the box of dress-up clothes. They enjoyed the brightly colored big clothes and bold accessories. The adults provided the children physical and verbal assistance as necessary for donning and doffing the chosen outfit. Each child "modeled" his or her outfit and received praise from the others.

All of the children were encouraged to sing the "clean up song," which is a familiar routine at the preschool. They returned items to the box. Occasionally, Shawntionya gathers new clothing to provide novelty to the group (see Figure 8-9 A and 8-9B).

SPECIAL OCCASION GROUPS

Colvin is an OT practitioner who works with four to six students weekly to improve fine-motor and handwriting skills. At the end of each quarter, Colvin plans a special topics (**special occasion**) group, allowing each student to take home a project as a sample of his or her progress in OT. The second quarter of the school year is at the end of January. Colvin communicates with the resource teacher on possible topics because the activity will be completed in her classroom. They are considering the following projects:

- Decorate a landscape with snow.
- Make Valentine's Day cards for parents or peers.
- Make St. Patrick's Day shamrock collages.

They discuss materials and supplies needed. Colvin offers to analyze each activity, including performance abilities (motor, cognition, social-emotional) needed for completion, sequence and timing, activity demands, cost, and the contexts. After exploring these aspects of the activity, they will decide how to proceed.

TIPS FOR LEADING PEDIATRIC GROUPS

Working with children in small groups offers opportunities for socialization, communication, sharing of materials and supplies, and a variety of experiences to enhance a child's developmental skills. Children learn negotiation, communication, sharing, turn-taking, and problem-solving when working on projects in small groups. They learn to assert themselves, read others' cues, and compromise with others. Working in groups can provide children with same-aged peer models from whom they can learn. Planning the sequence of activities is required for a successful intervention. Having the necessary materials and supplies is equally important.[5]

An alternative plan is helpful in the event that the activity ends early or children do not wish to engage. Alternative activities that can easily be incorporated into the current activity work well because children may change their minds quickly or perform differently than expected. Practitioners who consider additional related activities are better able to "think on their feet" and adjust the activity quickly so that children remain engaged. Practicing adjusting to a variety of conditions allows practitioners to be ready when necessary.

To provide inclusive therapy in the classroom, the teacher has to be willing to share space with the OT practitioner. Practitioners who take the time to build relationships with teachers and consider their educational goals are more likely to be successful. Working together to meet educational goals while

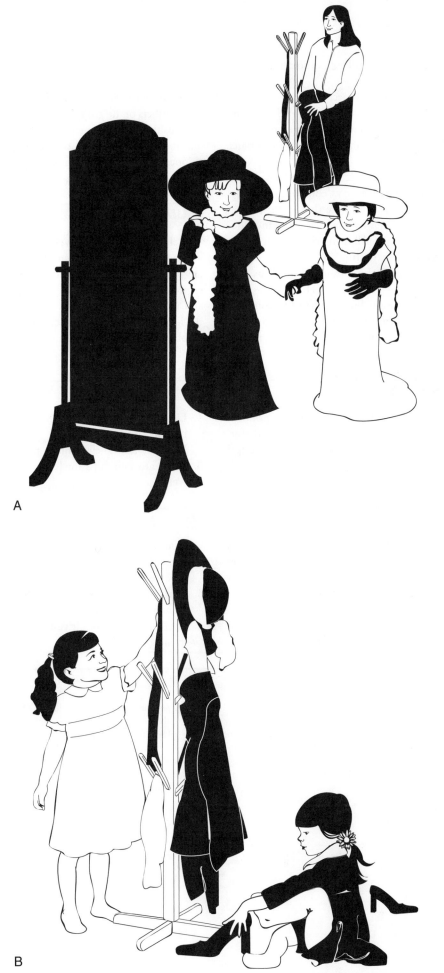

Figure 8-9 A, Playing dress up can help children develop important fine-motor skills. **B,** Singing the "clean up song" can help children wind down and get ready to leave.

allowing children to remain in a regular classroom is beneficial to students and teachers.

Certain children may require special equipment (e.g., swings or trampoline) to meet their OT goals. Although this may require a direct-service (pull-out) model, the practitioner makes an effort to integrate therapy into the classroom as much as possible.

Providing children with a sample of the end product is helpful. The practitioner should always complete the activity prior to leading the group to be sure that it can be successful. Children enjoy activities that involve a product they can share with family or friends. Allowing children to engage in short projects (rather than waiting) is preferred. Involving children in picking out and choosing as much as they can benefits them and makes the project feel more like their own. OT practitioners strive to allow the child to complete as much of the project as possible in the group. Thus, the goal is not a perfect product, but rather the goal is for the child to complete as much of the project on his or her own as possible.

Importantly, group activities must match the skill levels of the members of the group. Therefore, when planning the group composition the OT practitioner considers the client factors and individual goals and objectives for each child. OT practitioners target individual goals in group sessions. A thorough activity analysis is required.

SUMMARY

This chapter presents the types of groups and provides tips for leading groups with children. A variety of examples of groups are provided. The developmental sequence of the acquisition of prewriting skills is discussed. The proper mechanics of letter and number formation is presented. The differences between the inclusive and direct service (push-in versus pull-out) models of service delivery are described.

REVIEW QUESTIONS

1. What are the classifications and types of pediatric groups?
2. What are the differences and similarities of task-(performance component) and occupation-based pediatric groups?
3. List and explain the developmental sequence for the acquisition of prewriting skills.
4. List and describe the proper mechanics of letter and number formation.
5. What are critical elements in planning a pediatric group?
6. What are some tips for leading groups with children and youth?

SUGGESTED LEARNING ACTIVITIES

1. Visit a daycare center and observe in a classroom. Discuss planning a group for the following week with the daycare staff. Plan and implement the group. Analyze what went well and what could have been done differently after implementing the group.
2. Visit a day camp for children who have special needs and observe several children. Discuss planning a group for the following week with the day camp staff. Plan and implement the group. Analyze what went well and what could have been done differently after implementing the group.
3. Create a box of dress-up clothing that you can use to implement activities in the groups for 1 and 2.
4. Create a fine-motor kit you can use to implement activities in the groups for 1 and 2.

REFERENCES

1. Cermak S A, Marr D, Cohn E, Henderson A: Fine motor activities in Head Start and kindergarten classrooms, *American Journal of Occupational Therapy*, 57(5), 550-557, 2003.
2. Folio MR, Fewell RR: *Peabody developmental motor scales*, ed 2, Los Angeles, 2000, Western Psychological Services.
3. Olsen JZ, Knapton EF: *The print tool manual: handwriting without tears*, ed 3, Cabin John, MD, 2008, Western Psychological Services.
4. Pickett JP: *The American heritage dictionary of the English language*, ed 4, New York, 2000, Houghton Mifflin Company.
5. Solomon J, O'Brien J: *Pediatric skills for the occupational therapy assistant*, ed 3, St Louis, 2010, Elsevier.

Occupational and Group Analysis: Adolescents

Kerryellen Vroman, Jane Clifford O'Brien

CHAPTER OUTLINE

Psychosocial Developmental Tasks of Adolescents

Advantages of Group Interventions for Adolescents

Types of Groups and the Frames of References that May be Used to Structure Them

    Talk-Based Therapy Groups
    Social Learning Theory as a Frame of Reference
    The Model of Human Occupation as a Frame of Reference
    Psychoeducational Groups with Adolescents
    Strength-Based Groups—Activity Groups
    Community-Based Support Groups for Adolescents

Strategies for Group Interventions for Adolescents

Summary

KEY TERMS

cognitive-behavioral therapy	psychoeducational groups
developmental tasks	psychodynamic therapy
early adolescence	self-determinism, hope, and
habituation	empowerment
late adolescence	social learning theory (SLT)
middle adolescence	social participation
Model of Human Occupation	social skills
(MOHO)	talk-based therapy
perceived efficacy	volition
(self-efficacy)	applied behavioral analysis
performance capacity	psychiatric rehabilitation model
personal causation	self-actualization
projective activities	

CHAPTER OBJECTIVES:

1. Outline the developmental tasks of adolescents as they relate to group interventions.
2. Identify group needs specific to adolescents.
3. Describe strategies for working with adolescents.
4. Discuss group interventions and frames of reference for adolescents.

Adolescence, unique as a time of physiologic changes and psychosocial development, is characterized by exploration, experimentation, and the development of one's sense of identity. Relationships with parents are redefined, while those with peers are strengthened. Participation in peer activities increases, progressively greater independence is established, and competency in the skills for adult roles are gained. Many adolescents find this time in their lives stressful and there is an increased vulnerability for mental health disorders.

Practitioners need to consider the **developmental tasks** associated with adolescence. These include exploring intimacy, sexual and gender orientation, and sexual expression. In middle and high school "fitting in" is important, because identifying with a peer group as friends provides a sense of belonging that is key to successfully navigating the developmental tasks.[28] However, there are also pressures from peers, parents, and society to perform and conform. The pressures from peer groups to experiment can include engaging in risky behaviors and expressing group membership through actions such as choice of clothing, drinking, and interests that may create conflict with parents. Although other peer groups may create fewer tensions with parents, the need to follow peer trends and belong is perceived as paramount (Figure 9-1).

Adolescents report feeling stressed as a result of the pressure they feel to succeed academically and in areas such as sports and the arts, and to assume greater responsibilities for themselves. These responsibilities include managing finances. Some adolescents work not only for discretionary spending money, but to help support their families. They are increasingly expected to manage their time and to complete their self-care, to self-regulate emotions and behaviors, and to make sound judgments about their new freedom. All these expectations occur while they are still developing cognitive skills and exploring their values and beliefs. Irrespective of the specific group goals, the group-based interventions that occupational therapy practitioners provide to adolescents address the development of the performance skills required to participate successfully and to meet the demands of this developmental stage to assume the roles of adult life.

This chapter reviews the psychosocial milestones that are fundamental to adolescent development and underpin all groups conducted with this population in therapy and recreational settings. The chapter outlines strategies to assist practitioners in leading group interventions for adolescents. The authors

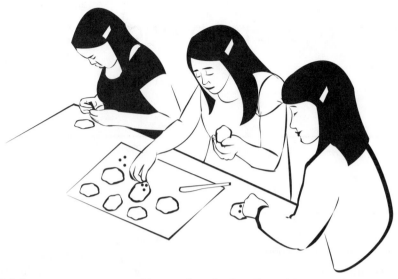

Figure 9-1 Peer groups are important to adolescents who seek to fit in. These adolescents are hanging out and decorating cookies, all dressed in similar fashion.

provide sample group templates that serve to organize intervention planning.

PSYCHOSOCIAL DEVELOPMENTAL TASKS OF ADOLESCENTS

In adolescence there is a psychosocial vulnerability that can result in behavioral difficulties (e.g., delinquency, participation in criminal activities, social failure, or participation in gangs) or psychopathologic conditions such as the onset of depression, eating disorders, drug and alcohol abuse, self-harming behaviors, and anxiety disorders.[11] In contrast, with supportive family, school, and community environments, which include validating adults, healthy psychosocial development results in **self-actualization**, namely a healthy self-concept, self-esteem, and sense of one's identity as an autonomous individual.

There are three stages of adolescent development (Table 9-1; Figure 9-2). **Early adolescence** encompasses the middle school years (11 to 13 years old) and the majority of young people in this age group experience puberty (the maturation of the reproductive system with the development of primary and secondary sex characteristics). **Middle adolescence** includes the high school years between the ages of 14 and 17. This is the period of the most intense psychosocial development, when the salient relationships with friends and other peer-mediated influences displace parental relationships and opinions. **Late adolescence**, between 17 and 25 years, is a time of consolidation of values, self-identity, and self-efficacy in performance skills required to meet the choices and demands of the roles of early adulthood such as work and forming a stable intimate relationship.

ADVANTAGES OF GROUP INTERVENTIONS FOR ADOLESCENTS

Research studies empirically support the effectiveness and importance of group interventions (counseling, social skills training, psychotherapy, and preventive programs) for adolescents.[16,17,28,29,33]

Adolescents prefer group settings; it is where they learn, develop, and seek support. Their lives are structured around formal, informal, and virtual groups, such as the classroom, the sports team, Facebook, and friendship groups. Group interventions assist adolescents to develop peer relationships in a structured, safe environment and to express themselves without fear of criticism, ridicule, or bullying. In therapy groups, structure and activities that are appropriate for age and development assist adolescents to find their voice, articulate their concerns, and receive support from peers and adults.

Adolescents with special needs or disabilities engage in fewer social activities and friendships outside of school. Even adolescents with friends at school report they have less contact with friends outside of school in comparison with their peers.[10] Reasons for this discrepancy include not participating in or not excelling in the activities such as sport. During adolescence, social participation and stereotypical characteristics of "physical attractiveness" and interpersonal skills are primary factors of high social status.[25,32] Adolescents with disabilities seldom have high social status and those with physical disabilities deal with additional challenges of mobility and community access. The negative consequence of limited participation with peers results in less engagement in the broad range of activities and tasks that promote role and skill development in adolescence (Figure 9-3).

Adolescents may be referred to occupational therapy because they are experiencing psychoemotional or behavioral problems. They are often reluctant attendees in the group sessions because they perceive that occupational therapy makes them "different." At this age teens want to conform to the "typical" image for adolescents in their community, culture, and particular peer group. Already challenged emotionally and lacking in the skills to articulate their thoughts, feelings, and needs, they may demonstrate their reluctance and ambivalence in their behavior rather than verbally express their concerns about being stigmatized. They fear what therapy will involve and mean for them. However, group interventions can also

TABLE 9-1 Psychosocial Developmental Tasks of Adolescents to Integrate into Group Interventions

PSYCHOSOCIAL DEVELOPMENTAL TASKS OF ADOLESCENCE

The developmental tasks in adolescence accumulate:
- The ability to establishing healthy relationships
- A sense of identify that includes a healthy self-concept and body image, and positive self-esteem
- Gender identification and the capacity for intimacy and expression of one's sexuality
- An occupational identity

Early Adolescence In middle school and early high school, a practitioner will find that adolescents in the groups are:	■ Egocentric: engrossed with self and relate most things to themselves, especially their physical attractiveness. They compare their bodies and appearance with those of other teens. ■ Interested in: ■ Own concerns and seldom consider other perspectives. ■ Their personal appearance and how others, especially peers, view them. ■ Separating emotionally from parents, less overtly affectionate and preferring to do fewer activities with their parents. ■ Less compliant with rules or limits set by adults (i.e., parents, teachers, and coaches). This includes questioning and challenging adults' authority. May challenge advice and expectations of parents, and find fault with adults in their lives. ■ Having changeable moods. ■ Cognitively able to differentiate between feelings and label them. ■ Inconsistent in their behavior, which is related to the development of their ability to self-regulate emotional expression, mostly influenced by immediate wants or needs and being susceptible to peer pressure. The occupational therapy group can be influential in shaping behavior and attitudes. ■ Mostly in same-sex friendships. ■ Demonstrating abstract thinking and can engage in group activities that promote self-awareness and insight. ■ Fantasize idealistically about careers; think about possible future self and roles. ■ Wanting privacy (e.g., write in diaries, have private telephone conversations, and secrets with friends and disclosing activities openly). ■ Developing interest in experiences related to personal sexual development and exploration of sexual feelings (e.g., masturbation). ■ Self-consciously displaying modesty. May blush, be awkward about self and body. In groups, a practitioner will avoid situations that draw attention to the adolescents in a manner that will heighten this acute self-consciousness. ■ Experiment with drugs (cigarettes, alcohol, and marijuana).
Middle Adolescence In the middle years of adolescence (the high school years), a practitioner is likely to find that adolescents are:	■ Moving toward psychological and social independence from parents. ■ Accepting the changes and growth of their bodies that have occurred. ■ Engaging with greater interest in grooming and appearing attractive and less preoccupied with the physical changes in their bodies. ■ Increasingly involved in *their* peer group culture. This will be displayed by adopting a peer value system, codes of behavior, and style of dress and appearance, all of which manifests in overt individualism. ■ Spending their discretionary time in formal and informal peer group activities, such as sports teams, clubs, gangs, and socializing while sharing interests (shopping, skateboarding, listening to music, or computer-mediated games). ■ Experiencing stress related to expectations and demands for academic performance. ■ Accepting changes in their body, engaging in sexual expression and experimentation with intimate (sexual) activities. ■ Exploring and processing their feelings and those of other people. ■ Becoming increasingly focused on realistic options for a career, vocation, or job. ■ Showing further development in their creativity and cognitive abilities. This includes pursuing recreational activities that offer opportunities for use and expression of these abilities (music, art, writing, advancing computer skills, and other academic pursuits). ■ Likely to use risk-taking behaviors to minimize or alleviate feelings. Risk-taking reflects feelings of omnipotence (sense of being powerful) and immortality (e.g., reckless driving, unprotected sex, and drinking or drug use). These behaviors reflect the immediacy of their decisionmaking with minimal consideration of potential consequences or rewards. ■ Accessing and experimenting with drugs (cigarettes, alcohol, marijuana, and other illicit drugs).
Late Adolescence In the latter years of adolescence (late high school, starting work or college) a practitioner may observe the adolescents in groups are:	■ Developing a stable sense of self and having consistent opinions, values, and beliefs that inform behavior. ■ Strengthening emotional relationships with parents (e.g., seek out and value parental advice and assistance). ■ Increasing independence in decision making and demonstrating an ability to express their ideas and opinions independent of peer pressure. ■ Interested in their future and consider the consequences of current actions and decisions, delaying gratification and planning for long-term outcomes, setting personal limits, monitoring their own behavior, and reaching compromises. ■ Resolving their earlier angst with issues such as gender and sexual orientation, and physical appearance to have a stable sense of self-concept. ■ Feeling a diminished peer influence and increased confidence in personal values and sense of self. ■ Interacting within an intimate relationship and preferring one-on-one relationships. ■ Starting to or already selecting a worker role and financial independence. ■ Developing an increasingly stable value system (moral and spiritual).

Table modified from Vroman.[32]
Sources of data: Radizik, Sherer, and Neinstein.[28]

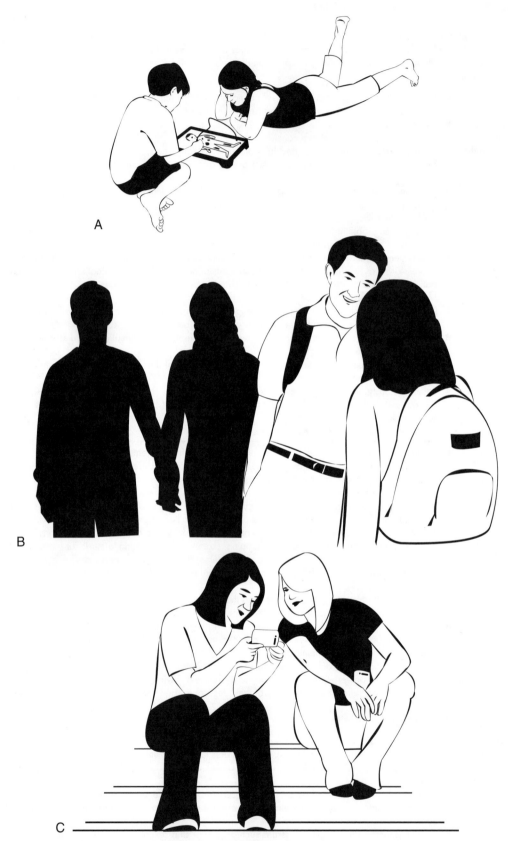

Figure 9-2 A, Young teens enjoy playing games with rules. **B,** High school students become interested in developing close relationships with peers as they begin to express their sexuality. **C,** Older teens begin to develop goals for their future and a sense of identity apart from their peers.

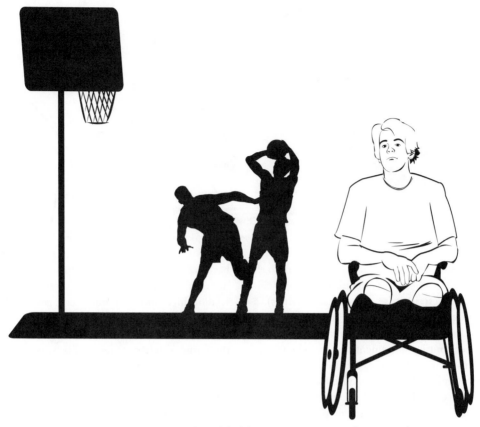

Figure 9-3 Adolescents who have physical disabilities may miss out on social activities with peers.

reduce their isolation by challenging the myths that one's emotions and experiences are unique. They can find peer acceptance, perhaps for the first time, and receive adult guidance and support in a context that also offers avenues to assert power and gain independence.[6]

TYPES OF GROUPS AND THE FRAMES OF REFERENCES THAT MAY BE USED TO STRUCTURE THEM

By using a **frame of reference**, a practitioner has a clear understanding of his or her role and a practical template to develop group interventions. Each frame of reference has assessments and strategies, including a perspective for interpreting adolescents' occupational performance. It defines outcomes that can be expected when therapy adheres to the frame of reference's evaluation and intervention process. In this section, we have selected frames of reference and paired them with common adolescent group interventions. The group and frame of reference illustrate one example of a group that a practitioner could employ for a given need or problem.

The choice of a frame of reference is based on many factors: the population characteristics, needs, performance skills, and capacity of group members; the occupational therapy goals; and the expertise of the practitioner. Although best practice recommends basing the choice of frame of research on evidence of its effectiveness, the choice may be influenced by the policies, resources, and philosophy of a setting. For example, a

residential school setting for adolescents with behavioral problems may have instituted a positive behavioral support [PBS] approach. The practitioner would need to incorporate PBS into his or her practice and therefore might select an acquisitional frame of reference for groups because it meets the needs of the adolescents in the occupational therapy group and it is compatible with PBS.

Occupational therapy group interventions for adolescents occur in many settings. Groups are offered in schools to enhance school performance or to facilitate transition from high school. Groups providing mental health or behavioral interventions may be based in health, justice, or educational settings. Other groups are delivered in the community, including summer camps, city-supported initiatives for youth, and programming that is an extension of school services. Any of these frames of reference–based groups, outlined here, can be provided in these settings.[32]

TALK-BASED THERAPY GROUPS

Occupational therapy with adolescents in mental health multidisciplinary settings is often provided in talk-based groups, such as **cognitive-behavioral therapy** or **psychodynamic therapy**. Social workers, psychologists, and youth workers also use these frames of reference.[24,32]

Adolescents involved in **talk-based therapy** benefit from structure. A practitioner uses structure to help adolescents manage their anxiety and lessen their resistance to participating

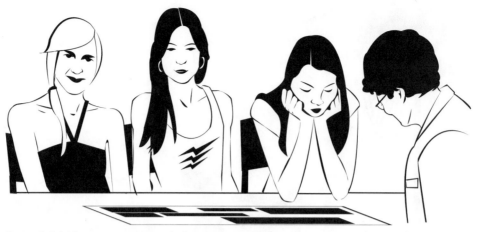

Figure 9-4 Adolescents may experience body image issues related to intense pressure to physically "fit in" with peers.

in therapy. Self-disclosure and sharing of experiences and feelings to promote insight and self-understanding can be facilitated using **projective activities** (self-awareness activities), a strategy that an occupational therapy practitioner brings to talk-based therapy. In projective activities, a variety of media such as art activities, music, movement, or sociodrama are vehicles for self-exploration and self-expression. Through an activity, adolescents express themselves and by talking about the theme of the activity they begin to give a voice to their feelings and concerns. For example, the magazine picture collage, a projective activity used to assess adolescents in mental health settings, provides insights into how they perceive themselves and describe their interests (Figure 9-4).[12]

Practitioners using projective activities need to be skillful at facilitating groups, because through these techniques adolescents may begin to access painful experiences and difficult emotions. The practitioner leading these groups must ensure that the group process proceeds at a rate that is appropriate to the participants' emotional and cognitive skills to cope. Self-disclosure is not the primary goal of projective activities. The primary goal is for the activity to provide the adolescents an opportunity to explore and gain insight into their experiences, values, beliefs, interests, and personal causation. From these insights they learn to self-regulate their emotions and reframe painful experiences so that trauma or emotional difficulties do not continue to undermine their occupational performance in areas such as social participation and education. It is integral to the therapeutic process of talk-based groups that issues raised in the session are addressed within the group through mutual support, sharing, and learning coping strategies. Therefore, time management is very important to ensure that an appropriate level of resolution of issues is achieved before the group session finishes and no member leaves the group unduly distressed.

SOCIAL LEARNING THEORY AS A FRAME OF REFERENCE

Life and social skills are two common areas of occupational performance addressed through group programs. In skill-based programs, goals must clearly delineate the area of occupational performance being addressed.[24] The label **social skills**

has become an umbrella term for the interpersonal and communication skills necessary for successful social participation, relationships, and community engagement. However, the performance skills (e.g., social interaction skills, communication skills, and social skills) consist of distinctive areas. Similarly, the frame of reference selected is based on the evidence of its effectiveness to promote development of the targeted skills. The context of the group program is also critical to the facilitation of the skills and the generalization of the learning to adolescents' everyday occupations. For example, a practitioner planning a group program to develop functional community mobility skills would select an occupation-based frame of reference so that the skills are acquired in the naturalistic setting (the adolescents' community). Although occupation-based learning in the natural context is optimal, practitioners addressing a limited performance skill frequently select a frame of reference that works on **acquisition** of the components of skills in a simulated context. Therefore, the **psychiatric rehabilitation model** may be the choice for a group of late adolescents who need to acquire activities of daily living skills to transition to a group home. We have chosen the category of social skills to illustrate a communication group program that would focus on acquisition of component skills in a simulated context.[24,29,33]

Social skills group programs may focus on the techniques of conversing and the mechanics of communicating. Other group programs within this broad area of skills may focus on the more complex principles of interacting that involve understanding interactions and developing multidimensional performance skills that support maintaining relationships through skillful communication.

Box 9-1 provides a description of the aspects of social skills. Selected subareas may be identified and expanded into a specific group program such as assertiveness, anger management, or self-regulation strategies for the classroom setting. This list emphasizes the importance of focusing on a comparable level of social skills and building a group program that is congruent with the performance capacity of the group participants. It is better to limit the focus and achieve skill competency, because the adolescent's self-efficacy (belief in one's ability to perform) in social skills builds self-esteem and increases the likelihood of **social participation**.

| **BOX 9-1** | **Group Interventions that Build Social Skills for Social Participation** |

Communication Skills
- Listen—includes attending and nonverbal body language congruent with attending such as eye contact.
- Initiate interaction, including information seeking and exchange.
- Use rapport-building strategies.
- Maintain and reciprocate verbal exchanges.
- Clarify information heard or given.
- End conversations.

Interpreting Social Interactions and Situations
- Show empathy, using sympathy appropriately.
- Accurately recognize emotions.
- Respond accurately and with the correct intensity of emotions.
- Use and understand humor.
- Organize thoughts and communicate message clearly in response to contextual cues.

Managing Social Interaction and Self-Regulation
- Manage conflict.
- Compromise.
- Be assertive.
- Accept and respond to compliments and feedback.
- Give compliments and feedback constructively.
- Apologize.

Self-Regulation and Expression (Emotions and Cognitive Processes)
- Regulate emotional responses (e.g., anger management)
- Self-monitor.
- Self-disclose.
- Manage difficult social exchanges.
- Be self-aware.
- Problem-solve.

AOTA, 2008[1]; Stein and Culter.[30]

Practitioners planning to implement social skills groups with adolescents are strongly encouraged to make use of resources available in the health and education literature. Practitioners use task analysis to identify the components of the skills to be addressed. The skills listed in Box 9-1 are divided into behavioral units according to the performance capacity of the adolescent group participants. For example, a group working specifically on communications skills might have sessions on conversing using verbal and nonverbal interactions such as greeting, initiating a conversation, and asking questions.

The predominant frame of reference used for many social skills interventions by occupational therapy practitioners is **social learning theory (SLT)** (more recently referred to as *social cognitive theory*). SLT groups are used to decrease behavioral problems, improve social behaviors and social skills, and to improve adolescents' self-efficacy in their performance. This approach is employed in groups that provide assertiveness training, anger management, or seek to change behaviors (e.g., stop smoking and develop healthy eating patterns).

SLT focuses on learning that occurs within social contexts and how people learn from one another through observation, imitation, and seeing other people model behaviors. In keeping with adolescents' need for a sense of autonomy, this frame of reference recognizes adolescents as self-determining—as able to make choices about their behaviors, and able to understand the importance of choices. It uses reciprocal interaction among them and their peers to foster vicarious learning. A fundamental concept of SLT is that adolescents will most likely learn new behaviors by watching other adolescents *like themselves (especially a person they hold in high esteem)* who can competently perform the desired skill or behavior. Vicarious learning can also inhibit undesirable behaviors. When an adolescent observes adverse consequences associated with behavior, this may lead to an inhibition of similar behaviors to avoid an unpleasant outcome.

Social skills groups following the SLT frame of reference employ strategies for learning and rehearsing new behaviors including activity analysis, role modeling, coaching, and role playing.

Ⓒ Clinical Pearl: Using Role-Play Techniques

Role play is useful in providing situations to try out or practice new behaviors. Safe and appropriate use of this learning and therapeutic technique follows a protocol of explicit steps and the practitioner's role as a "director and facilitator" is delineated. The practitioner leading a role play in a group session clarifies the objectives of role play for group members, describes the roles and tasks of participants who will perform the role play, and the tasks of the audience (other group members). Then he or she prepares role-play participants and coaches individual participants or models skill or behavior through the role play. At the end of the acting, the practitioner facilitates feedback to participants, debriefs the participants, and then integrates learning through discussion related to the role play and the session's goals. Before using role playing, a practitioner *must* learn how to use this technique correctly. Poorly executed role playing can be ineffectual or, worse, cause distress or harm to participants and observers, especially if the level of emotional intensity or demands exceed the emotional integrity or skills of the group members. Resources can be found in the educational and therapy literature and, depending on whether one's use is primarily educational or therapeutic, it is best to refer to material in that domain. Advance training in action techniques is available from sociodrama and psychodrama workshops.

THE MODEL OF HUMAN OCCUPATION AS A FRAME OF REFERENCE

Groups for adolescents based on the **Model of Human Occupation (MOHO)** frame of reference assist adolescents to develop strategies that support the developmental process associated with **occupational identity** and performance skill acquisition. Developing and leading groups based on MOHO begins by exploring the adolescents' **volition** for occupational performance.[18] Given that adolescents' development focuses on self-identity, identifying their values, interests, and **personal causation** is fundamental to therapy and contributes to the development of self-concept and self-esteem. Exploration of volition that occurs in groups engages adolescents in *value clarification* activities, exploring new or affirming current interests and developing mechanisms to realistically evaluate one's own performance to facilitate the development of personal causation. A practitioner may have group members complete *The Volitional Questionnaire*[8] or its pediatric version, *The Pediatric Volitional Questionnaire*[5] as a group activity in cognitively intact adolescents. Understanding the adolescents' goals, volition, and interests enables practitioners to focus intervention that is personally meaningful and will engage adolescents in the group process to achieve their therapeutic goals. Other assessments are *The Occupational Self Assessment,*[4] which is a self-report measure of a teen's values and **perceived efficacy** (**self-efficacy**; how well the adolescent feels he or she accomplishes a given occupation), and *The Interest Checklist,*[13,20,23] which assists adolescents to identify activities that the adolescent may want to explore or develop. These self-report measures and values-clarification exercises can help adolescents understand themselves and stimulate discussions to assist in the setting of individual and group goals.

Adolescents receiving occupational therapy services may experience difficulties structuring their time, developing constructive patterns of behaviors, and engaging in healthy habits and consistent routines. The **habituation** subsystem of MOHO examines whether the adolescent's roles, habits, and routines are functional or dysfunctional (lacking or poorly constructed). Group interventions aimed at improving habituation help adolescents develop routines and explore how current habits support daily activity and environmental demands. Identifying and describing their roles and the expectations associated with those and future roles help adolescents understand the performance skills they have and will need to develop. Irrespective of the reason for referral, occupational therapy intervention with adolescents prepares them to succeed in both current roles and those they will assume as adults. *The Activity Configuration*[26] is an effective tool to help adolescents identify patterns; *The Adolescent Role Assessment*[15] and *The Role Checklist*[27] provide a guide to examining the roles adolescents perform and desire. After the teen completes these tools, a practitioner is likely to discuss which factors support or hinder performance.

The **performance capacity** subsystem directs the practitioner to examine the status of adolescent physical and mental components and his or her related subjective experience.[18] Examining adolescents' physical and mental strengths and deficits provides data about the adolescents' capacity to perform. The practitioner considers each adolescent in the context of his or her environmental influences and its effect on occupational performance. This practice also extends to the group climate of therapy, ensuring that it supports problem solving, skill development, and the integration of the skills of adolescents' occupational performance in naturalistic contexts.

In *Model of Human Occupation: Theory and Application,* Kielhofner and Forsyth[18,19] identify therapeutic strategies (Table 9-2) that are universally accepted as useful when working with adolescents. Occupational therapy practitioners employ these strategies while engaging adolescents in activities in a group context with the goal that they will continue to develop their identity and recognize their competencies.

The following case illustrates a practitioner's clinical reasoning using the MOHO to gather an occupational profile and determine with the adolescent his group interventions.

TABLE 9-2   Strategies for Working with Adolescents in Groups[18]

Structure the therapeutic environment to:	■ Allow adolescents to take risks and experiment safely. ■ Offer ongoing opportunities and resources to identify interests and to support engagement in interests. ■ Challenge skill ability and practice newly acquired skills. ■ Allow adolescents to experience using their physical abilities within meaningful occupational tasks.
Validate:	■ Appropriate thoughts and feelings concerning performance capacities. ■ How difficult it can be to do things and that anxiety is experienced and managed.
Identify:	■ With adolescents their strengths and weaknesses in occupational performance. ■ Resources in the adolescents' social environment to support identified interests. ■ Conflicts between values and performance capacity.
Give feedback:	■ To support a positive reinterpretation of their experience of engaging in an occupation. ■ To shape and promote skill development. ■ Regarding adolescents' values and standards to foster constructive self-evaluation.
Advise adolescents to:	■ Engage in occupational tasks within performance capacity to ensure high degree of success. ■ Seek out environments consistent with occupational goals. ■ Seek social environments that support performance skill development. ■ Avoid social environments that encourage unhealthy habits or deviant roles.
Encourage:	■ Sustained effort until the person is able to complete the occupational task or routine. ■ Adolescents to sustain performance when they are showing signs of fatigue or difficulty.
Physically support:	■ When necessary to ensure success when motor skills are impaired.
Coach:	■ When appropriate to ensure success. ■ Adolescents in role enactment and routine development.
Negotiate with adolescent concerning:	■ Priorities and occupational goals. ■ Values and standards to be applied in therapy. ■ Group norms and rules as a collective agreement.

CASE STUDY

Kevin, a 17-year-old boy and high school senior, is diagnosed with depression. He is admitted to the hospital following a suicide attempt. He and his current group of friends are frequently in trouble with the law and with teachers; they skip school, engage in risky behaviors (e.g., drugs, alcohol, and petty crime). He reports the relationships with his parents have deteriorated over the last 12 months. Kevin has no plans after graduation, has not been sleeping, and broke up with his girlfriend; his grades have dropped significantly. The occupational therapy practitioner sees him for an assessment in the acute psychiatric ward.

The OT practitioner invites Kevin to participate in an assessment group with other recently admitted adolescents and young adults (Figure 9-5). The session's focus is on completing simple projects and exploring interests. In this group, the occupational therapy practitioner will gather an occupational profile and begin assessing his performance capacity. The practitioner encourages Kevin to get dressed and groomed to attend the group sessions in a timely manner. Coaching and negotiating with Kevin, the practitioner encourages him to participate and develop rapport with the other group members. Although he remains quiet and sullen in the first session, the practitioner recognizes his resistance as anxiety about the group and shame about his admission to hospital. She reinforces him when he engages, providing opportunities for him to voice his experience and validates his feelings. In these initial group sessions, the practitioner works with Kevin to identify his values, interests, and personal causation (volitional subsystem). She seeks to understand what his patterns, routines, and roles have been and how these are related to his motivations and desires (volition) and to his ability to engage in occupations (performance capacity), and especially how his depression is affecting his physical and mental status. This information, along with a description of the sociocultural environment, assists the practitioner and Kevin in setting therapy goals and determining which groups he will participate in to meet these goals.

As the group sessions continue, the practitioner discovers that Kevin enjoys physical activity although he is not involved in sports. The practitioner advises the group to plan some physical activities and brainstorm a variety that may be possible. Group members identify hiking, walking, swimming, skateboarding, rock wall climbing, and basketball as possibilities. Other members provide details on community settings near Kevin that offer these activities (Figure 9-6). The practitioner negotiates with Kevin that if he plans an activity, she will arrange for the group to participate, but Kevin must make all the arrangements. Kevin seems to enjoy the control he is afforded by this task. Together, the practitioner and Kevin develop a checklist of what he needs to consider. This organization skill will help Kevin in the future when he wants to engage in a new activity. The practitioner structures the tasks for Kevin so he is successful. She gives him feedback on his organization, group membership, and social participation in the group. The practitioner coaches Kevin on how to approach his peers, teachers, and parents. Because the occupational therapy practitioner has developed a therapeutic relationship with Kevin by empowering him to explore his interests, he listens to her coaching. When Kevin tests the boundaries of the group sessions, the practitioner skillfully redirects him. She continually gives him feedback on how his behaviors are interpreted by others and provides him with opportunities to succeed. Over time, Kevin begins to develop his identity as a physically active adolescent who enjoys being outside. He notices that others find him amusing and good at organizing. He also begins to articulate how some of his choices (e.g., friends who take drugs) are not supporting his future goals. This example illustrates how using the MOHO guides the practitioner through the complexity of working with adolescents in groups.

PSYCHOEDUCATIONAL GROUPS WITH ADOLESCENTS

Psychoeducational groups have become popular in health and education settings because research has demonstrated them to be a highly effective frame of reference.[16,17] In more than 30 studies of psychoeducational groups with adolescents who have been identified as at risk of severe mental illness and their families, research found improvement in adolescents' mental

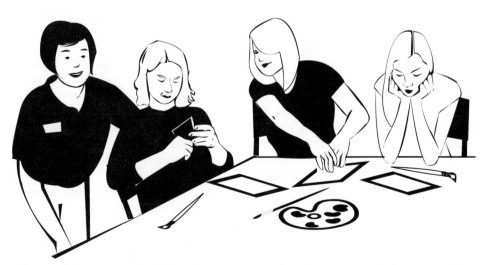

Figure 9-5 Teens may struggle with low self-esteem, anxiety, or depression as they try to develop a sense of self.

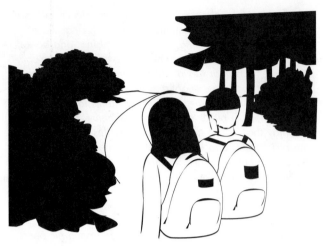

Figure 9-6 Peers and a supportive environment help teens develop a healthy sense of self.

health, fewer relapses, and improvement in family relations and well-being.[23] Therapeutic outcomes included improvement in academic performance, communication skills, problem solving, crisis management, and social relations. Psychoeducational group programs are used to address illness management (e.g., substance abuse, schizophrenia, and other major mental health disorders) to facilitate behavior change, develop social skills, and learn problem-focused coping skills. Using this frame of reference, occupations are acquired and occupational performance skills can be developed through education, experiential learning, and the power of sharing and learning with others who have similar issues, interests, and values.[16,17]

The core premise of this frame of reference is that through knowledge come healing, empowerment, and adaptive skills. The sessions of a psychoeducational group program integrate the developmental stage of the group into the therapeutic process. For example, in the beginning, when the group is at the initial (forming) stage of group development, the group engages in activities that highlight a sense of belonging and similarities among the adolescents to reduce anxiety and build group cohesiveness. Psychoeducational groups, which can have as many as 25 participants, are closed and time-limited, and consist of a set number of structured sessions designed to educate participants and assist them in skill development. In the safety of the group, adolescents learn and apply their new knowledge by practicing skills in life situations. The support of learning and sharing with others who are similar is a powerful component of the psychoeducational group. Janice Delucia-Waack[9] provides a comprehensive text, *Leading Psychoeducational Groups for Children and Adolescents,* for practitioners who wish to implement psychoeducational groups.

A symptom management group is an example of a psychoeducational group program for adolescents with mental illness. This group program integrates the recovery model of **self-determinism, hope, and empowerment** by assisting them to understand their illness and to learn strategies to manage their disorder. This type of psychoeducational program helps adolescents develop skills necessary to live with a psychiatric disorder while reinforcing that illness is not an identity. Box 9-2 presents the format of a psychoeducational group. Note that the

educational component has a primary role in the session and that there is homework to encourage transfer of learning to the adolescents' everyday lives. The components in this session are present in all psychoeducational groups.

STRENGTH-BASED GROUPS—ACTIVITY GROUPS

Research strongly supports the benefits of providing vulnerable adolescents with stimulating and supportive environments.[22] Most groups are designed to capitalize on the performance skills and attributes of the adolescent group members. Capitalizing on the adolescent's ability, activity demands can be adapted to provide the "just-right" challenge. This is particularly important, because most adolescents who enter the mental health, social welfare, or juvenile justice system and even the health system have had too many experiences of failure. The essential strategy of strength-based groups is that the practitioner uses the adolescent's strengths to work on areas of weakness.

Mosey[26] outlined a group activities taxonomy of groups that are designed to assist individuals who share common concerns or problems in relation to the acquisition or maintenance of occupational performance skills, patterns, and participation in occupations. Because labeling groups by the main activity does not convey goals or the process (e.g., cooking group, healthy living, or goal setting), she introduced six categories of activities. They are evaluative, task oriented, developmental, thematic, topical, and instrumental activities (Box 9-3). The categories of groups influence the group goals and outcomes, and the frame of reference used to achieve them. This taxonomy is important when selecting the type of activity group that will use adolescents' strength and meet therapeutic goals from a strong occupational therapy perspective. Box 9-3 provides a brief outline of the principles of each activity group category and its purpose. Activity groups are beneficial for adolescents because most prefer doing something rather than sitting and talking. The taxonomy assists practitioners in matching the adolescents' abilities and needs to the most appropriate activity group. Identity is shaped and affirmed through doing, and performance skills are developed and integrated into habits and routines.

COMMUNITY-BASED SUPPORT GROUPS FOR ADOLESCENTS

Occupational therapy practitioners working with adolescents who have chronic illnesses, physical disabilities, or psychosocial disabilities often initiate peer support groups in the community. Research studies' findings support the value of these groups that address disease management, managing emotional and behavioral issues associated with chronic illness, social support, health promotion, and health prevention.[17] These group programs can take many forms: participation in summer camps that target children with chronic illness, community groups that focus on education and peer-sharing, or social support groups that seek to reduce the isolation some teens experience as a result of their difficulties with social interactions (e.g., adolescents on the autism spectrum or young adults who are developmentally delayed).

BOX 9-2	Examples of an Individual Psychoeducational Group

Psychoeducational Group Program—Managing Symptoms and Maintaining Health
Session 3: Its All about Medication
Title
Let's Talk about Medication

Purpose of Group Session
Educate adolescents about how medications work and help them understand why medication regimens are important to the therapeutic outcome of taking medication.

Goals for Group Session
By the end of the session group members will be able to:
1. Describe how their medication works and name any contraindications.
2. Outline how and when their medication needs to be taken.
3. Identify strategies that assist in taking medication independently as prescribed.
4. Examine individual challenges and feelings to taking medications.

Materials
Medication fact sheet
Weekly medication containers

Introduction
Group leader welcomes members and outlines the agenda for this week's session. He or she introduces the topic of medication and briefly mentions the challenges of taking medication.

Warm-up (5 to 10 minutes)
Name that medication. Divide members into small groups. Using PowerPoint presentations, show common advertisements from TV or magazines for mental health medications and have teams identify as many as they can. This can be made into a competition or have teams take turns calling out the medication. This exercise will energize but also highlight extensive use of psychiatric medications.

Intervention
Group stage of development is considered in planning intervention for psychoeducational groups.

Education Session (30 minutes)
The inclusion of an information session is an essential component of psychoeducational groups.

Topic: Common Medications
Group leader introduces the guest speaker, a psychiatric nurse practitioner, who will provide a 20-minute overview of how common medications work, and their benefits and side effects (e.g. weight gain, dry mouth, photosensitivity). In addition, the nurse will discuss the dangers of discontinuing medication abruptly, the risks of sharing medications with friends, the need to take medications consistently because of the need to maintain a therapeutic level in the bloodstream, and other relevant issues such as the interaction and risks associated with drinking and medication.

Processing: Experiential Learning Component
1. Members are asked to take out their homework (a list of their medications and daily chart of the times they took their medication). In small groups, members discuss their personal experiences of taking medication and groups can develop questions they would like answered. A question-and-answer session will follow with the guest speaker.
2. Members discuss the challenges of taking medication and brainstorm strategies to improve their reliability.

Homework
Each member receives a medication container to organize medications for the week and to keep a daily journal consisting of activities that made them feel happier, relaxed, able to sleep at night, and so on.

Conclusion of Group
Members identify new information they learned about medications today. Leader reviews key points. Tell members next week's session is called *Beyond Medication* and will focus on other strategies for managing symptoms; this is the reason for noting what activities are helpful in managing symptoms and feeling well.

These groups are generally community based, have an ongoing membership, and provide support and social participation with peers. Ideally, the practitioner takes the role of initiating the group, but the members will eventually take responsibility. The practitioner's role then becomes one of mentor to a consumer-driven organization. Alternately, these community-based groups may be offered by other organizations and the practitioner's role is facilitating the transition from group-based interventions to successful participatory peer group activities. The Best Buddies program is an example of this type of community-based group. It is a group program that pairs adolescents with high school peers for friendship and social activities. Other examples of community groups can be found with organizations such as the National Alliance for Mental Illness or the Big Brothers Big Sisters program.

STRATEGIES FOR GROUP INTERVENTIONS FOR ADOLESCENTS

Practitioners who understand the issues of adolescents and apply this knowledge in their choice of groups and use of techniques are better suited to providing effective groups. The group therapy setting is ideal for adolescents; however, it can be difficult for practitioners.[29] In this section, we briefly identify strategies and issues that are specifically relevant for practitioners working with adolescents. Groups involving adolescents follow the same developmental process and have similar group dynamics as those observed in all groups; therefore, the universal strategies and techniques for facilitating groups are employed. Groups of adolescents are unique because they are experiencing the turmoil of significant psychological (cognitive) and social development along with physiologic maturation. Because interaction with and the opinions of peers are valued highly by adolescents and having a sense of acceptance and belonging is important, group climate needs to provide these psychosocial dimensions.

Because groups in therapy are a microcosm of everyday life, the characteristics that are common among adolescents are present in groups. They often assume their usual patterns of behavior and roles in the therapy group. Practitioners need to be aware of and manage these behaviors therapeutically. One characteristic is competition, which can be healthy.[33]

BOX 9-3   Activity Group Taxonomy

Evaluative

- The evaluative activity group is used to assess an adolescent's capacity to function, especially in a group. The practitioner observes while the group members interact and only intervenes when necessary. This type of activity group usually lasts between 45 minutes and 1 hour and has only four to six people. This is an opportunity for occupation-based assessment.

Task Oriented

- Task-oriented activity groups assist adolescents who have the capacity for insight and abstract thinking to become aware of their needs, values, ideas, and feelings, and how these factors influence their action. The overall goal is change through self-awareness or self-understanding.

Developmental

There are five activity groups in the *developmental* category and each is structured around abilities of the member based on the developmental level of their psychosocial capacity.

- *Parallel* groups are designed for the adolescents to work side by side either without or with minimal interacting. The practitioner takes an active, directive leadership role and reinforces positive behavior, makes eye contact, engages in conversation, and ignores inappropriate behavior, while fostering appropriate social behaviors and communication. This is an activity group for adolescents with limited cognitive abilities or social skills, or who are presenting with acute serious mental illness.
- *Project* groups are designed for the practitioner to work with the adolescents on short-term tasks using a directive but somewhat facilitative leader style. The purpose is skill development. These are adolescents who cannot interact in groups for a long period. Activities might include practical instrumental activities of daily living, such as making a meal, playing card games, creating craft activities, or participating in physical exercises.
- *Egocentric* groups are designed to encourage a group of adolescents to function semi-independently of practitioner direction. The practitioner facilitates the activities and interactions or group process as needed. Members are not given immediate assistance, but they are not left in a situation in which members or group process fails. The practitioner may make suggestions, but the group has the responsibility of coming up with ideas and solutions to ensure every activity or project is being done. The process of working together and developing skills is central to this activity group.

- *Cooperative* groups are based on collaborative participation and are used to assist adolescents develop cooperative interaction and social skills. The practitioner has an advisor-participant role.
- *Mature* groups are activity groups in which the adolescents have self-awareness and the group is a setting for them to role-play, experiment, and engage in exploration. The practitioner is a facilitator and sometimes a participant. Adolescents from different backgrounds or with different interests are ideal for mature groups.

Thematic

- Thematic groups assist adolescents gain knowledge, skills, and attitudes necessary for mastery of occupational performance. The goal is to have group members engage independently. Common settings include residential facilities, transitional units, high schools, or community groups. The practitioner has various roles, depending on the skills and abilities of the adolescents in the group. Universally, the role is to be highly supportive and educational. Activities are developed around the theme of the group and the adolescents' interests.

Topical

- Topical groups use activities to develop performance skills to participate in activity outside of group. There are two types of topical groups: anticipatory groups that include discussions about participation in activities, and concurrent groups involving discussion about activities the adolescents are currently involved. An example of the difference between thematic and topical groups is that in a thematic group activities are used to develop work habits and skills, whereas a topical group uses activities to learn how to find a job.

Instrumental

- Instrumental groups are designed to meet health needs or to maintain function. The goal is to allow adolescents to function at the highest level possible. This group is not concerned with the need for change. An example is a daily group that uses current events and news to maintain participants' cognitive function and facilitate social interaction.

The seeking of social status within a group and the presence of a hierarchy resembles the social patterns among adolescents in the community. It can also be unhealthy and result in behaviors such as disruptiveness, clowning around, attention seeking, derision of others (bullying), self-denigration, or behaviors involving self-harm. Adolescents compete for socially desirable positions in the group or the positive attention of the group leader.[33] They may also seek the role of the sickest or the most needy person, or elicit negative attention as the troublemaker.

Adolescents like to be physically active. They seek out physical contact such as touching, pushing, and interacting in a playfully physical manner to express themselves and relieve tension in social settings. This is particularly noticeable among boys. Adolescents also express the tension in a group with increased physical activity and move around or even leave when they become too anxious. A practitioner needs to be responsive to physical cues and therapeutically introduce breaks and activities

to enhance group dynamics and goal attainment while reigning in physical activity that is unruly or counterproductive to the members' goals.

Another characteristic of adolescents that has implications for groups is that they are egocentric. Therefore, a practitioner needs to develop appropriate norms concerning talking. Sometimes this is done through structuring the interactions in groups to developing listening, taking turns, and fostering empathy. Otherwise, it is likely they will focus on themselves, interrupt each other, not listen, and therefore not gain the self-awareness required to self-regulate their behavior or develop a capacity to be supportive to others.

Assisting adolescents' engagement in occupations requires group strategies that provide the adolescent with a sense of control while setting positive limits and boundaries in a firm but gentle manner. Adolescents test boundaries. A skillful practitioner offers adolescents choices and perceived control without relinquishing total control, which is essential to the integrity and safety of the members of the group. This process involves being direct, honest, and upfront with the group members and following through consistently as a way to develop trust.

Setting positive limits and defining boundaries can be key to motivating adolescent performance. Self-regulation of emotions and behavior is difficult for many adolescents who are referred to occupational therapy both because of their age and disorders. Some are impulsive and do not understand the consequences of their actions because they live in the present. Other adolescents are angry, may have been abused, and, rather than trust others, push back and take an offensive stance. Adolescents act out and have outbursts, threaten to leave therapy, criticize therapy as "useless" or a "waste of time," use offensive language, violate other group or organizational rules, or deny their need to be attending the group. Therefore, establishing constructive limits; defining clear, reasonable boundaries; and avoiding getting into a power struggle by going with the resistance are necessary but not always easy to achieve.

◎ Clinical Pearl

When defining a consequence for a rule or action that is either unacceptable or desired, the group leader (practitioner) *must* implement the consequence. Inconsistency compromises relations with adolescents, especially their ability to trust. Furthermore, external limits can generate a sense of safety because the practitioner's word can be relied on and clients remember that external control when they feel "out of control." External limits that are rational, consistent, and understood by the adolescent and used constructively over time assist him or her in developing internal limit-setting and self-regulating behaviors.

PBS uses individualized strategies to support children and adolescents to achieve social behavior change, and is based on **applied behavioral analysis**. The use of these strategies is equally applicable to group and individual interventions, but the strategies are considered especially beneficial when working with children and adolescents who exhibit difficult behaviors.[3] Case-Smith and Arbesman[7] reviewed intervention strategies for children and adolescents with autism syndrome disorders and reported that PBS had moderate to strong positive outcomes, and reduced problem and maladaptive behaviors such as aggression, destruction, disruption, self-injury, and stereotypical behaviors and tantrums. It is also within the guidelines of the Individuals with Disabilities Education Act, which included the concepts of PBS and functional behavioral assessment in the 1997 amendments to the Act.

The premise of PBS is to develop performance skills (often social or self-management and regulation skills) through the systematic redirection of an adolescent's attention away from the behaviors that are not functional and by providing stimuli and reinforcement for desired behaviors. Therefore, the identified problem behavior has few rewards, is less effective and efficient, and is no longer meaningful to the child or adolescent. Concurrently, the desired behaviors that increase their function yield more rewards and become part of their behavioral repertoire. Strategies also include modifying the adolescents' social and physical environment. For example, in the group environment the practitioner works on reducing or removing antecedents (triggers) to problem behaviors and consistently reinforces behaviors that are appropriate or that approximate desired behaviors and relevant skills.[7] The strategies of PBS are consistent with occupational therapy practice guidelines; they are client centered, individualized to each adolescent, and designed to achieve meaningful outcomes.[21]

PBS as a behaviorally based systems approach can be used in groups within school and community environments to enhance learning and social development, and to manage problems such as bullying.[31] The use of PBS in occupational therapy group interventions is most effective when it is embedded in the environment that is also using PBS. Furthermore, the use of both functional analysis and environment modification strategies in PBS is integral to occupational therapy.[7]

Playfulness balanced with the work within group sessions is likely to engage adolescents in the group process and encourage subsequent attendance. The American Occupational Therapy Association's[2] *Tips for Living Life to Its Fullest: Building Play Skills for Healthy Children and Families* stresses the importance of playfulness in practice and provides tips for play from early childhood to adolescence. Play and playfulness are integral to interacting with adolescents at all stages. In play, interests are explored, skills are developed, and social rules are learned while enjoying an activity and taking pleasure in the moment. Play provides relief from stresses and through it adolescents can find flow (the ability to lose one's self) or connectedness with others. Play can involve the use of games, music, screen or computer activities; working on recreational projects in parallel play; or simply hanging out and goofing around with group members. Play is a venue for low-stakes experimentation and risk taking with roles and skills. It can also discharge energy or change the tone of the group.

SUMMARY

This chapter outlines factors that a practitioner considers when working with groups of adolescents. It addresses the types of groups frequently used with this population and discusses the frames of reference a practitioner might used to offer an effective group intervention. Finally, we offer strategies that are specifically relevant to leading groups of adolescents and finish with a simple checklist to reflect on practice (Box 9-4).

| BOX 9-4 | A Practitioner's Reflection on Practice Checklist for Groups with Adolescents |

Were the strategies, structure, and group process therapeutically appropriate for adolescents and their goals?
  Check those that were present or occurred in the group session.
- Opportunities for experimentation and risk taking within the constraints of a safe accepting environment
- Participation of most or all members
- Moments of playfulness, fun, and laughter
- Group climate that provided a sense of belonging and was supportive
- Validation of members ideas, feelings, and constructive actions
- Space for independence and personal choice within normative boundaries
- Environmental stressors that were addressed
- Task demands that were appropriate for performance skills
- Group capitalized on skills attained while providing the "just-right" challenge to promote further skill development

- Peer-based learning
- Exploration of roles
- Inclusion of time to express thoughts and feeling
- Age-related social media used
- Group goals met

Group Leaders
- Were clear about rules and expectations.
- Were consistent about expectations and followed through on their commitments.
- Avoided jargon.
- Avoided getting defensive when challenged.
- Managed behaviors such as distress, anxiety, or acting out behaviors respectfully (going with resistance and avoiding power struggles).
- Acknowledged successes and constructive behaviors.

REVIEW QUESTIONS

1. What are the developmental tasks a practitioner includes in a group of adolescents at the early, middle, and later stages of adolescence?

2. Choose a frame of reference and design a group session for adolescents based on it.

3. What are the components of social skills?

4. What are some frames of reference used with adolescents?

5. Describe strategies that you would use when leading a group of adolescents.

REFERENCES

1. American Occupational Therapy Association: Occupational therapy practice framework: domain and process, *Am J Occup Ther,* 62:625-683.

2. American Occupational Therapy Association: *Tips for living life to its fullest: building play skills for healthy children and families,* 2011. http://www.aota.org/Consumers/consumers/Youth/Play/Play-Skills.aspx.

3. Anderson CM, Freeman KA: Positive behavior support: expanding the application of applied behavior analysis, *Behav Anal* 23:85-94, 2000.

4. Baron K, Kielhofner G, Iyenger A, Goldhammer V, Wolenski J: *The occupational self-assessment (OSA) (Version 2.2.),* Chicago, 2006, Model of Human Occupation Clearinghouse, Department of Occupational Therapy, College of Applied Health Sciences, University of Illinois at Chicago.

5. Basu S, Kafkes A, Geist R, Kielhofner G: *The pediatric volitional questionnaire (PVQ) (Version 2.0),* Chicago, 2002, Model of Human Occupation Clearinghouse, Department of Occupational Therapy, College of Applied Health Sciences, University of Illinois at Chicago.

6. Carrell S: *Group exercises for adolescents,* Thousand Oaks, CA, 2000, Sage.

7. Case-Smith J, Arbesman M: Evidence-based review of interventions for autism used in or of relevance to occupational therapy, *Am J Occup Ther* 62:416-429, 2008, doi:10.5014/ajot.62.4.416.

8. De las Heras CG, Geist R, Kielhofner G, Li Y: *The volitional questionnaire (VQ) (Version 4.0),* Chicago, 2003, Model of Human Occupation Clearinghouse, Department of Occupational Therapy, College of Applied Health Sciences, University of Illinois at Chicago.

9. De Lucia-Waack JL: *Leading psychoeducation groups for children and adolescents,* Thousand Oaks, CA, 2006, Sage.

10. Frederickson N, Turner J: Utilizing the classroom peer group to address children's social needs: an evaluation of the "circle of friends" intervention approach, *J Spec Educ* 36:234-245, 2003.

11. Gunther M, Crandles S: A place called HOPE: group psychotherapy for adolescents of parents with HIV/AIDS, *Child Welfare* 77:251-272, 1998.

12. Hemphill-Pearson BJ: *Assessments in occupational therapy mental health: an integrated approach,* ed 2, Thorofare, NJ, 2008, Slack.

13. Henry AD: *The pediatric interest profiles: surveys of play for children and adolescents, [unpublished manuscript],* Chicago, 2000, Model of Human Occupation Clearinghouse, Department of Occupational Therapy, College of Applied Health Sciences, University of Illinois at Chicago.

14. Hoag MJ, Burlingame GM: Evaluating the effectiveness of child and adolescent group treatment: a meta-analytic review, *J Clin Child Psych* 26:234-246, 1997, doi:10.1207/s15374424jccp2603_2.

15. Huebner RA, Lynnda J, Emery LJ, Shordike A: The adolescent role assessment: psychometric properties and theoretical usefulness, *Am J Occup Ther* 56:202-209, 2002, doi:10.5014/ajot.56.2.202.

16. Jones KD, Robinson EH: Psychoeducational groups: a model for choosing topics and exercises appropriate to group stage, *J Spec Group Work* 25:356-365, 2000, doi:10.1080/01933920008411679.

17. Kibby MY, Tyc VI, Mulhern RK: Effectiveness of psychological intervention for children and adolescents with chronic medical illness: a meta-analysis, *Psych Rev* 18:103-117, 1998.

18. Kielhofner G: *Model of human occupation: theory and application,* ed 4, Philadelphia, 2008, Lippincott, Williams & Wilkins.

19. Kielhofner G, Forsyth, Kirsty: HYPERLINK "http://eresearch.qmu.ac.uk/986/" Therapeutic Strategies for Enabling Clients. In: Model of Human Occupation: Theory and practice, 2008, Lippincott Williams & Wilkins, pp. 185-203. ISBN 9780781769969.

20. Kielhofner G, Neville A: *The modified interest checklist [unpublished manuscript],* Chicago, 1983, Model of Human Occupation Clearinghouse, Department of Occupational Therapy, College of Applied Health Sciences, University of Illinois at Chicago. http://www.uic.edu/depts/moho/

21. Koegel LK, Koegel RL, Dunlap G: *Positive behavioral support: including people with difficult behavior in the community*, Baltimore, 1996, Paul H. Brookes.

22. Makekoff A: *Group work with adolescents: principles and practice*, ed 2, New York, 2004, The Guilford Press.

23. Matsutsuyu J: The interest check list, *Am J Occup Ther* 232:323-328, 1969.

24. McFarlane WR, Dixon L, Lukens E, Lucksted A: Family psychoeducation and schizophrenia: a review of the literature, *J Marital Fam Ther* 29:223-245, 2007, doi:10.1111/j.1752-0606.2003.tb01202.x.

25. McWilliam RA, Tocci L, Harbin GL: Family centered services: service providers discourse and behavior, *Topics Early Child Spec Educ* 18:206-221, 1998.

26. Mosey AC: *Activities therapy*, New York, 1973, Raven Press.

27. Oakley F, Kielhofner G, Barris R: An occupational therapy approach to assessing psychiatric patients' adaptive functioning, *Am J Occup Ther* 39:147-154, 1985.

28. Radizik M, Sherer S, Neinstein LS: Psychosocial development in normal adolescent. In Neinstein LS, editor: *Adolescent health care: a practical guide*, ed 4, Philadelphia, 2002, Lippincott, Williams & Wilkins.

29. Shechtman Z: Group counseling and psychotherapy with children and adolescents: current practice and research. In De Lucia-Waack JL, Gerrity D, Kalonder CR, Riva MT, editors: *Handbook of group counseling and psychotherapy*, Thousand Oaks, CA, 2004, SAGE, pp 429-444.

30. Stein F, Culter SK: *Psychosocial occupational therapy: a holistic approach*, ed 2, Albany, NY, 2002, Delmar Thomson Learning.

31. Sugai G, Horner RH, Child GD, Child MH, Lewis TJ, Lewis TJ, Nelson CM, Scott T, Liaupsin C, Sailor W, Turnbull AP, Turnbull HR III, Wickham D, Wilcox B, Michael Rue M: *Applying positive behavior support and functional behavioral assessments in schools*, San Luis Obispo, CA, 2000, California Polytechnic State University, Retrieved from, http://digitalcommons.calpoly.edu/cgi/view content.cgi?article=1031&context=gse_fac& sei-redir=1#search=%22positive%20behavioral %20analysis%22.

32. Vroman KG: In transition to adulthood: the occupations and performance skills of adolescents. In Case-Smith J, O'Brien J, editors: *Occupational therapy for children*, ed 6, St Louis, 2010, Elsevier, pp 84-107.

33. Wood D: *Group therapy for adolescents: clinical paper*, 2009. Retrieved from, http://www.mental-health-matters.com/index.php? option=com_content&view=article&id=99.

10 Occupational and Group Analysis: Adults

Elizabeth A. Moyer, Jane Clifford O'Brien, Jean W. Solomon

CHAPTER OUTLINE

Developmental Tasks of Adulthood

Designing Groups for Adults

The Planning Process

General Conditions and Populations

Occupational Strengths and Weaknesses

Client Factors and Body Functions

Contexts

Teaching and Learning

Sample Teaching and Learning Activity
    Activity Overview

Task Analysis: Analyzing Occupational Performance*

Context and Environments

Role Playing as a Tool to Practice Group Leadership Skills

Reflection and Self-Evaluation

Summary

KEY TERMS

activity analysis	middle adulthood
client factors	occupational performance
developmental tasks early	analysis
adulthood	occupational therapy practice
late adulthood	framework (OTPF)

CHAPTER OBJECTIVES

1. Describe the developmental tasks of adults.
2. Use the occupational therapy practice framework to analyze activities.
3. Develop group sessions for adults.
4. Develop skills to complete an occupational and task analysis for adult group sessions.
5. Identify teaching and learning strategies for adults.

Occupational therapy (OT) practitioners often work with adults in groups for a wide variety of purposes. Compared with individualized sessions, the group format promotes social participation and encourages self-directed active participation. Members support and serve as role models for each other. This process allows clients to engage in the therapeutic process to reach their individual goals. Groups also provide an opportunity for the practitioner to observe the individual's skills in action (Figure 10-1).

This chapter begins with a description of the developmental tasks of adulthood, followed by an overview of how to design groups for adults who have a variety of physical or psychosocial conditions. Using the **occupational therapy practice framework (OTPF)**[1] as a guide, the chapter provides examples of how to analyze areas of performance, occupations, client factors, and tasks. It describes the group process and outlines teaching techniques to help readers understand the group process when working with adults.

DEVELOPMENTAL TASKS OF ADULTHOOD

Adulthood is generally considered to comprise the ages of 21 to 65 years; clients who are older than 65 years are most commonly referred to as being in *late adulthood* (see Chapter 11). See Table 10-1 for an overview of the developmental tasks of adulthood. The developmental tasks of **early adulthood** include finding one's work, establishing intimacy, and living independently. The tasks of **middle adulthood** involve establishing one's family, being productive in work, and caring for self and others. At this stage, many adults may be raising children and taking care of their own parents, explaining why this stage is often referred to as the "sandwich generation." A recent phenomenon reports that many middle adults have young adult children returning home. **Late adulthood** includes such tasks as contributing to society, reestablishing one's goals, and concern over one's legacy. At this time, adults are productive workers who may be decreasing work time as they near retirement age and considering options. As they age, adults become aware of declining physical performance.

Understanding the developmental tasks of adulthood can help practitioners develop appropriate intervention plans. Practitioners realize that all adults progress through the stages differently and at different rates.[3]

OT practitioners work with adults who have experienced a disruption in occupational performance caused by illness, disease, or trauma related to physical or psychosocial conditions.[3]

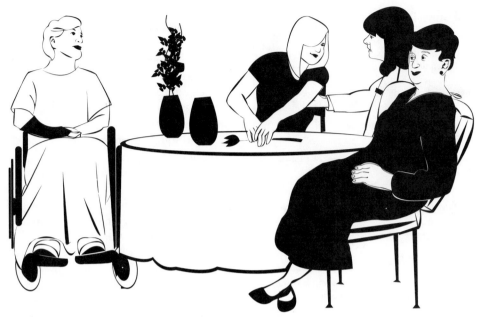

Figure 10-1 Group activities can provide an opportunity for the practitioner to observe the individual's skills in action.

TABLE 10-1 **Developmental Tasks of Adulthood**

	Psychosocial	Psychodynamic	Activities of Daily Living	Adaptive Skills
Early Adulthood	Commits to partnerships, develops relationships, searches for career or job.	Leaves home, establishes independence from parents, assumes responsibility for own development, identifies with other groups.	Completes personal grooming, manages home, selects mate, starts family, rears family (care of others).	Functions independently, able to control drives, practices self-efficacy, participates in intimate relationships.
Middle Adulthood	Guides the next generation, productive, established in career or work	Known as the "sandwich generation," ongoing financial responsibilities, economic independence, establishes a home.	Meets civic and social responsibility, assists teen children to become responsible adults, accepts and adjusts to changes of middle age, adjusts to aging parents.	Functions independently, sustains relationships, participates in a variety of activities.
Older Adult	Accepts one's own life cycle.	Accepts self, deals with loss of friends, examines one's life, manages retirement.	Adjusts to decreasing strength and health, retires; meets social obligations.	Adjusts to loss and establishing self in community, gives back to society.

Adapted from Llorens L: *Application of developmental theory for health and rehabilitation*, Rockville, MD, 1976, American Occupational Therapy Association.

Notably, the onset of many psychosocial conditions occurs in early adulthood requiring occupational therapy intervention. Practitioners may also work with young adults who have sustained a head trauma, spinal cord injury, or physical trauma resulting from high-risk activity (which are prevalent at this age). Additionally, Adults with chronic conditions may require the services of an OT practitioner.

DESIGNING GROUPS FOR ADULTS

Although common in mental health and some geriatric settings, intervention for persons with physical deficits has become almost completely individualized, primarily because of reimbursement systems. However, in 2012, Medicare revised its reporting and billing procedures to recognize group-based interventions in OT. This may lead to more interest in using groups for interventions.

OT practitioners begin designing groups for specific populations by first reviewing individual goals and objectives. This includes understanding the present functional levels and necessary accommodations of all members. Identifying group members based on individual needs and the goals of the group is necessary before designing the group. Once the group goals are identified, the practitioner schedules the group, implements the session, documents outcomes, and evaluates the session. The steps of group design help practitioners develop the necessary skills to lead effective group intervention (Box 10-1).

1. Review individual goals and objectives.

Conducting an **occupational profile** to explore the client's past history, goals, desires, environment, strengths, and weaknesses provides the practitioner with the foundation for intervention planning. Understanding the client's values, interests,

BOX 10-1   Steps of Group Design

1. Review individual goals and objectives.
2. Determine the areas of occupation to be addressed.
3. Identify present functional levels and necessary accommodations.
4. Identify group members based on individual needs and goals of group.
5. Schedule group.
6. Implement group.
7. Document and evaluate session.

TABLE 10-2   Sample Groups Based on Selected Areas of Occupation

Area of Occupation	Sample Group Theme	Session Example
Activity of daily living	Dining In	Feeding group using a variety of adaptive equipment, designed to help clients feed themselves independently.
	Makeover	Grooming using adaptive equipment, compensatory techniques. Members explore grooming techniques and learn how to adapt for physical limitations. (This group may also work with teens to help them develop self-confidence.)
Community Mobility	About Town	Members practice accessing the bus or subway system. They explore community resources.
Education	Back to the Basics	Members learn strategies to help them in school. They design organizational tools and explore their learning styles so they can develop accommodations for success in educational settings.

motivations, and beliefs about their abilities and competence, which Kielhofner[2] terms *volition,* is central to designing occupation-based intervention activities. Determining the client's physical, cognitive, and psychosocial strengths and weaknesses allows the practitioner to develop a whole picture of the client needed to develop goals and objectives (see Chapters 6 and 7). OT practitioners develop goals and objectives that are meaningful to the client and address an area of occupational performance.

2. Determine the areas of occupation to be addressed.

Goals are designed to address areas of occupation. **Areas of occupation** include activities of daily living (ADLs; feeding, dressing, bathing, toileting, grooming), instrumental ADLs (IADLs), work, leisure and play, sleep, community mobility, and education.[1] These areas form the domain of OT. Groups may be focused on specific areas of occupation. See Table 10-2 for sample groups addressing specific areas of occupation.

3. Identify present functional levels and necessary accommodations.

The OT practitioner identifies each client's present level of function and determines possible accommodations that may be necessary for the client to be successful. The practitioner may have to adjust the degree of difficulty to enable the client to succeed. Developing a list of possible accommodations prior to the group activity allows the practitioner greater opportunity for adjusting the activity quickly for clients. Being prepared is key to successful group sessions.

4. Identify group members based on individual needs and the goals of the group.

The practitioner identifies group members who will benefit from the goals of the group. Often practitioners design groups for a variety of clients who have similar goals. This allows the practitioner to engage members in groups that support and move all members toward their goals.

In circumstances in which members have varied goals, the practitioner skillfully moderates how members are progressing toward individual goals. The practitioner adjusts tasks or performance requirements to challenge the client at the right level (not too difficult or not too easy). Identifying group members who will support each other while meeting their own goals requires careful analysis.

5. Schedule group.

Scheduling groups involves determining the optimum duration and meeting time. For example, dining groups are best scheduled during meal times and community group outings may need to be scheduled early in the day to avoid rush-hour traffic and allow clients time to return home. Some groups may have a predetermined number of sessions, whereas others are open ended.

6. Implement group.

Selecting group activities involves thoughtful analysis of clients' performance, the contexts of group, individual goals, group goals, resources, and schedule. Practitioners must consider the strengths and limitations of group members and select a group activity that promotes their participation.

OT practitioners carefully analyze activity to best understand how to modify or adapt tasks for individual clients. Many sample formats exist to analyze activity. The OTPF provides one such format[1] (Table 10-3). Practitioners become skilled at analyzing activity quickly and completely so that each client benefits from group activity. The role of the practitioner is to adjust the activity, method of performing, or client's ability so that each member is successful. Practicing analyzing activity with a variety of clients forms the basis for OT intervention. Understanding how conditions or **client factors** influence participation in a group activity serves to illustrate the complexity of activity.

Grading activities refers to adjusting the activity (making it easier for the client to accomplish or more difficult to challenge clients). For example, requiring a client to button only one button of a shirt is easier than having to button all buttons. The practitioner has graded the activity for success. Requiring the client to button the entire shirt while being timed is an example of grading the activity to make it more challenging. **Adapting** activities refers to changing how the activity is completed by changing the steps (e.g., putting on a shirt with a hook and loop closure instead of buttons). Adapting often involves using equipment to change the activity requirements. Feeding one's

BOX 10-2 Literature Search on Assigned Population

Student: T. Jones *Date:* 10/28/11
Population: Stroke (hemiplegia)
Definition of Client Factors involved: Adult has limited use of right arm and hand.

Characteristics of this population: Characteristics of a stroke will vary with each individual, however there are a few classic signs that have been reported as being universal signals of a stroke: trouble walking or standing; sudden dizziness, confusion, weakness in the legs or be unable to coordinate the movements; muscle weakness; trouble with communication; slurred speech, an inability to express what is happening to them or a complete loss of voice are all characteristics of a stroke; numbness; damage to the nerves of the body can present as a feeling of numbness throughout the extremities. This numbness can prevent the stroke victim from being able to control general movement in the affected areas. In some situations, it can cause the victim to be paralyzed completely on one side of her body.

Visual disturbances, such as blurred or double vision, has been reported by stroke victims. In rare cases, complete loss of vision occurs.

One of the characteristics of a stroke that has been reported by victims is a sudden and severe headache that is not controlled by medication. This type of headache is often referred to as a stabbing sensation that prevents the stroke victim from completing basic tasks. This type of headache may be accompanied by muscle pains around the neck and face, nausea, vomiting as well as an altered state of consciousness.

Read more: http://www.livestrong.com/article/78558-characteristics-stroke/#ixzz21oeaRlWKPatients with stroke were older and more often had hypertension, diabetes, peripheral vascular disease, and atrial fibrillation (Saif et al). The authors found that paresis, speech, and sensory deficits were common among subjects hospitalized with confirmed stroke events. Male subjects were more likely to experience gait disturbances, and blacks were more likely to experience paresis in any location. Subjects with ischemic strokes were more likely to experience paresis, speech, and sensory deficits, while headaches were most common with hemorrhagic stroke events. Our data suggest that the clinical characteristics of stroke may vary for different population groups. (Kassem-Moussa et al).

Characterization of Incident Stroke Signs and Symptoms Findings From the Atherosclerosis Risk in Communities Study
Saif S. Rathore, MPH; Albert R. Hinn, MD; Lawton S. Cooper, MD; Herman A. Tyroler, MD; Wayne D. Rosamond, PhDStroke. 2002; 33: 2718-2721
doi: 10.1161/01.STR.0000035286.87503.31
Am Heart J. 2004 Sep;148(3):439-46.
Incidence and characteristics of stroke during 90-day follow-up in patients stabilized after an acute coronary syndrome.
Kassem-Moussa H, Mahaffey KW, Graffagnino C, Tasissa G, Sila CA, Simes RJ, White HD, Califf RM, Bhapkar MV, Newby LK; SYMPHONY and 2nd SYMPHONY Investigators

Potential occupational limitations faced by members of this population:
Persons who have had a stroke affecting use of the right hand experience difficulty performing tasks that require the use of two hands (e.g., stirring batter, buttering bread, buttoning shirt, grooming). They often experience cognitive processing delays and may take longer to complete tasks.

Grading and adaptations that promote successful participation in group activities:
Adaptations: Use no-slide pad or stabilizer to keep bowl from moving while stirring batter, wear adapted clothing that does not require buttoning.
Gradations: Stir thinner batter, which requires less strength; require less walking around the kitchen; allow client to sit and perform.

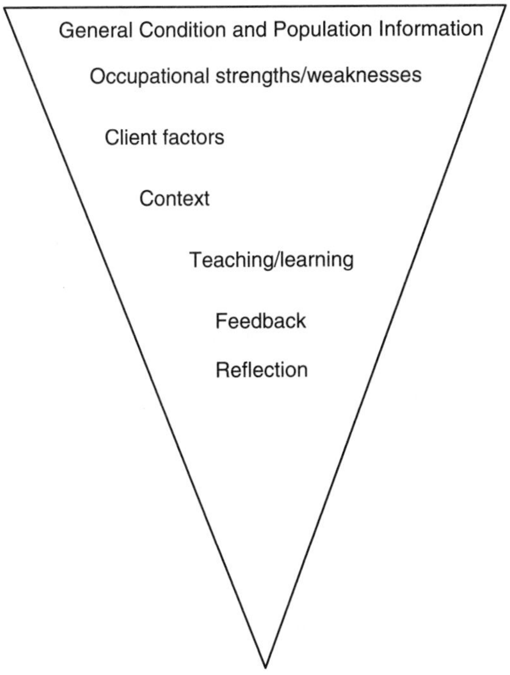

Figure 10-2 Process of group analysis.

(Triangle diagram text, top to bottom:)
General Condition and Population Information
Occupational strengths/weaknesses
Client factors
Context
Teaching/learning
Feedback
Reflection

self using adaptive feeding equipment (e.g., built-up handle spoon) is an example of adapting an activity.

THE PLANNING PROCESS

The planning process is essential for facilitating successful groups and attaining goals.

The process for planning group activities begins with a general analysis of the occupation by understanding the client's occupational strengths and weaknesses. A detailed review of the client factors along with the contexts in which the occupations occur provides additional information to inform the teaching-learning process. Reflecting on the process by evaluating the outcomes and seeking input from members allows the practitioner to plan future groups to promote learning. Figure 10-2 provides a schematic diagram of the process.

GENERAL CONDITION AND POPULATION

OT practitioners begin by understanding the population or condition needs, with particular emphasis on the influence the condition has on occupational performance. Achieving a general understanding of the population through a literature search serves as the foundation for specific intervention activities. Box 10-2 provides an example of the literature search findings of an adult population who has experienced the loss of the use of one hand after a stroke.

OCCUPATIONAL STRENGTHS AND WEAKNESSES

Once the practitioner understands the basic condition and possible occupational performance deficits, he or she can assess the client. The practitioner establishes the client's strengths and weaknesses through an occupational profile, evaluation, assessment, and clinical observations. Often, the practitioner observes the client performing occupations in the actual context. Observations help practitioners analyze the factors that may be interfering with performance. It may be possible to observe the client in a contrived activity to determine client factors to target for intervention.

CLIENT FACTORS AND BODY FUNCTIONS

Once an OT practitioner understands the population in terms of occupational performance, the practitioner examines the client factors and body functions that may require adaptations or modifications to help clients succeed. Analyzing activities at this level enables practitioners to use multiple, carefully designed activities to meet many individual needs. For example, the practitioner may focus on the loss of the use of one hand in the case of the adult population that experienced a stroke. The same activity may be used with clients who are trying to strengthen endurance for activity. Still further analysis of the body function of joint mobility and control of voluntary movement provides the practitioner with important information for intervention planning. Box 10-3 provides an example of a literature review on a client factor. Using research from the literature strengthens the findings to support intervention.

Because activities may target multiple client factors and body functions, identifying the goals and addressing them in intervention becomes paramount to effective intervention. The skilled practitioner remains mindful of the goals for each individual and uses activity to meet these goals. The process is systematic and deliberate, and the practitioner provides the proper amount of feedback, modification, and direction. The practitioner facilitates the motor, cognitive, or psychosocial goals through the planned use of activity. Table 10-3 provides an example of an analysis of client factor and body function from the OTPF.

CONTEXTS

The OTPF[1] identifies contexts as cultural, personal, temporal, physical, virtual, and social. Contexts influence activity and are examined as essential to the intervention process. For example, baking a cake in one's kitchen provides a very different context and social expectations as opposed to baking for a dinner party of 20. The temporal (time) context can show in the differences between participating in community exploration (mobility) activity between a young adolescent versus a retiree. Understanding the influence of context for each client is necessary before leading a group session.

BOX 10-3   Client Factor Analysis

Client Factor: Body function of joint mobility and stability and control of voluntary movement

Definition of Client Factor: Joint mobility: range of motion; joint stability: postural alignment or physiologic stability

Summarize at least two peer-reviewed journal articles about this client factor. Give proper American Psychological Association (APA) reference citations.

The authors examined a chart for motor capacity assessment modified after that of Fugl-Meyer et al. They found that the chart was useful in evaluating bilateral function and providing important information on the functional ability for patients with cerebrovascular disease, especially when the "non-paretic" side was also impaired.

Lindmark B, Hamrin E (1988) Scandinavian Journal of Rehabilitation Medicine, Evaluation of functional capacity after stroke as a basis for active intervention. Presentation of a modified chart for motor capacity assessment and its reliability, 20(3):103-109 (PMID:3187462).

Preliminary findings indicate the functional mobility assessment tool is reliable, thereby increasing the usefulness of this method for clinical assessment for clients who have had stroke, brain injury and spinal cord injury.

Badke MB, Di Fabio RP, Leonard E, Margolis M, Franke T (1993). Reliability of a functional mobility assessment tool with application to neurologically impaired patients: a preliminary report. Physiotherapie Canada, 45(1):15-20(PMID:10124336)

Discuss how limitations in this client factor may affect occupational performance:

Move Limitation up after: Limitations of bilateral motor control requires alternative approaches and adaptations for successful occupational performance.

OT practitioners must also consider in which context or environment the activity will be performed. Table 10-4 provides definitions and examples of each context.

Activities may be associated with cultural beliefs and expectations. The cultural significance of an activity may change the requirements or expectations required from the activity. Some clients may relate culturally to the activity, allowing them to be more invested in the outcome. Clients may have previous emotional reactions to activities that may support or hinder performance. Practitioners consider the cultural context of the activity as they analyze the requirements.

The personal context includes the client's age, gender, socioeconomic status, and educational status.[1] Participation in activities varies according to one's personal context. For example, a young boy views play activities differently than a middle-aged woman. The practitioner must consider this when planning activities for clients.

Temporal contexts refers to the time of the occupational performance in the client's life.[1] A young high school graduate differs in his or her expectations of work experiences than a retired person volunteering to help others.

The *virtual context* refers to using technology to communicate, such as telephone, computers, text messaging, e-mail, blogs, and so on. Practitioners examine how the person will complete the activity. Understanding how communication occurs, the standards of performance, and the skills required to be successful in this context help the practitioner design intervention.

TABLE 10-3 Client Factor Analysis

Name: T. Jones
Activity: Making pancakes
Brief description of activity: The group will make a breakfast, including pancakes, fruit, and coffee and tea.
Please describe how each client factor is used in the activity. (Some items may not apply to the selected activity)

Category	Client Factors	X Used	If Used, Describe Example
	Values, beliefs, spirituality		This activity may not address any values, beliefs or spirituality factors. However, it may be an activity that the client values or associates with values and beliefs. A client may associate making pancakes with family which they value.
Specific mental functions Higher-level cognitive	Judgment	X	Make judgments about the correct mix of ingredients, safety around the hot stove top, timing to flip pancake and remove from burner.
	Problem solving	X	Add more liquid, cook pancake longer, adjust amount to pour into pan.
	Learning	X	Measure and perform math functions: correct number of scoops for coffee (for number of people).
	Generalization	X	Understand that butter, margarine, and cooking oil are equal; realize different types of batter are still pancake batters.
	Cognitive flexibility	X	Understand that the ingredients can be added in any order, use hot water to make tea or coffee, understand different ways to make coffee.
	Metacognition	X	Analyze the results by exploring the steps that were taken and the outcome.
	Attention	X	Selective attention: Focus on the task at hand. Divided attention: Observe safety issues of a hot stove while performing different tasks.
	Memory	X	Procedural memory: Use cooking utensils in the intended manner for cutting, stirring.
	Visual perception	X	Figure ground: Find objects from background (e.g., identify box with pancake batter from other cereal boxes). Spatial relations: Determine distance between objects (e.g., keeping pancakes apart in pan). Depth perception: Identify amount of liquid in measuring cup.
	Position in space—proprioception	X	Be aware of one's position to move around the kitchen and not bump into others.
	Kinesthesia	X	Be aware of one's movement for voluntary movement (knowing that one is moving his or her hand up or down); ability to move around the kitchen.
	Sequencing complex movement	X	Reach, grasp, pour, use kitchen tools; adjust one's grip and modulate strength.
	Emotional expression and regulation	X	Be part of a group, negotiate tasks without becoming upset or frustrated, express desires in group setting, react to situations in a successful way.
Experience of self and time	Self-concept, self-esteem	X	Feel good about one's contribution to team effort, understanding one's strengths or weaknesses, identify how one participated in activity.
	Body image	X	One's reflection of his or her own body and experience, understanding of how one performed.
Global mental functions	Orientation	X	Orient to time, place, and event; know where, when, and what the activity involved.
	Temperament	X	Adjust to activity demands and group dynamics, manage one's self so as not to disrupt the group.
	Energy and drive	X	Participate in the group activity, showing energy and drive to complete tasks; exhibit self-directed behaviors (intrinsic motivation); be able to initiate tasks (e.g., help with clean up without being asked).
Sensory functions	Seeing	X	Identify supplies, materials, distance, shapes through sight.
	Hearing	X	Respond to verbal directions and communication.
	Vestibular	X	Sense changes in body position and movement.
	Taste	X	Identify food preferences (sweet, sour).

Continued

TABLE 10-3   Client Factor Analysis—cont'd

Category	Client Factors	X Used	If Used, Describe Example
	Smell	X	Acknowledge smell of food cooking and kitchen area.
	Touch	X	Discriminate between different objects through touch (e.g., spoon vs. spatula); be aware of features of objects.
	Pain	X	Respond to pain if touching hot stove or hot object.
	Temperature and pressure	X	Identify temperature of food, be able to gauge pressure required to hold objects.
Neuromusculoskeletal	Joint mobility UE	X	Grasp objects, hold and manipulate tools. Must reach for objects in cabinets. 1. Shoulder flexion and abduction ¼ AROM 2. Elbow flexion and extension full AROM 3. Wrist flexion and extension 4. Finger flexion and extension
	Joint mobility LE	X	Exhibit full AROM in LEs for walking, standing, and sitting.
	Joint stability (postural control and alignment)	X	Maintain an upright posture for walking, standing, and manipulating objects; sit with back aligned for feeding.
	Muscle power (primarily UE)	X	Possess adequate strength to walk and stand for 20 minutes.
	Muscle endurance	X	Must be able to maintain posture for 40 minutes, light physical activity for 30 minutes, and moderate activity when stirring for 5 minutes.
	Involuntary movement reactions		Not applicable
Control of voluntary movement	Fine motor control	X	Grasp and manipulate utensils, open packages, hold and stir, bring food to mouth.
	Gross motor control	X	Maintain upright sitting and standing, walk to gather supplies, sit for eating.
	Bilateral integration	X	Hold plate with two hands, stabilize plate with one hand and bring spoon to mouth, hold plate and stir.
	Crossing the midline	X	Reach for cooking materials across midline, pass objects (e.g., tea, fruit) to members.
	Ocular motor control	X	Follow moving objects (people), scan the room, use eye movements to monitor activity.
Body functions	Cardiovascular, hematologic, immunologic, and respiratory system functions	X	Cardiovascular : light physical activity (moderate when stirring), adequate respiratory functions for light activity; immunologic function to allow person to participate in 1 hour of activity around a variety of people.
	Voice and speech function	X	Communicate verbally with others during activity.
	Other functions (e.g., digestion)	X	Eating the food requires digestion.

AROM, Active range of motion; *LE,* lower extremity; *UE,* upper extremity.

Practitioners also consider the physical environment in which the activity occurs. Understanding such factors as the terrain (e.g., hilly or flat, rocky or sandy) and building characteristics, including wheelchair accessibility, helps the practitioner prepare and design intervention.

The social context of activities includes the relationships and expectations for a given activity. Some activities require individuals to act in a prescribed set of standards. Formal social environments differ from casual activities. Understanding the rules, expectations, and relationships helps practitioners prepare clients for activities. For example, consider the differences in social expectations of having lunch with two close friends versus dining at a large formal dinner party.

Context and environment help frame the activities in which people participate. As such, they change the requirements and may support or hinder success. OT practitioners who are able to thoroughly analyze the contextual requirements are better able to address client factors during intervention that will help clients successfully perform in a variety of contexts.

TABLE 10-4 Contexts of Activity

Describe what would be typical for this activity.

Cultural	X	Many cultures view breakfast and eating together as important. Pancakes may be specific to some cultures and evoke feelings.
Personal	X	Men and women of all ages with minimal educational status can complete this task. It is not associated with any socio-economic status.
Temporal	X	Adults typically make breakfast for themselves. Adults may be preparing food for others as part of a care giving role.
Virtual		Directions for making pancakes may be obtained on the internet.
Physical	X	The activity requires minimal strength and 40 minutes of light endurance (except when stirring). This activity is generally easily accomplished and often part of one's routine.
Social	X	Eating together allows members to interact, communicate, and socialize. Making the food together provides a common experience and promotes team work.

*Refer to *Occupational Therapy Practice Framework: Domain and Process*[1] for more details on these categories.

TEACHING AND LEARNING

Before teaching clients in a group, the OT practitioner considers the purpose of the group, as well as how the group activity can allow an individual's intervention goals to be addressed. This content helps inform the developmental level of the group itself. These **developmental levels** as described by Mosey[4] include:

1. Parallel: working side by side on the same or similar tasks without interactions among group members.
2. Project: working side by side on individual project without sharing of materials or supplies, although there may be some social interaction among group members.
3. Egocentric cooperative: sharing materials to complete a group project with members not sharing similar perceptions of process of outcomes.
4. Cooperative: sharing of materials and interactions to complete a shared or group project.
5. Mature: working together to reach goals and objectives.

Mosey believed that most individuals function at two developmental levels during their interactions with groups.[4] Practitioners help clients learn in different ways in groups. Practitioners use a variety of group leader roles to facilitate learning (Box 10-4).

OT practitioners may find themselves using all of the roles. The instructor role is frequently when explaining things to members or to help members learn or complete new tasks. Practitioners using this mode carefully provide clear directions, monitoring the pace adn performance of members. When the group leader assumes a participant role, he or she engages in the group as a member. This allows the leader to understand the group and process along with members. Practitioners must be careful to not devulge too much personal information when acting as a participant leader as this may take away from the clients' experience. The participant leader also remembers that the goal of the group is to address members' goals.

The chairperson role requires the leader remain neutral and not express opinions, but keep track of procedures and process. In this role, the leader presents material and allows members to work things out while assuring the group to follow necessary steps.

An OT practitioner may lead by acting as a consultant. In this role, the OT helps members when needed, and provides

BOX 10-4 Roles of the Group Leader[6]

Instructor	Talks at the group, informs them of what to do.
Participant	Acts as another member of the group and a resource to members.
Chairperson	Remains neutral and doesn't express opinions, but keeps group in order; keeps track of procedures.
Consultant	Helps when needed, provides insight as requested.
Facilitator	Stimulates members to keep moving and addressing goals, uses questioning or challenging techniques.

insight or advice as requested. When working as a consultant, the leader allows the group to make mistakes.

When facilitating, the practitioner pays attention to each member's goals and helps them address their goals in the session. Facilitators may use questioning or challenging techniques to help members progess. The facilitator role is the most commonly used role and it allows the practitioner to help clients meet their goals by challenging them physically or cognitively.

SAMPLE TEACHING AND LEARNING ACTIVITY

Cooking groups are common intervention groups for adults in many settings. The ability to prepare food safely is an important IADL addressed in OT (Figure 10-3). The practitioner can teach directly, such as to instruct low-functioning clients to cook from a picture cookbook, or indirectly, as illustrated when higher functioning group members rotate who plans and supervises each cooking session. The OT practitioner and clients may also problem solve together how to carry out familiar cooking tasks with new strategies and adapted equipment necessitated by the loss of body structure or function. The practitioner leading the group determines the amount of structure necessary to meet the goals.

A more recent use of groups stems from the motor control and motor learning theory, which requires frequent practice with variation for learning or retaining a skill. This has led to the use of stations; individuals in a group move from station to station to practice physical, cognitive, or perceptual skills (Figure 10-4).

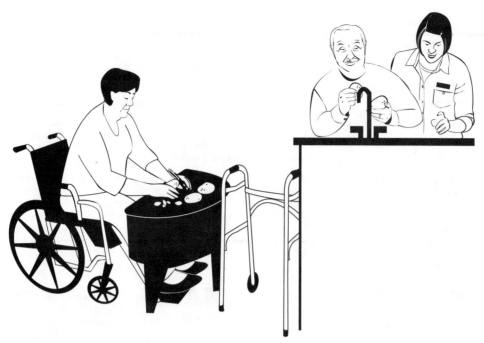

Figure 10-3 Cooking groups are common intervention groups for adults in many settings. The ability to prepare food safely is an important instrumental activity of daily living addressed in occupational therapy.

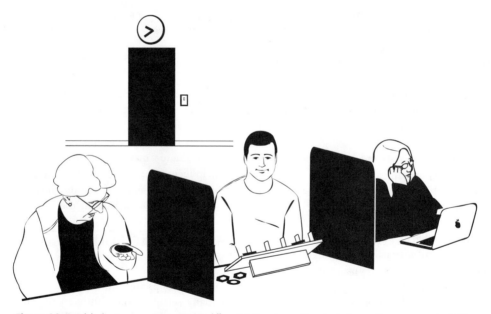

Figure 10-4 Adult clients may enjoy moving to different stations to practice physical, cognitive, or perceptual skills.

This approach, which is similar to the way people participate in fitness activities in a gym, emphasizes responsibility and self-reliance for the client. Consequently, this approach promotes independence and deemphasizes the traditional passive role of clients in therapy settings. Moyer has used this group approach successfully with community-dwelling persons with Parkinson's disease to work on motor, ADL, and perceptual skills.[5]

Practice designing and implementing activity helps practitioners understand the complexity of activity and prepare for group sessions. Allowing practitioners to preplan and gain experience in group structure and design helps them develop skills necessary for working with clients who are experiencing occupational performance deficits. The activity analysis based on the OTPF[1] provides a structure for designing a teaching and learning group activity (Box 10-5).

TASK ANALYSIS: ANALYZING OCCUPATIONAL PERFORMANCE

The activity analysis helps the practitioner prepare and make important decisions about possible group sessions. Practitioners critically analyze occupational performance to address client factors by detailing the requirements for the specific actions, skills, and movements. This process allows practitioners to become

BOX 10-5 Activity Analysis

Brief description of the activity: The group will make pancakes and serve a light breakfast of pancakes, fruit, and orange juice. They will have to gather all ingredients and supplies, mix ingredients, pour and cook pancakes, and flip them over. They will eat together (total time, 45 minutes).

After completing this activity successfully, the participants will have accomplished the following goals or objectives:

Cooperative cooking group: Group will communicate and collaborate to successfully prepare a simple meal.

1. Members will use both upper extremities to reach for and carry objects to the table.
2. Members will move around the kitchen.
3. *Tools and equipment (nonexpendable), cost, and source:* bowls, whisk, spoon, pan, spatula, fork, knife, oven mitt
4. *Materials and supplies (expendable), cost, and source:* Pancake batter, cooking oil, eggs, butter and syrup, orange juice, fruit
5. *Space and environmental requirements (room needed, chair and table set up):* Fully equipped kitchen (oven, refrigerator, water), table, and chair
6. *Sequence and time required for each step in the activity:*

- Introduce activity: 1 minute
- Members decide on tasks: 2 minutes
- Gather ingredients, tools, and equipment: 3 minutes
- Measure ingredients, mix: 5 minutes
- Heat greased pan
- In small groups, but at the same time, members will (15 minutes):
  - Pour pancakes onto pan
  - Cook and flip pancakes
  - Set table—butter, syrup, silverware, napkins, plates
  - Pour orange juice into cups
  - Wash fruit and place on table
  - Place pancakes on plate
  - Repeat until enough pancakes for all
- Eat and enjoy: 10 minutes
- Clean up and wrap up: 5 minutes

7. *Precautions (sharps, toxins, etc.):* Hot pan and stove will be on; knives will be sharp
8. *Special considerations (age appropriateness, educational requirements, cultural relevance, gender identification, other):* None
9. *Criteria for successful completion:*
   The group will make edible pancakes for each person. Members will all contribute to the process. All members will use both upper extremities and move around the kitchen during the activity. Members will state that the pancakes are tasty.
10. *Identify special population considerations for this activity. Indicate if the activity would be inappropriate or if the activity would need to be modified for successful participation. Describe these modifications in detail for each of the following populations:*
    a. *Visual deficits (low vision, visual field loss):* Members may require large-print directions, tactile cues, contrasting plates or place mats on the table.
    b. *Motor control deficits (apraxia, dyspraxia, neuromuscular or skeletal issues):* Members may need weighted utensils, larger bowls (requiring less accuracy), longer time to complete steps, adapted equipment (e.g., nonslip pad, built-up handle utensils).
    c. *Mental functions:* Members may benefit from one-step verbal directions, partnering with one other group member, and close supervision around safety (hot stove top).
    d. *Sensory functions:* Members may not like tactile sensations of the pancake or taste. Members may experience tactile avoidance or oversensitivity and require that members not stand too close. Members may show aversions to smell.
11. *In what area of occupation is the activity?*
    Instrumental activity of daily living—cooking group.
12. *What developmental level is this group (Mosey[4])?*
    Egocentric cooperative—Each member will complete an individual task that will lead to a common outcome.

---

skillful at quickly evaluating the challenges to occupational performance. Sometimes making simple adaptations or modifications enables clients to be successful. This process may become automatic for experienced clinicians; yet, the process of exploring activity by analyzing each task is an essential feature of OT practice.

Table 10-3 serves as a guideline to systematically analyze the client factors involved in occupational performance.

ROLE PLAYING AS A TOOL TO PRACTICE GROUP LEADERSHIP SKILLS

OT students and practitioners benefit from practicing leading groups. Role playing can help facilitate this. The following assignment provides an example of how to use role playing to teach group leadership skills. The leader picks a client factor to address in the session and he or she develops a group goal. Leaders develop a 20-minute group activity, prepare the activity, and conduct an activity analysis. They introduce the activity and lead the session. The leaders are required to articulate the goals and facilitate members' participation in the group session as if they were in a clinic session See Box 10-6.

Class members role play specific conditions to help the leaders learn to "think on their feet" and simulate how to adapt, modify, or change activities according to the clients' needs. To simulate a variety of clients, student members role play a different condition or population. The group leader may select an assistant if necessary. The assistant can serve as an intern, volunteer, or certified OT assistant, depending on the specific needs of the client. The assistant helps the client during the activity, but does not lead the activity (e.g., the assistant may need to read instructions to a client who is unable to read or who has low vision). The leader may also enlist the help of a student observer if more help is needed. The leader concludes the group and engages members in clean up, adhering to the time constraints. This requires that the leader be prepared and structure the session as one may have to do in a clinical setting (Table 10-5).

At the conclusion of the role play, the entire group discusses what went well and what could have been better. The leaders reflect on the experience.

REFLECTION AND SELF-EVALUATION

Group leaders learn through careful reflection. Students and practitioners benefit from evaluating group performance. Even well-planned activities sometimes go less well than expected. The process of reflecting on and evaluating one's own performance

Box 10-6   Feedback on Role Play

Name of Group Leader:
Goal of Session:
Your role in group: Participant/Observer
Provide feedback on the following items (Be specific and provide examples):
a. Content/interest of the activity
b. Organization of the environment and materials
c. Delivery and therapeutic use of self
d. Temporal awareness
e. Ability to control the group
f. Ability to modify activity to meet individual needs
g. Ability to answer questions
h. Eye contact with participants
i. Materials and organization/preparation
j. Visual Aid

TABLE 10-5   Grading Rubric for Teaching and Learning Activity

2 = excellent; 1 = okay; 0 = poor

Preparation: Enough materials, organized	2	1	0
Structure of group: Interesting introduction, clear sequence of steps, nice conclusion	2	1	0
Creativity: Interesting, creative, met goals, novel, appropriate levels of difficulty and interest	2	1	0
Therapeutic use of self: Voice, humor, speaking skills, professional, engaging, answered questions	2	1	0
Conclusion: Facilitated clean up and conclusion, met time limit	2	1	0
Materials: Written materials professional, neat, and clear; activity materials suitable for project or activity	2	1	0
Comments:			
Total points:			

Box 10-7   Self-Evaluation of Group Experience

Leader's Name:
1. How well prepared were you?
   a. Were there enough supplies, materials?
   b. Did you feel organized and knowledgeable?
2. How well did you provide directions to the group?
   a. Were you respectful towards members?
   b. Did you clearly describe the steps?
   c. Were written directions or a sample provided?
3. Was the activity interesting?
   a. Was the goal of the group clear?
   b. Did you meet the goal?
4. Overall impression of the group:
5. How did you do at grading and adapting the activity for the different populations?
   a. Was there anybody that was more difficult in the group?
   b. What would do differently?
6. Suggestions for improvement for next time:
7. Summarize your strengths and weaknesses:
8. Idea

and the group members' performance can lead to changes that benefit the next session. For example, the leader may realize that the directions were too complicated even though he or she simplified them. The activity may take too long or clients may want more time to discuss the products. Much is learned during the evaluation and feedback phase of group activity. Gathering data from others and one's self is beneficial See Box 10-7.

SUMMARY

Each group has a different composition of clients, and therefore each group responds differently to activity. As practitioners and students practice leading a variety of groups, skills at organization, timing, teaching, and leading improve. Leaders establish clear and realistic expectations of the group, producing better outcomes. A well-designed group is interesting and rewarding for participants and helps them reach their goals. This chapter provides an outline of how to analyze and design groups for adults.

REVIEW QUESTIONS

1. What are some developmental tasks of early, middle, and older adulthood?
2. What are some client factors observed during occupational performance?
3. What are the contexts for activity?
4. What are the cognitive, motor, and psychosocial factors involved in group activity?
5. What are the developmental groups as defined by Mosey[4]?
6. What does an OT practitioner consider when developing and implementing groups with adults?

REFERENCES

1. American Occupational Therapy Association: Occupational therapy practice framework: domain and process, ed 2, *Am J Occup Ther* 62:625-683, 2008.
2. Kielhofner G: *Model of human occupation: theory and application*, ed 4, Baltimore, MD, 2008, Lippincott, Williams & Wilkins.
3. Llorens LA: *Application of a developmental theory for health and rehabilitation*, Rockville, MD, 1976, American Occupational Therapy Association.
4. Mosey AC: Legitimate tools of occupational therapy. In Mosey A, editor: *Occupational therapy: configuration of a profession*, New York, 1981, Raven, pp 89-118.
5. Moyer E: *The effectiveness of occupational therapy intervention for persons with Parkinson's disease [unpublished manuscript]*, Portland, ME, 2008, University of New England.
6. Trowbridge R: *Teaching and learning in small groups: Part one. Lecture notes from MMEL 620*, Portland, ME, 2011, Department of Medical Education, Maine Medical Center, University of New England.

Analyzing the Effect of Aging on Occupations with an Emphasis on Cognition and Perception

Regula H. Robnett

KEY TERMS

adaptation	senescent changes
conductive hearing loss	sensorineural hearing loss
endurance	sensory changes
global mental functions	agnosia
locus of control	anosmia
memory	categorical fluency
perception	episodic memory
postural control	fluid intelligence
praxis	procedural memory
presbycusis	prospective memory
presbyopia	quality of life
resiliency	semantic memory

CHAPTER OBJECTIVES

1. Identify common aging stereotypes.
2. Describe the changes associated with aging.
3. Describe the effect of age-related changes on occupational performance.
4. Hypothesize factors contributing to fall risk.
5. Analyze cognitive and perceptual abilities in activity.
6. Differentiate between activity-, client-, cognition-, perception-, and sensation-focused activity analyses.
7. Explain grading and adapting activities for older adults.
8. Develop activities for older adults.

This chapter on working with older people provides learning opportunities interspersed throughout to promote the learner's occupation-based critical thinking and clinical reasoning. Readers may want to reference the occupational therapy practice framework (OTPF),[4] which facilitates understanding of the chapter contents and assists readers in transforming the OTPF into clinical and community practice.

AGING AND FUNCTIONAL PERFORMANCE

Life and change are invariably linked. However, the tendency is to believe that all early change in life is good (e.g., growth, development, and maturity) and all late change in life is bad (e.g., decay, decline, and ultimate death). This chapter explores some of the changes in late life related to occupational performance, specifically in the realm of cognition and perception. Although the stereotypes point to inevitable bad news, the reality is not so dire.

Levels of specific client factors change throughout life based on genetics, context, lifestyle, and various other reasons. The first exercise in thinking about aging involves brainstorming. Look over the client factors of the OTPF[4] (pp 634-637) and think about how we anticipate or expect that these will change as one heads into old age. For this exercise, think about how society or the general population would predict change (e.g., aging stereotypes). Do this before reading the rest of the chapter (Table 11-1).

Most readers find that the list is composed of more negative changes and traits than positive changes and traits. People anticipate more problems as they age (e.g., increased forgetfulness, decreased endurance). Occupational examples (right column of Table 11-1) are important to consider because they focus on the stereotypes of aging, many of which are only partially true; some are patently false. There are no right or wrong answers, because expectations are based on cultural norms and ideas that become ingrained over time. Levy,[31] who studied the stereotypes of aging extensively, found negative stereotypes about aging among children as young as preschool age, who

TABLE 11-1 Aging Stereotypes—Anticipated Changes

Client Factor (or Subfactor, Other Function, Trait, or Skill) Examples	Occupational Example of What is Anticipated
Decreased short-term memory	Person forgets to take medications.
Slower movements	Person walks slowly and needs more time to do things.
Poor balance	Person falls more often.
Hard of hearing	Person has trouble hearing what is said.
Cognitive decline	Person gets confused easily.
Sensory changes	Person gets cold more easily or puts the heat up higher.

already describe older people as more helpless and less capable of taking care of themselves. By the time people reach old age, these perceptions are often internalized and are even more negative than ever.

Using the list and the OTPF, brainstorm adjectives or traits that we tend to attribute to older people in this country. For example, a commonly mentioned trait is being hard of hearing (HOH). Feel free to go beyond the realm of political correctness. What is important is to list what our society tends to think about aging. (We will correct the misconceptions and stereotypes later. The first step is awareness, so list anything that comes to mind.) Complete the list before reading further.

Now you have a list of many traits, many of which are likely to be less than flattering, and most are based on what you may have learned to expect as you age. Consider which of these traits are caused entirely by the passage of time. For any change to be considered a **senescent change** (caused solely by aging) it must fulfill the following criteria. The trait must be:

- Developmental
- Intrinsic
- Progressive
- Irreversible
- Occur universally (at some point in time if people live long enough, it would happen to everyone)

Look at the list to determine if they really are caused by aging (i.e., meet the criteria for senescence) or if possibly they could be caused by other factors. Are the traits based on fact or stereotypical expectations? A few key examples are provided, but readers can ask crucial questions and analyze the rest of the list on their own.

- **Hard of hearing**

Becoming HOH is an expected fate for older people, but surprisingly, many older people do not have hearing loss to the point that it interferes with daily functioning. Nonetheless, changes definitely do occur in the ear and within the aural system, which can rob an older person of the precise hearing of youth. The changes associated with hearing loss are described in detail later in the chapter. At this point, take a moment to

consider what else besides aging could cause decreased hearing? (There are at least three reasons, which will be revealed later in the chapter.)

- **Gray or white hair**

Loss of pigmentation of the hair shafts is common, but not all people lose their hair coloration as they age. For many, dying and bleaching the hair hide the true color, so although loss of luster or rich color may be associated with age, even this common age-related trait is genetic.

- **Poor memory**

Memory is a construct that has many facets. *Short-term memory* refers to what one can remember for just a few seconds or minutes. Several other causes beside old age can affect memory performance, either temporarily or permanently, in both younger and older people. Think about what factors might cause poor memory performance.

- **Muscle weakness**

It is generally expected that people will become weaker over adult life. Studies demonstrate that this is a valid expectation. However, this expectation is based on a lack of strength training. Doing nothing, or not regularly using one's muscles, can easily result in a significant loss of muscular ability. Age can exacerbate the situation because of the increased prevalence of disease that occurs as one gets older. Again, many reasons beside chronologic age can cause muscle weakness.

SENESCENT CHANGES

As people age, changes that influence functional and occupational performance tend to occur. Some of these changes are truly senescent, or unavoidable; others are due to various factors often related to lifestyle. This chapter explores these changes, starting with a brief review of sensory and physical changes, and later examining cognitive and perceptual changes in more depth.

Sensory Changes

Several **sensory changes** occur as people age. Vision is affected early in life, beginning in one's 20s, and this sensory change is one that is considered to be senescent (or caused by aging). Predictable changes occur in the structures of the eye, including the cornea and the lens, both of which are important for focusing images on the retina at the back of the eye. The cornea becomes thicker and less transparent, and the lens also becomes more opaque and less elastic, resulting in difficulty accommodating to new visual stimuli. Already in middle age the majority of people have the condition of **presbyopia**, or farsightedness, resulting in the need for reading glasses to compensate for these structural changes. The *iris*, or colored portion of the eye, which regulates the amount of light entering the eye by dilating and constricting as needed, contains a set of muscles that atrophy over time, resulting in more constricted pupils, which then require additional lighting to focus on visual stimuli. In addition, the structures in the retina—cones associated with fine, close, and color vision and rods associated with vision in dim circumstances—also undergo gradual cell death.[44] Therefore, it is little wonder that older people have poorer night vision as well as poorer close vision. However, under normal circumstances, corrective lenses can bring visual acuity up to a level such that impaired sight will not interfere with day-to-day tasks, even for those in their 80s and beyond.[45] Generally speaking, occupational therapy practitioners can assist people who have low vision by increasing the size of stimuli, increasing the contrast between the visual stimuli and the environment, and by improving the lighting (brighter task lighting and less glare).

Beyond the normal, presbyopic visual changes, abnormal or disease-related visual impairments are more common in older people as well. The primary diseases of the eye that occur as people get older are:

■ Macular degeneration, which particularly impairs central vision
■ Glaucoma, which affects peripheral vision
■ Cataracts, which decrease visual acuity
■ Diabetic retinopathy, which is associated with spotty and fluctuating vision

Intervention on the part of the occupational therapy practitioner requires an assessment of the effect of decreased vision on function. The general principles of better lighting, higher contrast, and larger size tend to fit for these conditions as well. Total blindness, which occurs in approximately 10% of those who are visually impaired,[13] obviously requires different tactics, including using other sensory systems to compensate, organizing the environment, setting up routines not dependent on intact vision, educating the client and his or her family, and referrals to vision specialists (Figure 11-1).

Presbycusis is defined as an age-related decrease in the sense of hearing. There are two types of hearing loss: conductive and sensorineural. **Conductive hearing loss** is easier to manage because it involves problems with the outer or middle ear; examples include a buildup of cerumen (ear wax) or the ears becoming stopped up because of an upper respiratory infection. **Sensorineural hearing loss** is more permanent and more difficult to compensate for or to correct. It involves damage to or death (apoptosis) of the hair cells (cilia) in the inner ear. This hair cell loss also is associated with a higher prevalence of vertigo as people get older, with 18.4% of those 85 and older reporting bouts of dizziness.[41] The density of hair cells in the inner ear decreases as people age, and these sensitive sensory cells can also be damaged by loud noise, especially, but not exclusively, of extended duration.[17] Occupational therapy practitioners can work with people who have hearing loss to help them compensate for and adapt to the environment for improved ability to understand the spoken word. For example, older people have more difficulty tuning out background noise and hearing consonants, and men especially tend to lose the ability to hear higher-pitched voices.[44] To improve an older person's ability to understand, speaking directly to the person in a lower pitched (though not necessarily louder) voice can be helpful, along with ensuring that the environment in which conversations take place is not overly distracting. For example, it will be more difficult to enjoy dinner conversation with an older person in a noisy restaurant. Hearing aids are only useful if they are worn and

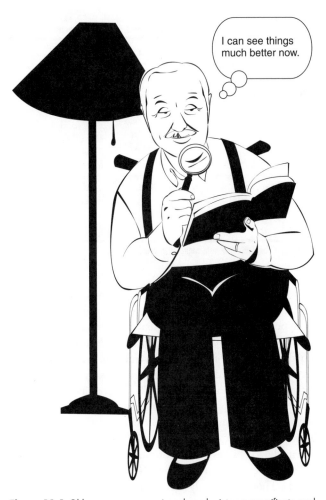

Figure 11-1 Older persons may require enlarged print or a magnifier to read.

working, which is perhaps an obvious detail, but one that is often ignored in day-to-day life.

In old age people often develop **hyposmia**, which is a decrease in sense of smell, or **anosmia**, which is the absence of olfactory or smell sensation. Older people are less sensitive to odors in general, and men are more significantly affected than women. Different odors are differentially affected by age. For example, sensitivity to banana or rose scents is more likely to be maintained, whereas sensitivity to vanilla or musky odors is more likely to decrease from decade to decade.[42] The loss of smell sensation is generally insidious, and quite often older people are not aware of the loss. Nordin, Monsch, and Murphy[38] found that 77% of the older people who were found to have significant olfactory sensory losses, but otherwise had no disease, reported that their sense of smell was normal. Beside age itself, disease states, medications and drugs, airway obstruction, and environmental pollutants can all affect one's sense of smell. Hyposmia and anosmia can have a negative effect on independent living skills, and this loss may need adaptations to be appropriately managed. Table 11-2 allows the reader to spend time thinking about the effect of decreased olfactory sense. This table could be replicated for any of the senses and is provided as just one example.

TABLE 11-2	Olfaction and its Effect on Performance	
Area of Occupation: Specific Activity	Give an Example of How Anosmia or Hyposmia Can Affect This Activity	How Can Occupational Therapy Help?
ADL: Eating	Unable to notice foods that have spoiled.	Provide ways to date food, look for signs that it is bad. Provide labels for food.
IADL: Safety and emergency maintenance	Unable to smell fire or noxious gas.	Provide fire alarms and gas alarms. Ensure proper ventilation of rooms.

ADL, Activity of daily living; *IADL,* instrumental activity of daily living.

Taste is closely related to the sense of smell. Not only does the number of taste buds decrease significantly over time, but the types of taste buds are differentially affected over time as well. The ability to detect salty and bitter decreases more rapidly than the ability to detect sweet and sour.[42] Therefore, older people tend to need higher thresholds of salty flavor to taste the saltiness, but their taste buds for sweet flavors are better maintained. This pattern of change with aging is one reason why older people may tend to over-salt their food and rely too heavily on sweets.

Finally, somesthesis (sense of touch), proprioception (sense of body in space), and kinesthesia (sense of movement of the body) are not significantly affected by aging per se. The number of corpuscles (e.g., pacinian and Meissner for pressure and light touch, respectively) does decrease, but overall touch sensitivity remains intact throughout typical aging. However, a significant portion of older people may lose sensory functioning in this realm. Acquired brain injury or cerebrovascular accidents (sustained by 795,000 people in the United States per year, three fourths of whom are 65 or older[27]) are often associated with decreased sensation, including discriminative touch, proprioception, and kinesthesia.[29] This is not normal aging, but a common problem found among those who are older. Even a slight decline in proprioception and vestibular sense (along with muscle weakness and other potential risk factors) can lead to increased risk of falls.

Pain is also associated with sensory functioning. It plays a valuable role in protecting the body from harm, but it can also be a nuisance and can significantly interfere with daily functioning. Some have contended that increased pain is just a part of the normal aging process, but others do not agree. Farrell[19] reported that, although studies have found a slightly decreasing mean for pain threshold over time, they also have found more heterogeneity among the older population, resulting in some 90-year-olds, for instance, having the same threshold for pain as typical 30-year-olds. One cannot assume that older people feel less (or more) pain than any other age group. The assessment of pain (using a 1 to 10 or a smiley face–sad face continuum) can be a valuable addition to occupational therapy intervention (Figure 11-2).

PHYSICAL CHANGES

Physical changes occur with age; some are chronologic, whereas others are due to extrinsic factors. The changes discussed in this chapter include range of motion (ROM), strength, endurance, and coordination. ROM, or how far each joint moves through space, does decrease slightly (mean range) as people get older, but when aging is typical, the older person's ROM remains within functional limits, meaning that the joint range is adequate to complete the tasks one needs to complete. Strength is related to ROM. Those who have good strength (4 or 5 out of 5) generally have full ROM, unless there is a joint problem, such as an obstruction. We need adequate strength to do our activities of daily living (ADLs) and instrumental activities of daily living (IADLs). Depending on the demands of the tasks, the amount of ROM and strength required can vary. For example, shoveling snow requires very good strength, whereas typing on a keyboard requires very little. Box 11-1 challenges readers to think of reasons why, other than old age, ROM or strength might be below what is considered normal (Figure 11-3).

Arthritis, perhaps the most common cause of joint problems, including decreased ROM and muscle strength, is likely near the top of the list. The Centers for Disease Control and Prevention estimate that approximately 50 million adults in the United States (or 22% of the adult population) report that they have diagnosed arthritis, and 21 million (9% of adults) report that they have arthritis to the level that it impedes their functional performance.[16]

Sarcopenia is the loss of strength in skeletal muscle as one ages, starting in middle age.[28] Using a large-scale national sample, Janssen, Heymsfeld, and Ross[28] found the majority of people older than 60 (52% of men and 69% of women) have a strength level at least one standard deviation below the average of those aged 18 to 39. Those who had losses in the range of more than two standard deviations below the mean of the younger group were more likely to have functional limitations affecting daily functioning (odds ratios twice as great for men and three times as great for women).

Disease states such as cerebrovascular accidents (which are more common in old age) can rob limbs, usually those contralateral to the lesion, of strength completely. However, generally strength is measured on a continuum, and in typical aging (with no disease states) weak muscles are amenable to strengthening through exercise programs or functional activities. In occupational therapy, the preferred method of strengthening is to use occupational engagement in tasks that challenge the current level of strength.

Endurance is the ability to sustain engagement in an activity that involves physical strength. Someone may be very strong but have limited endurance, or have good endurance for tasks that require only limited strength. Generally those with good endurance also have a functional level of strength. Not only is endurance less affected by age than strength, but a meta-analysis of 13 exercise training programs of 30 weeks or longer in duration demonstrated that aerobic exercise can improve endurance as well as strength and range of motion.[24]

Pain Intensity Scales

Simple descriptive pain intensity scale*

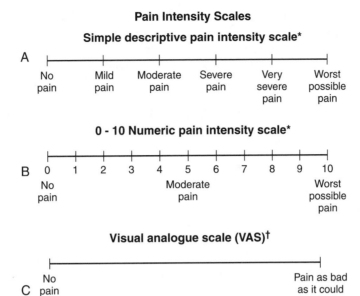

A

| No pain | Mild pain | Moderate pain | Severe pain | Very severe pain | Worst possible pain |

0 - 10 Numeric pain intensity scale*

B 0 1 2 3 4 5 6 7 8 9 10

No pain   Moderate pain   Worst possible pain

Visual analogue scale (VAS)†

C No pain   Pain as bad as it could possibly be

* If used as a graphic rating scale, a 10-cm baseline is recommended.
† A 10-cm baseline is recommended for VAS scales.

Which face shows how much hurt you have now?

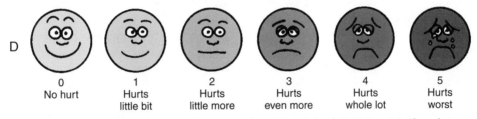

D

| 0 No hurt | 1 Hurts little bit | 2 Hurts little more | 3 Hurts even more | 4 Hurts whole lot | 5 Hurts worst |

Figure 11-2 (A-D) Pain scale provides a valid assessment of pain. (From Rothrock JC, McEwen DR: *Alexander's care of the patient in surgery*, ed 14, St Louis, 2011, Elsevier.)

BOX 11-1	**Potential Reasons for Decreased ROM or Strength**

1	Disuse
2	Strength
3	Bandages
4	Limited vital capacity
5	Disease process
6	Trauma
7	Pain
8	Perception or anticipation of pain
9	Edema
10	Muscle tone

ROM, Range of motion.

Control of voluntary movement, or fine and gross motor control, allows people to manipulate items and to smoothly move the body through space. **Praxis** is another way to describe purposeful motor actions. Fortunately, typical aging does not substantially affect coordination. Practicing tasks over the course of years generally allows people to improve or at least maintain performance. An example of this is Salthouse's[43] description of older secretaries who do not significantly lose typing speed. He theorized that through "anticipatory

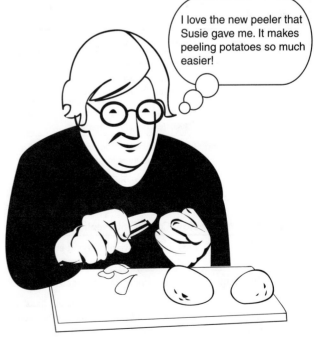

I love the new peeler that Susie gave me. It makes peeling potatoes so much easier!

Figure 11-3 Using one's hands to complete meal preparation can be challenging for clients with arthritis. The occupational therapy practitioner provides an adaptive knife to help the older person.

processing" and continued practice of their art, secretaries (and perhaps others who practice physical tasks) are able to maintain performance (even if speed does decrease for some). Once again, control of voluntary movement may decline as people get older, but the causes are generally disease related (e.g., cerebrovascular accident, arthritis) or associated with disuse.

One area of voluntary movement that does decline with age, for many, is **postural control** or occupational mobility. Nearly one third of people older than 65 fall every year, and falling even once increases the person's risk of falling again.[18] Falls are caused by many factors, both intrinsic and extrinsic. To improve safety, occupational therapy practitioners work to remediate the intrinsic factors that are amenable to intervention as well as to adapt to or compensate for extrinsic factors that cannot be fixed.[20] Table 11-3 requires the reader to list potential intrinsic (within the person) and extrinsic (outside of the person) factors potentially causing decreased postural control. For example, an intrinsic factor leading to falls could be muscle weakness, and a potential extrinsic factor could be uneven floor surfaces in the client's home. For each factor, think about how occupational therapy could help.

Sensory changes are inevitable. For example, visual changes generally lead to farsightedness, and a higher proportion of older people develop one of the diseases of the eye mentioned earlier. Sensory losses (especially if stimulation is not augmented through corrective measures [e.g., hearing aids, glasses] or replaced through another sensory system) can both lead to and be exacerbated by sensory deprivation in a sort of vicious cycle. The majority of older adults are likely to have one or more chronic conditions that can magnify the difficulties encountered because of sensory changes related to aging.

In 1999, 82% of Medicare patients reported having at least one chronic condition, with 65% reporting multiple chronic conditions.[49]

Yet in spite of the sensory losses and the chronic health conditions that befall many older people, the majority, indeed the vast majority, manage to function in everyday life quite well. Older workers, when compared with younger workers, have a lower absentee rate, incur fewer workplace injuries, and are considered more dependable.[37,39] Approximately 40% of those 65 and older report having a functional limitation affecting performance in everyday tasks (42% according to the *Long-Term Care Insurance Sourcebook,*[33] and 38% according to the Administration on Aging[2]). Most of these reported limitations are in one or two ADLs (18%), whereas 5% reported problems with three or four ADLs, and 3% with five or six ADLs.[33] Looking at these statistics as a glass half full or from a strengths, perspective, 71% of those 80 and older do not report needing assistance.[2]

PERSONALITY AND PSYCHOLOGICAL CHANGES

The OTPF[4] includes aspects of the client's psychological character such as coping and behavioral regulation, body image, self-concept and self-esteem, and emotional stability. In considering the typical aging process, no major changes in psychological functioning or emotional regulation are expected. A few studies are notable and worth considering when working with older people; on the other hand, it is also worth noting that they offer general considerations and each individual may or may not fit into the expected trends. The long-term Baltimore Longitudinal Study of Aging, which was instigated in 1958, found that as men age they tend to become more nurturing and more accepting of their feelings, whereas women tend to become more assertive and confident.[22] Erikson proposed eight stages of human personality development, with the final stage being wisdom in old age, during which a person becomes more reflective and may even gain, in a sense, a better quality of life.[50] With regard to the "big five" personality traits proposed by McCrae and Costa,[34] there is evidence of both personality stability over time, with potential accentuation of inherent traits and ongoing development or change over time.[6] For example, agreeableness and conscientiousness may increase into old age, whereas openness may tend to decline, especially after age 70.[50] However, little is known about the differences of personality change among different ethnic and racial groups. Ardelt[6] argues for the need to consider the context in which persons find themselves, including the social environment and life events that may bring about successful adaptation (resilience) or succumbing to stressful life events. When working with older people one has to consider that personal change and growth are possible and probable, and also that positive personality traits may be obscured by various events such as the influences of medication, pain, fear, and various medical procedures.

Bandura[11] has written extensively about **locus of control**, with people generally falling into one of two camps: those with

TABLE 11-3	**Factors Contributing to Fall Risk and Potential OT Interventions**
Intrinsic Factors	**How Can OT Intervention Help?**
Muscle weakness	Increase muscle strength through engagement in valued occupations, including exercise if client desires.
Poor postural control	Provide core strengthening activities or external supports.
Poor coordination and timing	Increase coordination and timing; provide visual cues to assist client.
Visual perceptual	Provide cues to help client navigate; use assistive technology.
Extrinsic Factors	**How Can OT Intervention Help?**
Uneven floors	Provide home evaluation and education regarding safety in the home.
Barriers in the house	Remove barriers, provide hand rails if necessary.
Environmental hazards (i.e., wet, icy, and snowy surfaces)	Provide assistance removing environmental hazards; provide technology (e.g., railings, lifts).

OT, Occupational therapy.

an internal locus of control who believe they are masters of their own fate, and those with an external locus of control who believe they are merely pawns under the control of others (or fate). There are several domains of control: health, finances, transportation, friends, families, and living arrangements. One might expect that, as the number of chronic conditions increases and older people have less control over their living arrangements, the locus of control would become more external as people age. However, overall this has not been found to be the case. The diagnosis of depression rather than age is associated to a greater degree with a decreased sense of internal locus of control.

High degrees of self-esteem and self-efficacy are associated with resiliency, or the ability to successfully cope with change. **Resiliency** is a personality trait considered to be a part of aging well.[47] Those who are resilient in the face of losses tend to rate their health as better subjectively, be more independent in instrumental ADLs, and practice more health-promoting behaviors.[50] Engaging in creative endeavors may increase resilience and have a positive, neuroprotective effect on the aging brain, according to a study by McFadden and Basting.[36] This is important information for the profession of occupational therapy as we promote engagement in meaningful creative ventures as part of the therapeutic process.

Quality of life is an overarching aspect of everyday living that also is expected to decline with age. As losses are incurred through an increasing number of conditions and decreased physical functioning (at least to a degree), one might assume that a general quality of life score would decline with age. Surprisingly, the opposite is true, resulting in what has been termed "the paradox of aging."[14] As people get older, they actually tend to rate their quality of life higher, if they have a minimum standard of living and are aging typically. Baltes and Baltes[10] suggested that the reason may be "selective optimization with compensation" during which older people focus on those activities most important to them and learn to compensate for any loss of performance.

COGNITION AND PERCEPTION

COGNITION

Cognition and perception are client factors addressed in occupational therapy practice. Cognition includes thinking, learning, remembering, and perceiving. All conscious thought processes fall under the realm of cognitive performance. Client factors related to cognitive performance skills include:

- *Global mental functions:* levels of alertness and orientation, energy, motivation, and emotional stability
- *Attention:* sustained, selective, alternating, and divided attention
- *Memory:* of various types as explained later in this chapter
- *Thought functions:* recognition, categorization, generalization
- *Higher level cognitive functions:* insight and judgment, awareness, concept formation, metacognition, and mental flexibility (list adapted from the American Occupational Therapy Association [AOTA],[4] p. 635).

In considering these factors in relation to aging, many changes can occur, but relatively few are the inevitable outcomes of the aging process. **Global mental functions** refer to basic cognitive skills and emotional stability, and these are deemed to be more crystallized or fixed, and are not altered significantly through the typical aging process. Crystallized intelligence, as first proposed by Cattell,[15] involves language comprehension, occupational qualifications, acquired knowledge, expert decision making, and the cognitive ability to use one's experience and knowledge, what overall might be termed *wisdom.*[9,30] These aspects of crystallized intelligence tend to remain stable or even improve throughout life for those without neurologic conditions.

Included in global mental functions is orientation to person, place, and especially time, the last of which is more likely to be negatively influenced by a retirement lifestyle than just old age, especially if one's days are quite routine and indistinguishable from one another. There seems to be no evidence that levels of mental alertness and mental energy decline in those who are aging well. Evidence of well elders continuing the lifelong learning process is provided by an American Council on Education report,[3] which states the majority of adults at least up to age 79 remain engaged in work, education, learning, or a community service role.

Basic attention, or mentally being able to focus on a task, also does not decrease significantly with age, remaining intact in healthy aging. However, more complex attention skills such as alternating or divided attention (switching back and forth between tasks or multitasking) that also require increased speed of processing, or selective attention (which requires one to tune out distractions while focusing on a task) do decline with age even under typical conditions.[46] Driving is one example of a task that does require higher levels of attention, especially in high-traffic areas and with passengers in the vehicle.

Memory describes a myriad of constructs related to remembering. The various types of memory are affected differentially by aging. Short-term memory (e.g., the name of a person one just met, what one had for breakfast, and other recent episodes in one's life) does decline with age. Primary or immediate memory (e.g., repeating up to several digits immediately after hearing them) does not seem to change much over time in well older people.[23] Long-term memory such as autobiographical information is well retained through old age, although retrieving information may become more difficult (as it is encoded in the brain but not always available on demand).[12] **Episodic memory** is the memory of experiences we have had in our lives. This type of memory is significantly affected by age. Cross-sectional studies demonstrate that younger respondents outperform older ones.[7,23] Logically this makes sense if one considers that experiences are cumulative; the brain may run out of storage capacity, especially for experiences that are not particularly emotionally engaging. Another working hypothesis about memory impairment in old age is that it may be less about faulty memory and perhaps more associated with decreased sensory processing.[35]

Semantic memory is remembering information about the world in general. It may involve remembering basic math facts or one's primary language (including grammatical rules). This type of memory is associated with crystallized intelligence or thinking that is solidly grounded and not easily lost through the typical aging process.[7]

Prospective memory refers to the ability to remember to do a task in the future, such as taking medication or doing a homework assignment. Older people may be better able to compensate when this type of memory is impaired. They tend to spontaneously compensate, perhaps because over time they have grown used to making adaptations as their memories decline.[8] **Procedural memory** is one's memory for motor performance skills. For example, driving safely involves several types of memory (e.g., rules of the road, finding your car, using the car's instruments). The procedural memory portion of driving involves basic over-learned, motoric aspects such as shifting the gears, inserting the key, and turning the steering wheel. Because procedural memory is also deeply ingrained, often automatic, and therefore less affected by the aging process per se, this type of memory can be viewed as a strength for many older people.[18] This has a downside, however, for example when someone who has dementia remembers the motor aspects of driving but cannot problem solve or remember the rules of the road to drive safely (Figure 11-4).

Thought functions listed in the OTPF include recognition, categorization, and generalization. **Recognition** is simply recognizing and identifying items and other aspects of the world. Recognition is a type of memory that is usually less difficult than free recall.[8] Upon identification, any item or idea can also be categorized or related to a broader grouping based on past experience or developed for a new set of stimuli. **Categorical fluency** is the skill of naming items in a category, such as naming as many animals as possible in a minute, or as many words beginning with a certain letter. Older people do tend to show decreases in speed of categorical fluency tasks and in ability to generate as many items in any given category. Significant decreases in the skill of categorical fluency are associated with the development of Alzheimer's disease and other disorders of executive functioning.[5] **Generalization** involves expanding learning or the transfer of skills. Skills are learned, and then maintained, through practice. Older people may need more practice or a little longer to learn new skills and to transfer the learning to new situations. Prompts from occupational therapy practitioners, for example, can be gradually decreased as the person is able to complete the task on his or her own.[21]

Higher level cognitive functions, according to the OTPF, include insight and judgment, awareness, concept formation, metacognition, and mental flexibility, all of which are influenced by the common cognitive diseases of aging (e.g., Alzheimer's disease). Researchers found that interindividual variability of performance on cognitive tasks increased among an older cohort (versus a younger cohort).[5] Some maintained or even improved their functioning, whereas the cognitive functioning of others declined precipitously. Generally this heterogeneity (i.e., the severe decline) is due at least in part to the onset in old age of various neurologic conditions, including acquired brain injury, dementia, Parkinson's disease, and mild cognitive impairment (MCI).[25] Typical aging does not have nearly as large an effect on high-level cognitive performance as these neurologic conditions. Decreases in judgment and insight are associated with gray matter reduction specifically in the prefrontal cortex areas.[40] **Fluid intelligence**, which is less reliant on experience and more dependent on genetics, includes both speed and accuracy of processing information. Old age is associated with a decrease in fluid intelligence, especially speed of processing.[5] However, well elders are often fully capable of completing tasks that involve both crystallized and fluid intelligence skills. Baltes[9] draws an interesting analogy about this relationship between aging and cognitive performance. Imagine a younger person and an older person walking together along a road; the older person keeps up just fine, but when the two approach a steep hill, it may be more difficult for the older person to keep up the pace (Figure 11-5).

PERCEPTION

Perception is the ability to make sense of and interpret in-coming sensory information. Visual perception relates specifically to the ability to interpret sensory information coming in through the eyes. Following the visual pyramid developed by Warren,[48] the assumption is that before sensory information can be interpreted it must first be properly sensed. An analogy is cooking. One may be a wonderful cook and be perfectly capable of interpreting even the most complex of recipes. However, if the ingredients are inaccurate, the recipe cannot be expected to turn out correctly. With regard to aging, the visual system is the first sensory system to undergo age-related changes and

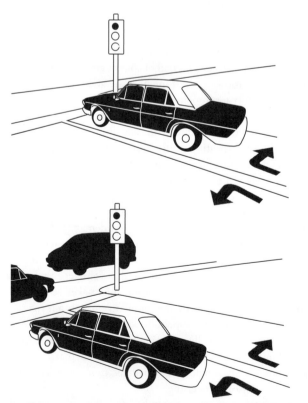

Figure 11-4 Older persons may have difficulty driving through intersections. They may sway over the yellow line when turning but be able to correct when driving straight.

also is often affected by disease processes associated with aging, including glaucoma, macular degeneration, diabetic retinopathy, and cataracts. These diseases of the eye can influence how visual information is perceived and interpreted. One outcome of macular degeneration, for example, is visual hallucinations in a significant portion of those who have the diagnosis (i.e., a 40% prevalence rate).[1] Although this is a visual perception problem, those who experience it can understand that it is due to the disease of the eye and not mental illness.

Visual perception skills do not tend to uniformly decline in healthy aging. There is even some evidence (e.g., Lindfield[32]) that older people may be better able than their younger counterparts to complete visual closure tasks (e.g., interpreting the whole when viewing only part of an object) perhaps because they are more familiar with objects from years of viewing and use. Another perceptual loss is termed **agnosia**, in which people cannot recognize formerly familiar objects (e.g., people, faces, body parts, etc.). Agnosias are not a part of normal aging, but once again are associated with neurologic impairments such as acquired brain injuries.

SUMMARY OF COGNITIVE AND PERCEPTUAL CHANGES RELATED TO AGING

Thinking, learning, remembering, and perceiving are all skills needed every day for successful completion of occupations. Although some aspects of these skills do demonstrate relatively small declines in those who are aging well, much larger declines are associated with conditions that become more frequent as people age. Particularly visual perception and executive or high-level cognitive functioning are affected greatly by both dementia and acquired brain injuries, such as stroke. The greatest challenge to overcome with regard to cognitive functioning and aging is the common societal expectation that aging (often alone) causes a severe decline in cognition. Older people do show somewhat slowed performance as in longer reaction times, and taking longer to learn new tasks. However, in typical aging, which the vast majority of older people experience, at least for the greatest proportion of their lives, cognitive and perceptual functioning does not decline enough to significantly

affect daily life. Moreover, taking concrete steps to combat the potential losses through physical and mental exercise and engagement in meaningful, challenging occupations can significantly improve cognitive performance in nearly everyone, even those who may have sustained a degree of neurologic impairment. Greater losses in the realm of cognition may be caused by the lived experience, or "self-fulfilling prophecy" of the expectations of loss at a given age, rather than by the reality of what will occur as a result of the marching forward of time into old age.[31]

Table 11-4 relates cognition, perception, and aging. It provides a format for the reader to briefly explain in the middle column his or her expectations of aging prior to reading the chapter and to record in the right column what was learned after reading the chapter.

ACTIVITY ANALYSIS

The next section of this chapter explores the activity analysis process integrating the information on cognition, perception, and aging. Activity analysis is an occupational therapy tool used to thoroughly examine the properties of an activity. Although it can be completed on any activity, generally it is done as an academic exercise to ensure that the practitioner is considering all aspects of the activity for ultimate client success. This section of the chapter starts with a basic activity analysis from the perspective of the activity as it is usually completed (making an egg salad sandwich and managing a monthly budget). We then consider some of the basic changes of aging and how these changes might affect the ability to do these tasks. The author then uses activity analysis of a specific client (in this case, George, who has mild dementia) to illustrate the concepts. Again this section uses reader exercises to stimulate the thinking process. The case examples are offered to help convert the general knowledge base gained to specific interventions. Although the cases are individual and specific, the process used for task analysis is more far reaching, and readers, through these initial exercises, can use the process for any specific client they encounter at any time. Boxes 11-2, 11-3, and 11-4 provide formats for activity-based; client-centered; and cognition-, perception-, and sensation-focused activity analyses.

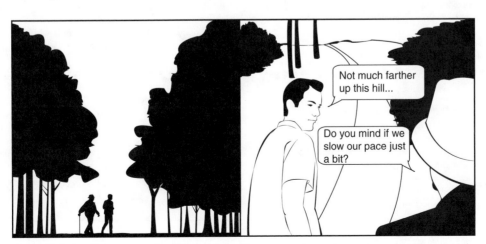

Figure 11-5 An older person may be able to continue with past occupations as long as some adaptations are made. For example, taking one's time going up a steep hill may allow the older person to succeed.

TABLE 11-4   Cognition, Perception, and Aging

Skills and Traits	Expectation of What Occurs in Old Age	Empiric Evidence (Support for or Against)
Orientation (alert and oriented to person, place, and time)	People can become disoriented to person, time, and place as they get older.	Medications, head trauma, or disease process may cause orientation difficulties.
Energy and endurance	People slow down with age.	Physical activity helps people continue to have the energy and endurance for movement. Generally those with good endurance have functional level of strength.
Emotional stability	People become wise with age. They may become depressed due to the loss of friends.	Erickson proposed the final stage being wisdom in old age, during which the person becomes more reflective and may even gain a better quality of life.[49]
Motivation	As people age, they want to leave something behind and influence future generations.	This follows Erickson's stage of development.
Attention	Older people pay less attention to details.	Visual deficits may make visual attention difficult.
Short-term memory	Older persons may forget things that occurred earlier in the day.	Evidence shows that many things, such as medication, head trauma, anxiety, and stress may cause short-term memory loss.
Long-term memory		
Prospective memory		
Procedural memory		
Thought functions		
Insight and judgment		
Awareness		
Mental flexibility		
Visual perception		

BOX 11-2   Activity Analysis—Making an Egg Salad Sandwich

1. Name of activity: Making an egg salad sandwich
2. Essential steps (up to 10), including usual time for completion
   a. Determine if all ingredients are available (egg, mayonnaise, bread, salt, pepper, saucepan, and water)—5 minutes
   b. Get egg out of refrigerator—1 minute
   c. Get out small sauce pan—1 minute
   d. Fill pan approximately half way with water—1 minute
   e. Turn on stove to high—<1 minute
   f. Put egg in pan—<1 minute
   g. Boil water and egg for 10 minutes—10 minutes
   h. Cool and then peel egg—5 minutes
   i. Chop up egg, and add mayonnaise and salt and pepper to taste—2 minutes
   j. Spread on bread—2 minutes
   k. Cut sandwich in half—1 minute
3. Precautions and contraindications (if any): Allergies to eggs, dietary restrictions
4. Age ranges (children, adolescent, young adult, adult, older adult): Adolescent and older; younger children need supervision for knife and stove use
5. Contextual consideration—Environmental (physical): Kitchen area with stove top

6. Contextual considerations—Other (cultural, temporal, virtual, social): Cultural—eating eggs and in this fashion; temporal—may have this sandwich for lunch
7. Activity demands—objects and their properties (typical for activity): Tools—pan, fork, spoon or knife; materials—egg, mayonnaise, pepper and salt, bread; equipment—stove top, countertop, sink
8. Activity demands—space demands—lighting for cooking, small counter space for sandwich making
9. Activity demands—social demands—NA
10. Successful outcomes: Sandwich tastes good and is eaten for lunch
11. Degree of being amenable to change (is activity rigid or flexible): Could use alternate ingredients for sandwich; make sandwich without stove use
12. Potential transfer of learning—list small to large changes for consideration: To make easier—make sandwich with simple noncooked ingredients such as peanut butter or cheese; use sliced bread, not toasted; to increase complexity make several course meal using eggs; include grocery shipping and meal planning

NA, Not applicable.

Note: Remember there is often more than one right answer for any one section.

BOX 11-3 Activity Analysis—Client-Centered: George M.

1. Name of activity—Making an egg salad sandwich
2. Essential steps (up to 10)—see activity-centered activity analysis in Box 11-2.
3. Steps to be analyzed (form can be used for one or more applicable steps): Peel egg, chop up egg, add mayonnaise and salt and pepper to taste, spread on bread
4. Client factors—values, beliefs, and spirituality if applicable: George is agreeable to eating eggs, enjoys egg salad sandwiches—chose this for lunch; has enjoyed fixing his own (simple) meals
5. Client factors—Mental functions (global—see activity analysis, cognition and perception focus): Must be conscious, alert, have attention for at least 15 minutes, able to initiate and terminate task, memory to know when to turn off stove. May need to set timer.
6. Client factors—Sensory functions and pain (global—see activity analysis, cognition and perception focus): George can see the egg, pan, water, etc. Has good awareness of sharp and hot objects.
7. Client factors—Neuromusculoskeletal—functions of joints and bones
   a. Which joints are involved? (unilateral U/bilateral B) B use of hands to fill pan, get egg out of pan.
   b. Mobility required (WNL, WFL, or approximate measurements): approximately ⅓ ROM of shoulder, ½ ROM of elbow, ¾ ROM of fingers, and generally walking around kitchen.

   c. Muscle power required—per joint (UE—approximate muscle grade 2-5): Shoulder 3+/5; elbow 2/5; fingers—grasp 3+/5.
   d. Muscle endurance required: Only a few minutes, can take breaks.
   e. Control of voluntary movement—eye-hand and eye-foot coordination, unilateral or bilateral, gross motor or fine motor: Bilateral coordination to peel egg, open mayonnaise jar, spread on sandwich, cut sandwich; unilateral to mix egg salad.
   f. Control of voluntary movement—oculomotor (fixation, accommodation, binocularity, saccades, pursuits): Basic vision only required.
   g. Mobility—level of mobility required, LE function: Generally done ambulating around kitchen.
8. Is activity amenable to alteration (focus on item 7, neuromusculoskeletal)? Describe: Could be done at wheelchair level, most tasks could be done unilaterally with some difficulty.
9. Other applicable body functions (e.g., cardiovascular, hematologic, immunologic, respiratory, voice and speech, digestive, metabolic, endocrine, genitourinary, reproductive, skin, hair, and nail functions): Need to not be allergic to eggs
10. Body structures—if applicable, see p. 637 of OTPF.[4]

B,***; LE, lower extremity; *OTPF,* occupational therapy practice framework; *ROM,* range of motion; *U, ***; UE,* upper extremity; *WFL,* within functional limits; *WNL,* within normal limits.

BOX 11-4 Activity Analysis—Cognition-, Perception-, and Sensation-Focused

1. Name of activity—Making an egg salad sandwich.
2. Essential steps—see activity-centered activity analysis in Box 11-2.
3. Client factors—Specific mental functions—describe or NA
   Insight and judgment—Stove use, knowing egg is fresh enough to eat
   Concept formation—Understanding concept of sandwich and lunch
   Metacognition—NA
   Awareness—Awareness of time to know when egg is ready
   Cognitive flexibility—Ability to substitute one ingredient for another as needed
4. Client factors—Specific mental functions—Attention—describe or NA
   Initiation and Termination—Starting and ending project appropriately
   Sustained attention—Not getting distracted and leaving egg to boil too long
   Selective attention—Being able to concentrate on making sandwich even if distractions occur (e.g., telephone rings)
   Alternating attention—Not usually necessary for making sandwich
   Divided attention and multitasking—NA
5. Client factors—Specific mental functions—Memory—describe or NA
   Orientation (person, place, time)—Need to understand concepts of time (10 minutes) and place (kitchen)
   Immediate memory—NA
   Short-term memory—Remember to turn off stove
   Working memory—NA
   Long-term memory—Remembering the concepts of sandwich making and eating meals

   Semantic memory—NA
   Episodic memory—NA
   Procedural memory—Remembering the motor steps of sandwich making
   Prospective memory—Remembering to turn off stove in 10 minutes
6. Client factors—Specific mental functions—Learning—describe or NA
   Simple 1-2 steps—NA because client has done this task many times before
   Multistep learning—NA
7. Client factors—Specific mental functions—Communication—describe or NA
   Understanding of written language—NA
   Understanding of verbal language—NA
   Expression of written language—NA
   Auditory expression—NA
   Expression of nonverbal communication—NA
8. Client factors—Specific mental functions—Thought processes—describe or NA
   Recognition—Identifying the items needed for task: egg, mayonnaise, bread, etc.
   Categorization—NA
   Generalization—NA
   Logical, coherent, appropriate thought and awareness of reality—NA
9. Client factors—Specific mental functions—Sequencing—describe or NA
   Sequencing task—Retrieve egg, boil egg, peel egg, then make salad, spread on bread, eat
   Sequencing complex movement—Most complex movement is peeling egg and discarding shells

Continued

BOX 11-4   Activity Analysis—Cognition-, Perception-, and Sensation-Focused—cont'd

10. Client factors—Specific and global mental functions—
    Emotion—describe or NA
    Coping skills—Usually NA unless problem arises
    Behavioral regulation—Usually NA
    Emotional expression and stability—Usually NA
    Energy, motivation, and drive—Need to be motivated to eat
11. Client factors—Specific and global mental functions—
    Knowledge and skills—describe or NA
    Demonstration and copying—NA
    Language—NA (unless checking expiration dates for eggs, mayonnaise)
    Calculations—Calculating 10 minutes from current time
    Problem solving—Problem solving how to quickly cool egg by running under cold water
    Organizing and planning—Planning activity and organizing time so meal will be on time
    Creating—Building sandwich
12. Client factors—sensory functions
    Vision—acuity—Ability to see ingredients (egg, paper, salt, pepper, peeling)
    Vision—visual fields—Dependent on where items are (right, left, inferior, superior)
    Vision—fixation—Focusing on ingredients
    Vision—accommodation—Quick accommodation not necessary
    Vision—saccades—NA
    Vision—pursuits—NA
    Hearing—every-day conversation—NA unless using timer
    Hearing—background noise—NA
    Taste functions—NA (task does not include eating sandwich)
    Smell functions—Would be needed if food looks good, but is spoiled

Touch functions—tolerance of being touched or touching different textures—Touching egg and peelings, utensils, bread
Touch functions—stereognosis—NA although this helps with peeling egg and not squeezing it too hard
Touch functions—hot, cold, and pain—Careful with boiling water and very hot egg
Touch functions—pressure and vibration—NA
Proprioception—Needs to be intact for UE (at least for dominant side)
Kinesthesia—General movement patterns for task as described
13. Client factors—sensory functions—perception
    Visual perception—item recognition—Recognizing items needed: egg, bread, etc.
    Visual perception—contrast sensitivity—For everyday items (egg likely different color than pan, bread contrasts with egg salad)
    Visual perception—form recognition—Not confusing sauce pan with frying pan or mayonnaise with sour cream
    Visual perception—visual closure—Only if items are partially obscured
    Visual perception—depth perception—Using stove knobs for correct burner
    Visual perception—visual memory—NA for short-term visual memory
    Perception—discrimination of sensory input—Vision, touch, possibly smell and hearing
14. Client factors—planned movement
    Execution of learned movement patterns—Sandwich making pattern
    Execution of complex/novel movement patterns—NA

NA, Not applicable; UE, upper extremity.

CASE STUDY

George M. is an 84-year-old man who was widowed 6 months ago. During the past few months George's family has begun to worry about him, because his general functioning has declined and he is showing signs of dementia. He also has intention tremors, which are starting to interfere with his daily tasks. Once timely and organized, he now does tasks with little attention to detail and frequently seems to gets confused. He wants to continue to live at home, but does state that he really misses his "May," who took care of him so well. Family members have been bringing in nightly meals but George does need to make his own breakfast and lunch. Family members check on George at least once per day. Box 11-2 outlines the activity analysis for making an egg salad sandwich. Box 11-3 describes a client-centered activity analysis for George. Box 11-4 provides an in-depth analysis of the cognition, perception, and sensation required for the task of making an egg salad sandwich (Figure 11-6).

This activity analysis is based on one person's procedure for making a rather simple sandwich. Not all sections are definitive and many sections may have other answers than the ones provided. The process is worthwhile to understand the demands of any task, taking into account the strengths and limitations of the client. Given a typical aging pattern, making an egg salad sandwich would not likely place undo demands on the client.

However, considering George's probable dementia, the activity analysis highlights some cognitive aspects that need to be assessed. In this case, sandwich making is relatively uncomplicated, but areas of concern are stove use and specifically remembering that the egg should boil for only 10 minutes. Because memory, especially short-term memory, is often impaired in dementia, a meal preparation assessment would lead the practitioner to decide whether to recommend continued use of the stove. Other concerns would arise if any unusual circumstances or problems occur. For example, if the bread was moldy, the kitchen was out of the necessary ingredients, or the process of sandwich making was interrupted by someone knocking at the door, a well-learned automatic task could be transformed into a novel task, which is likely to be more difficult for someone who has dementia.

Normal age-related changes, which for the most part involve only slight alterations of sensory and functional performance, are not likely to affect this simple task, but diseases associated with aging (e.g., cerebrovascular accident, macular degeneration, severe arthritis) could negatively influence the ability to complete IADL tasks such as sandwich making. Investigating the functional implications of any impairment, when combined with activity analysis, can help the practitioner match the individual person with those occupations that are both meaningful to the person and have a high probability of success.

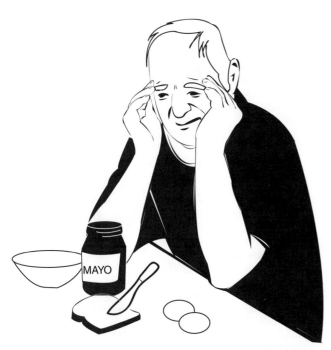

Figure 11-6 George makes an egg salad sandwich. There are many tasks involved in making a simple sandwich. Occupational therapy practitioners are skilled at analyzing the activity at multiple levels.

Rather than repeating the activity analysis with several more activities, the reader is invited to complete a higher level cognitive task: managing the monthly budget using the task analysis specifically for cognitive perceptual tasks (Box 11-5).

Although this is a tedious process, any task could be thoroughly examined using these processes. Activity analysis provides a way for the practitioner to methodically and exhaustively understand how specific clients, with their own personal strengths and areas needing improvement, match or mismatch their personally relevant occupations.

GRADING AND ADAPTING

The final section of this chapter considers those times when a mismatch occurs between the activity of meaning and the skills of the client as determined through client assessment and activity analyses. Although no recipe exists for grading and adapting to achieve a better match between task and client, the occupational therapy process can assist practitioners in developing adaptations and in grading to achieve optimal performance.

Adaptation is "a change in response approach that the client makes when encountering an occupational challenge" (AOTA,[4] p. 662). Adaptations can be instigated by the client;

BOX 11-5   Activity Analysis—Managing a Monthly Budget

1. Name of Activity—Managing a monthly budget
2. Essential steps
   1. Determining how much money is available and from which source
   2. Determining each monthly bill and how much is needed for other necessities
   3. Deciding which bill to pay and when
   4. Writing checks (this could be done online, but George does not use the Internet)
   5. Staying within budget for food, clothing, entertainment, other items
   6. Depositing and recording in-coming checks
   7. Deciding what is essential versus what he can live without
   8. At the end of the month, evaluating how well he stuck to his budget
3. Client factors—Specific mental functions—describe or NA
   Insight and judgment—Keeping in mind what is essential and what is superfluous
   Concept formation—Must understand money, the value of things, services, etc.
   Metacognition—Able to evaluate how well client met his own goal; what he did well and what changes in his budget are needed
   Awareness—Having a sense of appropriate spending compared with means
   Cognitive flexibility—Need to be able to find alternative ways to pay for necessities and other goods (e.g., using coupons, looking for sales, substituting less expensive items, waiting until one has the money or gets paid)
4. Client factors—Specific mental functions—Attention—describe or NA
   Initiation and termination—Not neglecting budgeting but also not being obsessed with the task
   Sustained attention—Focusing to plan monthly budget (<1 hour), and then periodically to pay bills and spend or save money throughout the month

Selective attention—Adhering to budget even when tempted to spend frivolously
Alternating attention—NA
Divided attention and multitasking—NA
5. Client factors—Specific mental functions—Memory—describe or NA
   Orientation (person, place, time)—Needed to understand concept of paying in a timely manner, whom to pay and when, and where to send a check
   Immediate memory—Recording amount spent in register
   Short-term memory—Remembering what one recently spent
   Working memory—Keeping running totals
   Long-term memory—Long-term financial goal kept in mind
   Semantic memory—Understanding numbers; language (bills); dollar signs; how banking, spending, and bill paying work
   Episodic memory—Remembering that one has paid a bill, spent a certain amount of money, deposited funds, etc.
   Procedural memory—Remembering how to write checks, make deposits, and other budgeting procedures
   Prospective memory—Paying bills in a timely fashion
6. Client factors—Specific mental functions—Learning—describe or NA
   Simple 1-2 steps—NA, budgeting has long been a part of the client's life tasks
   Multistep learning—Only likely if client decides to learn how to bank online
7. Client factors—Specific mental functions—Communication—describe or NA
   Understanding of written language—Reading bills, coupons, labels, price tags
   Understanding of verbal language—Comprehending stated prices; sales pitches
   Expression of written language—Writing checks, setting up budget

Continued

BOX 11-5   Activity Analysis—Managing a Monthly Budget—Cont'd

Auditory expression—Communicating with bank tellers, salespersons

Expression of nonverbal communication—NA

8. Client factors—Specific mental functions—Thought processes—describe or NA

Recognition—Recognizing different denominations of money, the value of items

Categorization—Could group into various ways (e.g., bills to pay immediately, bills that can wait; needed items and those that are not necessary; different types of coins and bills)

Generalization—NA

Logical, coherent, and appropriate thought and awareness of reality—Needs to understand economic status and what that means with regard to purchasing items

9. Client factors—Specific mental functions—Sequencing—describe or NA

Sequencing task—Paying the most important bills first, writing check, putting in envelope with stub, addressing envelope, stamping envelope, putting in mailbox

Sequencing complex movement—Writing, sealing envelope, opening bills (no movement that is overly complex)

10. Client factors—Specific and global mental functions—Emotion—describe or NA

Coping skills—Because client lives on a fixed income, he has to find ways to cope with less money than desired

Behavioral regulation—Client needs to demonstrate appropriate behavior with regard to money and spending (not gamble away his savings, steal, or rob)

Emotional expression and stability—NA

Energy, motivation, and drive—Client needs motivation and drive to complete budgeting task

11. Client factors—Specific and global mental functions—Knowledge and skills—describe or NA

Demonstration and copying—NA

Language—Both written and symbolic language is included

Calculations—Basic ability to calculate (add, subtract, multiply, and divide) needed, or ability to use calculator

Problem solving—Need to prioritize what is most important, how to pay for all necessities, making sure there is still money left at the end of the month

Organizing and planning—Planning when to pay for what and what amount

Creating—NA

12. Client factors—sensory functions

Vision—acuity—Viewing bills (or online statements), denominations of money, checks, banking slips

Vision—visual fields—Mostly central for reading (in all directions past midline)

Vision—fixation—Several-second fixation is needed

Vision—accommodation—Needed to refocus on next budget item or task

Vision—saccades—Needed for reading tasks

Vision—pursuits—NA

Hearing—everyday conversation—Needed for in-person or phone banking or purchasing

Hearing—background noise—May be a factor in a busy store, but generally NA

Taste functions—NA

Smell functions—NA

Touch functions—tolerance of being touched or touching different textures—Only touching everyday objects such as coins, bills, paper, and pen

Touch functions—stereognosis—Needed to identify coins in pocket possibly

Touch functions—hot, cold, and pain—NA

Touch functions—pressure and vibration—NA

Proprioception—Needed for writing

Kinesthesia—Fine motor kinesthesia needed for writing, handling money

13. Client factors—sensory functions—perception

Visual perception—item recognition—Need to be able to identify different denominations of money, items to purchase

Visual perception—contrast sensitivity—Needed for different denominations of dollar bills (cannot identify by color)

Visual perception—form recognition—Also needed for identifying bills and coins

Visual perception—visual closure—Ability to recognize bills or number amounts when only a portion is visible

Visual perception—depth perception—NA

Visual perception—visual memory—Remembering numbers long enough to record

Perception—discrimination of sensory input—NA

14. Client factors—planned movement

Execution of learned movement patterns—Used for writing, mailing, handling money

Execution of complex or novel movement patterns

NA, Not applicable.

for example, if the client gets fatigued easily, he or she can complete the bulk of the meal preparation in the morning when he or she has plenty of energy. On the other hand, adaptations can be designed and implemented by the occupational therapy practitioner, such as when one recommends the use of adaptive equipment (e.g., larger handled utensils or a reacher to pick up items off the floor).

Grading an activity or occupation involves changing one or more aspects of the activity to make it easier to accommodate for impairments or more challenging to direct the client toward improved performance. For example, an occupational therapy practitioner may modify any of the following features of the task:

1. Duration
2. ROM required (by the arrangement of objects)
3. Strength required (considering the assistance-resistance continuum)
4. Complexity (includes cognition and perception such as number of choices)
5. Graded cues (based on cognitive level)
6. Extent of physical handling (which needs to be at the client's level for safety)

Table 11-5 provides an outline for readers to grade and adapt the task of lunch preparation.

The occupational therapy practitioner has the professional tools, knowledge, and skills to thoroughly analyze any activity and subsequently adjust whatever is necessary into a just-right occupation considering the individual needs of the client. One of the key aspects of the ongoing, omnipresent assessment is being an excellent listener, not only to the stated words, but

TABLE 11-5   Grading and Adapting the Task of Lunch Preparation

Potential Steps	Potential Grading or Adapting (One or More Examples as Appropriate)
Determining what to make for lunch (steps all could be further delineated)	Offer two choices (grading to make easier) up to unlimited choices (even to the point of shopping for ingredients).
Planning steps of meal preparation	Provide simple directions in writing. Provide directions one step at a time. Provide verbal and written one-step directions.
Gathering ingredients	Arrange all ingredients in same area for client. Require client to find all ingredients throughout the kitchen. Provide the list of ingredients. Require client to make the list of ingredients and obtain them at the grocery store.
Appliance and utensil use	Provide direct supervision for safety. Provide adapted utensils for ease in handling.
Putting together main course	Require client to time meal so that all items are hot when it is ready. Require client to serve only cold foods so they do not have to worry about timing. Have a time limit for the meal.
Presentation of the food on the plate	Require client to make individual servings. Allow client to serve food buffet style.
Bringing meal to the table	Carry individual plates to table. Allow each person eating to serve themselves. Carry plates a short distance. Use paper or plastic plates versus fine china.

also to other modes of communication such as body language and the feelings behind the words (see Chapters 3 and 4). This is especially important when working with those, often older, people who cannot communicate as clearly because of some of the problems associated with the aging process.

SUMMARY

Occupational therapy practitioners focus on improving lives, to assist clients to "live life to its fullest." The focus on people's strengths, not just their impairments; on finding solutions to enhance daily life rather than on lamenting the problems associated with being alive; in celebrating reaching old age rather than wallowing in the problems that sometimes show up in our bodies and minds as we grow older. Difficulties do occur; that is life. But rather than blaming the problems on the aging process, practitioners help clients overcome problems that are surmountable rather than to succumb meekly to those expectations of decline. Hope resides in old age if one takes a full perspective, rather than focusing on the daily troubles that invariably get in the way.

REVIEW QUESTIONS

1. What are some stereotypes about aging?
2. How do age-related changes influence occupational performance?
3. What are some factors contributing to fall risks in older adults?
4. Define cognitive and perceptual abilities.
5. What are the differences between activity-focused, client-focused, and sensation-focused activity analyses?
6. What is meant by *grading* and *adapting*?
7. How could you change activities to help older adults be successful?

REFERENCES

1. Abbott EG, Connor JB, Artes PH, Abadi RV: Visual loss and visual hallucinations in patients with age-related macular degeneration (Charles Bonnet syndrome), *Invest Opthalmol Vis Sci* 48(3):1416-1423, 2007, doi 10.1167/iovs.06-0942.
2. Administration on Aging: *A profile of older Americans: 2009*, Washington, DC, 2009, Department of Health and Human Services. Retrieved 1/23/2011 from http://www.aoa.gov/aoaroot/aging_statistics/Profile/2009/16.aspx.
3. American Council on Education: *First report: reinvesting in the third age: older adults and higher education*, Washington, DC, 2007, author.
4. American Occupational Therapy Association: Occupational therapy practice framework: domain and process, ed 2, *Am J Occup Ther* 62(6):625-703, 2008.
5. Anderson E: Cognitive change in old age. In Jacoby R, Oppenheimer C, Dening T, Thomas A, editors: *Oxford textbook of old age psychiatry*, Oxford, UK, 2008, Oxford University Press, pp 33-50.
6. Ardelt M: Still stable after all these years? Personality stability theory revisited, *Soc Psychol Q* 63(4):392-405, 2000.
7. Bäckman L, Small BJ, Wahlin A: Aging and memory: cognitive and biological perspectives. In Birren JE, Schaie KW, editors: *Handbook of the psychology of aging*, San Diego, 2001, Academic Press.
8. Baddeley AD: The psychology of memory. In Baddeley AD, Wilson BA, Watts FN, editors: *The handbook of memory disorders*, Chichester, UK, 1995, John Wiley and Sons.

9. Baltes PB: The aging mind: potential and limits, *Gerontologist* 33:580-594, 1993.

10. Baltes PB, Baltes MM: Psychological perspectives on successful aging: the model of selective optimization with compensation. In Baltes PB, Baltes MM, editors: *Successful aging*, Cambridge, 1990, Cambridge University Press, pp 1-34.

11. Bandura A: *Self-efficacy: the exercise of control*, New York, 1997, WH Freeman and Company.

12. Birren JE, Schroots JJF: Autobiographical memory and the narrative self over the life span. In Birren JE, Schaie KW, editors: *Handbook of the psychology of aging*, Burlington, MA, 2006, Elsevier, pp 477-498.

13. Braille Institute: *Facts about sight loss.* Retrieved July 27, 2012 from http://www.brailleinstitute.org/About_Sight.Loss_aspx

14. Carstensen LL, Mikels JA, Mather M: Aging and the intersection of cognition, motivation, and emotion. In Birren JE, Schaie KW, editors: *Handbook of the psychology of aging*, Burlington, MA, 2006, Elsevier, pp 343-362.

15. Cattell RB: *Intelligence: its structure, growth, and action*, New York, 1987, Elsevier.

16. The Centers for Disease Control and Prevention: *Arthritis.* Retrieved 1/20/2010 from http://www.cdc.gov/arthritis/data_statistics.htm.

17. Cavanaugh JC, Blanchard-Fields F: *Adult development and aging*, ed 5, Belmont, CA, 2006, Wadsworth Thomson Learning.

18. Craik FIM, Bialystok E: Lifespan cognitive development. In Craik FIM, Salthouse TA, editors: *The handbook of aging and cognition*, ed 3, New York, 2008, Psychology Press, pp 557-601.

19. Farrell MJ: Pain and aging, *Bull Am Pain Soc* 10(4). Retrieved 1/19/2011 from, http://www.ampainsoc.org/library/bulletin/jul00/upda1.htm.

20. Ganz DA, Bao Y, Shekelle PG, Rubenstein LZ: Will my patient fall? *JAMA* 297(1):77-86, 2007.

21. Gardner MK, Strayer DL, Woltz DJ, Hill RD: Cognitive skill acquisition, maintenance, and transfer in the elderly. In Hill RD, Bäckman L, Stigsdotter Neely A, editors: *Cognitive rehabilitation in old age*, New York, 2000, Oxford University Press, pp 42-60.

22. Hayflick L: *How and why we age*, New York, 1994, Ballantine Books.

23. Hoyer WJ, Verhaeghen P: Memory aging. In Birren JE, Schaie KW, editors: *Handbook of the psychology of aging*, Burlington, MA, 2006, Elsevier, pp 209-232.

24. Huang G, Shi X, Davis-Brezette JA, Osness WH: Resting heart rate changes after endurance training: a meta-analysis, *Med Sci Sports Exerc* 37:1381-1386, 2005.

25. Hultsch DF, Strauss E, Hunter MA, MacDonald SWS: Intraindividual variability, cognition and aging. In Craik FIM, Salthouse TA, editors: *The handbook of aging and cognition*, ed 3, New York, 2008, Psychology Press, pp 491-556.

26. *Internet Stroke Center: About stroke*, Retrieved 7/26/2012 from http://www.strokecenter.org/patients/about-stroke/stroke-statistics/

27. Jacoby R, Oppenheimer C, Dening T, Thomas A, editors: *Oxford textbook of old age psychiatry*, Oxford, UK, 2008, Oxford University Press.

28. Janssen I, Heymsfield SB, Ross R: Low relative skeletal muscle mass (sarcopenia) in older persons is associated with functional impairment and physical disability, *J Am Geriatr Soc* 50(5):889-896, 2002.

29. Kim JS, Choi-Kwon S: Discriminative sensory dysfunction after unilateral stroke, *Stroke* 27:677-682, 1996.

30. Kim JS, Hasher L: The attraction effect in decision making: superior performance by older adults, *Q J Exp Psychol* 58A(1):120-133, 2005.

31. Levy BR: Mind matters: cognitive and physical effects of aging self-stereotypes, *J Gerontol B Psychol Sci Soc Sci* 58(4):P203-P211, 2003, doi:10.1093/geronb/58.4.P203.

32. Lindfield KC: Identification of fragmented pictures under ascending versus fixed presentation in young and elderly adults: evidence of the inhibition-deficit hypothesis, *Aging Cogn* 1(4):282-291, 1994.

33. American Association for Long-Term Care Insurance: *Long-term care insurance sourcebook*, 2009, Retrieved 1/24/2011 from http://www.aaltci.org/long-term-care-insurance/learning-center/long-term-care-statistics.php.

34. McCrae RR, Costa PT: *Personality in adulthood: a five factor theory perspective*, ed 2, New York, 2003, Guilford.

35. McDaniel MA, Einstein GO, Jacoby LL: New considerations in aging and memory. In Craik FIM, Salthouse TA, editors: *The handbook of aging and cognition*, ed 3, New York, 2008, Psychology Press, pp 251-310.

36. McFadden SH, Basting AD: Healthy aging persons and their brains: promoting resilience through creative engagement, *Clin Geriatr Med* 26(1):149-161.

37. Ng TWH, Feldman DC: The relationship of age to ten dimensions of job performance, *J Appl Psychol* 93(2):392-423, 2008.

38. Nordin S, Monsch AU, Murphy C: Unawareness of smell loss in normal aging and Alzheimer's disease: discrepancy between self-reported and diagnosed smell sensitivity, *J Gerontol B Psychol Sci Soc Sci* 50B:P187-P192, 1995.

39. Prenda KM, Stahl SM: The truth about older workers, *Business and Health May*: 30-38, 2001.

40. Rabin LA, Saykin AJ, West JD, Borgos MJ, Wishart HA, Nutter-Upham KE, et al: Judgment in older adults with normal cognition, cognitive complaints, MCI, and mild AD: relation to regional frontal gray matter, *Brain Imaging Behav* 3(2):212-219, 2009.

41. Rauch SD, Velazquez-Villasenor L, Dimitri PS, Merchant SN: Decreasing hair cell counts in aging humans, *Ann N Y Acad Sci* 942(1):220-227, 2001.

42. Rawson NE: Age-related changes in perception of flavor and aroma, *Generations* 27(1):20-26, 2003.

43. Salthouse TA: Age-related differences in basic cognitive processes: implications for work, *Exp Aging Res* 20:249-255, 1994.

44. Sandmire DA: The physiology and pathology of aging. In Robnett RH, Chop WC, editors: *Gerontology for the health care professional*, ed 2, Sudbury, MA, 2010, Jones and Bartlett, pp 53-113.

45. Schieber F: Vision and aging. In Birren JE, Warner Schaie K, editors: *Handbook of the psychology of aging*, ed 6, San Diego, CA, 2006, Elsevier, pp 129-161.

46. Tun P, Wingfield A: Does dividing attention become harder with age? Findings from the divided attention questionnaire, *Aging Cogn* 2(1):39-66, 1995.

47. Wagnild G: Resilience and successful aging: comparison among low and high income older adults, *J Gerontol Nurs*, 2003 Dec; 29(12):42-49.

48. Warren M: A hierarchical model for evaluation and treatment of visual perceptual dysfunction in adult acquired brain injury, part I, *Am J Occup Ther* 47(1):55, 1993.

49. Wolff JL, Starfield B, Anderson G: Prevalence, expenditures, and complications of multiple chronic conditions in the elderly, *Arch Intern Med* 162:2269-2276, 2002.

50. Woods B, Windle G: Personality in later life: the effects of ageing on personality. In Jacoby R, Oppenheimer C, Dening T, Thomas A, editors: *Oxford textbook of old age psychiatry*, Oxford, UK, 2008, Oxford University Press, pp 591-603.

Emerging Occupational Therapy Practice Areas

Jean W. Solomon, Jane Clifford O'Brien, Judith Clifford Cohn

CHAPTER OUTLINE

Centennial Vision

Emerging Occupational Therapy Practice Areas

Developing Creative Group Protocols in Emerging Areas of Practice

Creative Group Protocols for Emerging Areas of Practice

Summary

KEY TERMS

Centennial Vision

children and youth

creative group protocol

disability

emerging occupational therapy
  practice areas

ergonomics

evaluations

Fitness, yoU, and Nutrition
  (FUN) program

group design and protocol

health and wellness

implementation

mental health

needs assessment

participation

pet-assisted therapy (PAT)

productive aging

rehabilitation

work and industry

CHAPTER OBJECTIVES

1. Describe the American Occupational Therapy Association's *Centennial Vision* and the importance of the vision to the practice of occupational therapy.
2. Identify traditional occupational therapy practice areas and describe the role of the occupational therapy practitioner in these areas.
3. Identify emerging occupational therapy practice areas and describe the role of the occupational therapy practitioner in these areas.
4. Describe a variety of creative group activities addressing emerging areas of practice.

By the year 2017 . . . We envision that occupational therapy is a powerful, widely recognized, science-driven and evidenced-based profession with a globally connected and diverse workforce meeting society's occupational needs."

American Occupational Therapy Association *Centennial Vision*, 2008[1]

Occupational therapy (OT) practitioners are responsible for understanding the meaning of this vision as a way to move the profession forward. In this chapter, we describe the meaning of the **Centennial Vision** statement and how it directs practice. The chapter provides an overview of **emerging OT practice areas** along with creative examples of group programs.

CENTENNIAL VISION

Vision statements are developed to lead organizations or professions. They are designed to help members, consumers, and stakeholders understand the purpose or meaning of the organization or profession. Often the very process of developing a vision statement allows members of the organization to understand the purpose more clearly. Articulating the vision allows all members to work toward the same end goal.

The profession of occupational therapy will be 100 years old in 2017. In preparation for this landmark and in response to society's changing needs, the American Occupational Therapy Association (AOTA) developed its Centennial Vision.[1] AOTA's Centennial Vision statement describes the future of the OT profession as powerful, widely recognized, science driven, and evidence based. A variety of strategies are being implemented to reach this vision.

Powerful: OT practitioners are encouraged to seek leadership roles in health care, education, and policy making to help the profession meet society's needs. The leadership positions will help to move the profession of occupational therapy forward as a powerful profession to better serve clients and their families.

Widely recognized: An image-building campaign has been launched by AOTA to promote the profession such that it will be widely recognized globally. Members are encouraged to promote the profession locally, regionally, nationally, and internationally. The profession will be better able to meet society's health care needs as it becomes more recognized.

Science driven: The profession seeks scientists to engage in research to develop new and effective intervention methods to be used by OT practitioners. The profession will benefit from scientific evidence to support evaluation and intervention.

Evidence based: Using research to support the efficacy of practice benefits the profession, clients, and stakeholders.

Practitioners are urged to use the evidence to provide the best practice. Furthermore, practitioners are encouraged to contribute to the evidence base.

AOTA's Centennial Vision provides direction for the future of the profession considering changes in society. The population is aging, health care costs are rising, and limitations are being placed on reimbursement. There is an increased focus on primary or preventive medicine. The areas of technology and assistive technology are expanding significantly. Universal design for active living is more of the norm rather than the exception. The need for evidence to support best practice continues as clients and consumers search for answers. Lifestyle values are changing and there is growing diversity in the workforce. All of these forces influence the delivery of OT in current and emerging areas of practice.

EMERGING OCCUPATIONAL THERAPY PRACTICE AREAS

A *practice area* refers to a field of work within a profession. Traditional or current areas of practice refer to those areas in which services have been provided for a significant period. AOTA has identified pediatric, psychosocial, and physical rehabilitation as traditional areas of practice. These areas of practice are conducted in school systems, acute care and rehabilitation hospitals, psychiatric centers, skilled-nursing facilities, home health, and private practice clinics.

AOTA in its Centennial Vision has identified six emerging areas of practice. These areas represent practice arenas in which OT practitioners may expand or creatively provide services to better meet society's needs. Following is a brief description of each area and some possibilities for service provision.

- Mental health
- Productive aging
- Children and youth
- Health and wellness
- Work and industry
- Rehabilitation, disability, and participation

Within the **mental health** area there is an increased need to address the psychosocial needs of children and youth. The profession has identified a need to explore areas of mental health in community and school settings rather than traditional hospital settings. For example, children may benefit from services from OT practitioners that focus on behaviors that interfere with educational goals. OT practitioners, who are trained to address the physical and psychosocial issues affecting occupational performance, are in a unique position to address these concerns in school systems or community environments.

Productive aging refers to helping older adults remain in their homes or on their own. As more people age and live healthier lives, services are required to allow them to remain independent. OT practitioners can provide services that allow older persons to live productive lives. For example, the profession has identified the need for low-vision services. OT practitioners can provide support and adaptations to help the older person with low vision continue to engage in a variety of occupations. Identifying specific needs of older adults and helping them remain safely at home are part of the domain of occupational therapy. Refer to Chapter 11 for detailed information on the needs of older persons who wish to remain in their own homes (Figure 12-1).

Although OT practitioners work in early intervention settings and school systems, AOTA has identified the need for practitioners to explore practice with **children and youth** and,

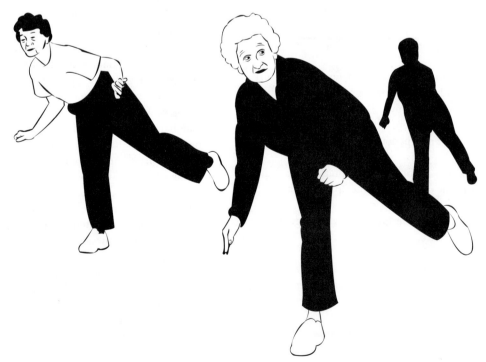

Figure 12-1 A group of older persons doing aerobics at a senior center.

in particular, the area of training in the use of assistive technology. OT professionals can play important roles in assisting children using assistive technology, and helping children transition into the work force (Figure 12-2). Furthermore, practitioners can play a role in facilitating healthy physical and nutritional activity to prevent childhood obesity. An example of a fitness and nutritional group is described at the end of this chapter.

Health and wellness trends are prevalent in the United States. OT practitioners can play a key role in helping people stay healthy and well. Examining habits and routines and designing individualized plans while considering the unique health needs of clients are all within the domain of OT practice. The vision statement views OT practitioners as contributing to this area of practice in creative ways. For example, practitioners may decide to conduct health and wellness classes in skilled-nursing facilities or at community centers.

Exploring opportunities for practitioners to help clients continue to engage in **work and industry** provides a new avenue for the profession. The need for **ergonomics** consulting to promote health and wellness in the work environment continues to evolve. Evaluating and designing effective work environments that promote productivity are all within the realm of OT practice (Figure 12-3).

As science and technology evolve, OT practitioners continue to be involved in **rehabilitating** clients so that they can reengage in desired occupations. This important role is observed as practitioners work with veterans returning from Iraq, Afghanistan, and wars in other parts of the world. Helping service men and women return to their desired occupations is essential and a part of OT's core values. Helping people with **disability participate** in occupations is fundamental to

OT. The profession urges practitioners to explore this area and expand the opportunities for all.

The previous examples are not exclusive and practitioners are urged to explore areas in which OT may be beneficial. Conducting practice that is supported by research promotes the profession and increases the availability of services for clients. Therefore, practitioners are encouraged to describe the findings from these programs and disseminate the results.

DEVELOPING CREATIVE GROUP PROTOCOLS IN EMERGING AREAS OF PRACTICE

Creating innovative programs in emerging areas of practice often provides the first step in developing a scientific base. The steps for developing group protocols include:

- Needs assessment
- Group design or protocol
- Implementation
- Evaluation

A **needs assessment** includes the reasons for the group and often includes a description of the gap that the group is addressing, the rationale for the group, and cost effectiveness of the proposed group. Needs assessments can be formal (complete with a literature review and data) or informal (local need expressed). Many times a needs assessment includes interviews or focus groups with stakeholders or surveys to understand the issues more clearly. Understanding the need is key for effective group intervention. To further provide evidence of the influence of the group on the members and stakeholders, practitioners should document the need prior to implementing the group. This documentation can become part of the group evaluation process.

Once the need for the group is established, the practitioner designs the group protocol. The **group design and protocol**

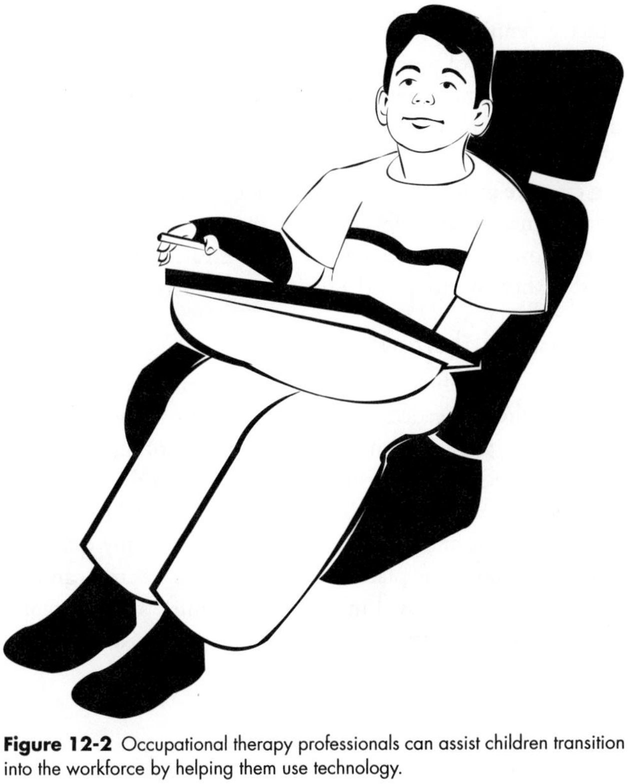

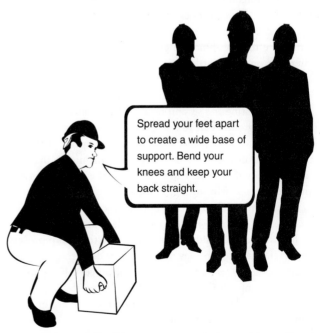

Figure 12-2 Occupational therapy professionals can assist children transition into the workforce by helping them use technology.

Figure 12-3 Occupational therapy practitioners evaluate and design effective work environments to promote productivity.

TABLE 12-1   Group Design and Protocol

Therapist's name: _____	
Title of group	
Overall purpose	
Sample goals	
Time	
Optimal size of group	
Location	
	Directions to location
	Precautions regarding location
	Supervision
Costs	
Equipment needs	
Supplies	
Sequence of events (include time)	
Physical requirements	
Precautions and special considerations	
Notes	
Evaluation methods (survey, outcome)	

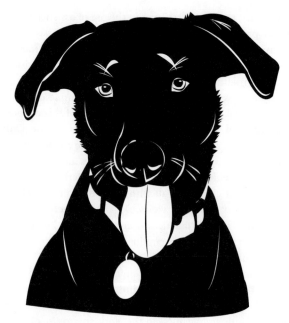

Figure 12-4 A family pet requires training to take part in pet-assisted therapy.

provides the specifics of the group and includes such things as group membership, time, duration, location, purpose, goals, costs, and specific activities. Often budget, supplies, equipment, and supervision are included in the protocol. See Table 12-1 for a template of a group design and protocol. Importantly, practitioners decide in this phase how they will measure the group outcomes. This may be a group evaluation form (survey) or include postdata of client performance, depending on the purpose of the group. However, each group should include a measure to determine the group's effectiveness with special attention on how participation in the group closed the gap identified in the needs assessment.

Implementation of the group involves leading the groups and documenting the session results. Practitioners use knowledge of the group goals to address individual member's goals. They facilitate performance and oversee all aspects of the session. Practitioners understand the group dynamics so that they can intervene if necessary to ensure that the group runs well and members benefit from group sessions.

After completion of each group intervention, practitioners evaluate the process. Practitioners reflect on the success of each session and consider ways to improve the group process. However, practitioners may need to realize that groups struggle (storming stage) as part of the normal process. Refer to the stages of groups in Chapters 1 and 6. During the implementation phase, OT practitioners consider how the group could be more effective and explore alternative ways of leading the group. The practitioner analyzes feedback from members of the groups while examining the goals.

Evaluations can be conducted as focus groups, written surveys, formal evaluations (of performance measures), or through observation. Some administrators may require financial reports. Documentation of the results of the group may provide data to justify additional groups or funding. Importantly, the practitioner evaluates how well the group addressed the needs of the members.

CREATIVE GROUP PROTOCOLS FOR EMERGING AREAS OF PRACTICE

The Centennial Vision encourages OT practitioners to explore emerging areas of practice and develop science supporting this practice. Disseminating the results of group protocols or the design of groups helps practitioners seeking to conduct similar programs and supports the profession's evidence base. Designing **creative group protocols** and conducting program evaluation promotes the profession while serving a variety of clients. The following examples describe two creative groups: a pet-assisted therapy group and a fitness and nutrition group.

Pet-Assisted Therapy*

A goofy black Labrador puppy named Remmy came into my life just when I needed him. As my children went off to college and my youngest entered her senior year of high school, I wondered about my own life transition. "What do I do now?" I pondered on my walks with Remmy. He wagged his tail and explored. Then he looked at me as if to answer my question, "Just keep taking me places, especially places where I can play ball." My family advised me to share Remmy with the world and this series of events led me to explore **pet-assisted therapy** (**PAT**; Figure 12-4).

_____

*By Judith Cohn, MEd

Whether you grew up with or without a pet, everyone remembers wanting a dog, wanting to ride a horse, or admiring that adorable fluffy kitten at the pet store. It is difficult not to respond to an animal. The animal-human bond is unique and it brings out one's compassion. Animals may elicit memories from childhood and they can be calming. When working in a therapeutic field, such as OT, there are many approaches to developing relationships, including PAT. PAT can help individuals work on a variety of skills.

In the 1950s, Dr. Boris Levinson, a New York psychologist, was working with a troubled teenager. The boy attended several sessions but he would not talk. One afternoon, Dr. Levinson went into the waiting room to get the boy for his weekly appointment. The doctor heard talking and was surprised when he realized that the teenager was talking to Jingles, Dr. Levinson's pet dog. The doctor included Jingles in therapy sessions from that point on and found that Jingles presence somehow gave the teenager the courage to share and talk. Dr. Levinson documented the success of including his pet in therapy and he is credited as the founder of PAT.[12]

Since that time, others have documented the influence of pets in prisons, hospitals, mental health facilities, schools, and skilled-nursing facilities.[2,5,9] PAT has been successful in helping people with disabilities, older people, people who have endured abuse, and students. Katcher and colleagues[5] found that interacting with a pet lowered blood pressure, whereas interacting with a person, even in one's own family, raised blood pressure. In another study, Martin examined the influence of a PAT program on children with pervasive developmental disorders and found that those children exposed to PAT exhibited a more playful mood, were more focused, and were more aware of their social surroundings.[7] Within a year of the program, there were visible changes in many depressed nonverbal patients.[7] Studies suggest numerous psychological benefits from interacting with pets, including increased positive affective state, humor, play, self-esteem, need to be needed, independence, motivation, education, and sense of achievement.[2,5,7] Others have found social and physical benefits from a PAT program, namely social cohesion, cooperation with caregivers, recovery from illness, and increased ability to cope with illness.[7,9,11]

OT practitioners may choose to work with a pet facilitator or to become certified themselves as a way to introduce pets to clients served in OT practice.

PAT programs are designed to maintain a healthy, safe, and appropriate therapeutic environment for the pet, client, and facilitator. To ensure that this happens, the pet guardian (owner) is educated in the field of PAT and family pets are involved. The therapy pet must be up to date on all immunizations, see a veterinarian, be groomed regularly, and be in good health. It is important that the therapy pet be well mannered and practice obedience skills daily. Because the pet needs to be healthy, he or she will participate in socialization time (with and without other dogs) and recreational activities such as playing fetch with a ball.

Clients are specifically referred for PAT in their intervention plans. They must be oriented to the pet and provided time to feel comfortable with the pet. The pet guardian must possess

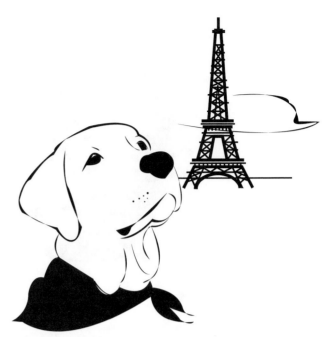

Figure 12-5 Viewing pets at recognizable places may help clients engage in conversations that stimulate cognitive processing.

adequate insurance and supervise the pet at all times. The pet facilitator monitors the session to determine the length of the visit based on the current situation and interaction.

Session Standards

The pet, client, and facilitator meet in a safe and appropriate location. The therapy pet and client are given time to adjust to the new situation, become comfortable with each other, and build a relationship. The pet facilitator instructs the client in ways to approach the therapy pet and treat the animal with respect.

Each session is unique, depending on the needs of the client, the number of clients in the group, and the setting. Sessions should not last more than one hour and may be shorter if the client and pet are tired. Professionals using PAT use their creativity to accomplish the therapeutic goals of the clients. The presence of the pet drives the session. However, the pet is not "performing" but is present and often a member of an interdisciplinary team that might include a social worker, physical therapist, occupational therapist, or other professional. The activity is focused around the pet and the needs of the client.

The facilitator makes sure that his pet is safe, secure, and treated kindly. Once the guidelines are in place, the therapy pet is introduced to the clients and the session begins.

PAT is driven by the human-pet bond. For example, if the client is an older person living in isolation, the pet's presence may encourage the client to talk about what he or she knows about pets, recollections of past pets, or experiences around animals. Caryl Freedman, a certified professional PAT facilitator, designed an arts-based program called "Paws Four a Hug."[3] Freedman uses photo editing software to place images of her dog within images of famous places (e.g., Paris, France) (Figure 12-5). These photos elicit memories of traveling or spark conversation about a movie or book. When working in

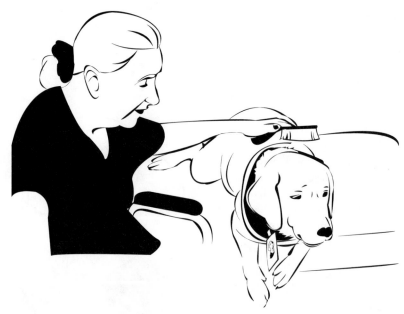

Figure 12-6 Occupational therapy practitioners may choose to engage clients in pet-assisted therapy to help them prepare for caring for their own pet. Caring for one's pet is an instrumental activity of daily living.

skilled-nursing facilities or assisted-living residences, the presence of a dog might be enough to bring smiles to clients. Sometimes people just need a connection.[3]

OT practitioners may include the presence of a pet to achieve a variety of goals. Petting, brushing, feeding, and walking a dog are all ways to incorporate motor skills. Brushing the dog provides the opportunity to practice many skills, including dynamic balance, posture, sequencing, timing, holding, grasping, manipulating, and bilateral hands skills. Making dog biscuits ties into the life skills of following a recipe, measuring, and baking, and incorporates a variety of motor and cognitive abilities. OT practitioners can work with a client to teach him or her how to be a responsible pet owner. Pet responsibility is considered an instrumental activity of daily living (IADL) and as such part of the domain of occupational therapy. Practitioners may choose to engage clients in PAT to help them prepare for caring for their own pet (Figure 12-6).

Clients, along with the pet facilitator, can walk with the pet in public settings to encourage social participation. Walking a dog is a quick way to urge clients to interact with others because people cannot resist asking someone about a furry dog. Clients who are isolated or working on communication skills may interact with others more easily when the dog is present. Taking clients to the dog park may help them converse more easily. Furthermore, there are many writing and reading activities that clients can do in relation to pets. For example, clients can write letters, cards, poems, and memories of their pets. They can read stories, poems, and information about pets.

Each pet facilitator plans activities to help clients reach their goals and objectives with the pet as the focal point. The facilitator can be creative while planning activities considering the client's and pet's needs. PAT can work in many different settings from prisons to schools and with many different populations from preschoolers to older persons. OT practitioners are in a unique position to use this modality as a creative option for therapy.

PAT is an emerging profession and OT practitioners may benefit from become facilitators and including pets as part of therapy. Involving pets in a therapeutic setting stimulates the human-animal bond and can bring out the best in people.

The presence of a fluffy white kitten or lanky black dog makes everyone smile. Remmy is a great therapy pet. He is gentle, smart, and fun. He loves to play and he is happy sitting quietly and being petted. He loves to go to new places and although at times can be skeptical, he soon opens up. As a therapy pet, he has helped our family progress through life changes. Therapy is most effective when the participants (human and nonhuman) enjoy it.

Sample Lesson Plan for a Pet-Assisted Therapy Group Session

The following lesson plan illustrates how OT practitioners may use PAT to address client goals.

Group Members: Six teenaged students who have various behavioral issues, the OT practitioner, PAT facilitator, and pet dog (Remmy) will be present (Figure 12-7).

Group Goal: Students will establish a sense of caring and the ability to connect with others through engaging in the pet therapy sessions.

Objective: The students will express pleasure when practicing basic obedience skills with the pet. Students will interact with others by using positive communication. Students will show kindness and caring behaviors with the pet.

Method: The practitioner and pet facilitator begin by introducing the session, stating the guidelines for how to treat the pet, and demonstrating basic commands with Remmy. They emphasize that the pet is always treated kindly and positive behaviors are reinforced (with a dog treat or through petting). The adolescents are encouraged to respect others at all times.

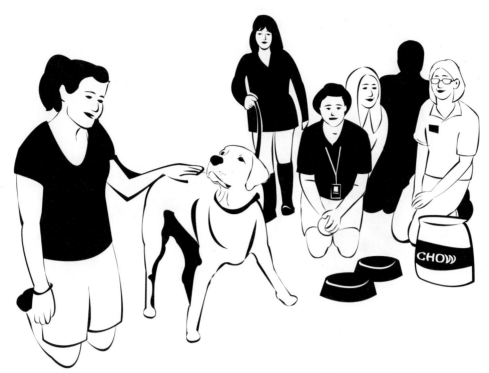

Figure 12-7 Pet-assisted therapy allows clients to interact with pets as part of their occupational therapy intervention plan.

Each teen takes a turn practicing a basic obedience skill. One at a time, the students instruct the dog to sit, stay, down, leave it, watch me, or come. The students are educated regarding proper hand techniques and commands. While one student works with the pet, another student takes photos using a digital camera.

Each adolescent gets his or her photo and is asked to write about the experience working with the dog. The students share their papers and discuss questions, such as "How do you think the pet did? Why do you think he was able to do so well? Why is it important as a pet owner to teach your dog basic obedience?"

The OT practitioner emphasizes the positive behaviors and communication skills that the adolescents displayed. The pet facilitator reminds the members that the dog practices every day and he has been to a lot of classes. They review the responsibilities required of pet owners. The teens discuss caring for pets and the things they like about pets.

   Conclusion: The session provides teens with the opportunity to succeed and interact with an animal. Teens are able to communicate with others about the experience and receive feedback from the animal. The response from the dog is reaffirming to children who may bond and feel a connection with the animal.

Fitness, yoU, and Nutrition (FUN) Program[†]

Childhood obesity is a growing national problem with one third of all youth falling into the category of overweight (body mass index between the 85th and 95th percentiles) or obese

[†]Jane O'Brien, PhD, OTR/L Courtney Craib, MS, OTR/L Lindsey Holmes, MS, OTR/L Kira Keough, MS, OTR/L Loren LePage, MS, OTR/L Erin O'Brien, MS, OTR/L

(body mass index over 95th percentile). Obese and overweight children are at risk for developing serious health problems such as diabetes, heart disease, sleep disorders, apnea, and asthma.[8] AOTA[1] recognizes programs to prevent childhood obesity as an emerging area of practice.

Multiple factors contribute to childhood obesity; these include deprivation, low socioeconomic status, prolonged television viewing, poor leisure facilities, low consumption of fruits and vegetables, poor school meals, and low expenditure on food.[4,10] Thus, programs that use a multifaceted approach to wellness by incorporating diet, exercise, and family involvement are more effective than those targeting weight alone[10,13]

Importantly, OT practitioners are interested in the routines and habits for physical activity as well as the child's motivation toward healthy activities. Increasing children's values, interests, and motivation toward a variety of physical activities may lead to lifelong participation or engagement in activities.[6] One's values, motivations, and interests as well as how the child perceives his or her skills and abilities are referred to as *volition.*[5] Children who are obese frequently suffer decreased volition, which leads to more eating or poor choices of foods, which may then lead to lower self-esteem and in turn a more sedentary lifestyle. Helping children and families participate in volitionally oriented activities enables them to feel empowered and motivates continued involvement. Therefore, programs that stimulate a child's volition or motivations can serve to increase one's sense of self and lead to wellness.[6]

The **Fitness, yoU, and Nutrition (FUN)** program uses a multilevel approach to improving health and wellness in children and families. The FUN program, designed by OTs and based on the Model of Human Occupation (MOHO),[6] provides

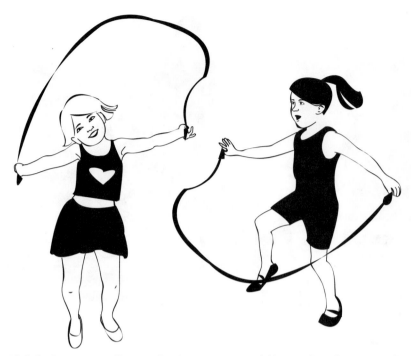

Figure 12-8 The Fitness, yoU, and Nutrition (FUN) program engages children in volitionally motivating physical and nutritional activities.

children with a variety of physical and nutritional activities to explore and discover, which they find motivating, interesting, and valuable. The FUN program stresses changing one's habits and routines for a healthy lifestyle through fun and interesting activities.

This program was based on the MOHO and specifically addresses each subsystem.

Volition: Develop interesting and fun activities so that children will continue to engage in them after the program is finished. Activities are designed to allow children to explore a variety of noncompetitive games. The leaders encourage children to create new activities for themselves. For example, some children enjoy playing outside. The leaders might challenge the children to make a snowman in the winter and find as many different leaves as possible in the fall.

Habituation: Children complete weekly nutritional and physical activity journals. As a way to encourage healthy habits and routines, children are reminded about goals. The group leaders continue to bring up the weekly goals. Parents and family members are advised to engage in the healthy routines as well. To help everyone participate, the team provides a booklet describing weekly sessions and goals.

Performance Capacity: Children are encouraged to participate in the games and play to their level. All activities are designed to be fun and structured so that all children can participate. The group leaders intervene in subtle ways to playfully help children achieve. The focus of the FUN program is on allowing all children to engage in physical and nutritional activities. Games and activities are easily modified so that all children are successful.

Environment: The program takes place at the children's school and in their community. Parents are invited to participate in activities if they want. Helping the children participate in healthy physical and nutritional activities in their own environment may increase carryover. The group leaders incorporate community events into lesson plans. For example, in one program the leaders played a "fishing game" during the same week as the local fishing tournament and reminded the children to participate in the fishing tournament. The leaders provided a healthy hot cocoa recipe and discussed the importance of getting outside even when it is cold. The leaders reinforced environmental opportunities as they arose throughout the sessions. Some children invited classmates to join them. By becoming aware of environmental opportunities, the FUN program helps sustain ongoing healthy habits.

FUN Program Design

All children are invited to participate in the after-school program that meets for 10 weeks at the school. Parents sign consents and complete demographic information, and children are measured on height and weight. Children complete pre- and post-program surveys, an interest checklist, and weekly activity and nutrition journals.

Each week, children participate in 40 minutes of physical activity followed by 30 minutes of a nutritional snack and activity (Figure 12-8). The group leaders emphasize a healthy habit for the week (e.g., drink plenty of water, not soda) and a physical activity goal (e.g., do something outside for one hour every day). Each session is developed around a theme (Table 12-2). Children receive an incentive

TABLE 12-2   FUN Sample Weekly Lesson Plans

Theme	Physical Activity	Physical Goal	Nutritional Activity	Nutritional Goal
Food Pyramid	Relay races through the food pyramid	2 hours of activity a day	Make a plate of food using all the food groups.	Eat a variety of foods.
Pajama Day (healthy breakfast)	Wake up stretches and walking and running games	Start morning active	Make a breakfast snack of fruit, yogurt, granola cups.	Start your morning with a healthy breakfast.
Pioneer Day (whole grains)	Old fashioned games: Red Light–Green Light Hopscotch Jump rope Simon Says	Fun nonexpensive ways to be active	Make your own trail mix with nuts, berries, raisins, pretzels, seeds.	Replace two favorite foods with whole grains. Eat more whole grains.
Beach day (fruit and water)	Hula hoop games, beach ball games, get the "fish in the water"	Moving and getting ready for summer	Make fruit kabobs.	Drink water instead of soda drinks. Eat a fruit a day.
Out of This World (vegetables)	Large ball games, relay races "around the solar system"	Activity for 2 hours a day.	Name the vegetable and food (fruit). Children try new and different foods.	Eat a vegetable a day. Try new foods.
Farm Day (milk)	Animal races—walk like an animal (e.g., bear, crab, cow, horse)	Jump rope games to be active	Make milk shakes—add flavors to milk and shake!	Drink 2 cups of milk a day.
Strength (protein)	Soccer games, lifting balls, and doing aerobic activity to music	Noncompetitive ball games to make you strong	Make peanut butter or soy butter sushi (see recipe), (Box 12-1) meat and protein platter.	Eat more protein snacks.

to continue the physical activity at home. For example, they receive things such as a hula hoop, jump rope, ball, and Frisbee. They bring home healthy snacks such as fruit, vegetables, cheese, trail mix, and water.

Parents receive a booklet describing the weekly activities and emphasizing the weekly goals. Families are encouraged to participate in the healthy activities. The children are encouraged to have fun and be active during the session (Figure 12-9). The focus of the group session is on having fun with peers. Table 12-2 provides an outline of the weekly sessions.

SAMPLE LESSON PLANS FOR THE FUN PROGRAM

The following lesson plans provide the OT practitioner with ideas on how to develop creative groups to promote healthy physical and nutritional activities for children.

Theme: Beach Day (fruit and water)
Goals
- Play outside for one hour a day.
- Replace soda and sugar drinks with water.

Physical Activity
Children played beach ball games and hula hoop to beach music. They were shown a variety of ways to play with the hula hoop.

Nutritional Activity
Children made fruit kabobs and talked about summer fruit. They discussed the sugar content in soda and fruit drinks.

Box 12-1   Banana Sushi

Wheat bread
Banana
Peanut butter, soy butter, Apple butter or nutella

1. Roll out wheat bread into thin slice with a rolling pin.
2. Spread with peanut butter, soy butter, nutella and/or apple butter.
3. Place banana on edge and roll bread around it.
4. Press tightly so bread stays around banana.
5. Cut into small 'sushi' sized bites

The leaders showed bottles full of sugar to illustrate the amount of sugar in soda drinks.

Take-Home Incentives

Children brought hula hoops, water bottles, and fresh fruit home. They were encouraged to play and see if they could hula hoop in different ways.

Theme: Out of this World (vegetables)

Goals
- Eat a serving of veggies with every meal.
- Play active, outdoor games.

Physical Activity

Children played "out of this world" Frisbee games. Children tried to throw Frisbees at "space" targets. Children were

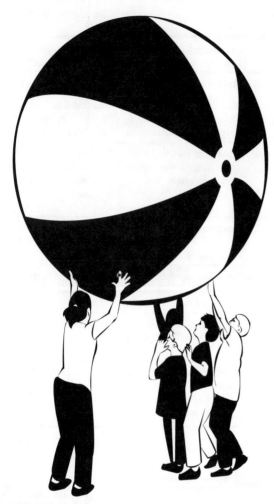

Figure 12-9 Children enjoy playing games with peers and are more inclined to continue to participate in fun and interesting activities.

asked to run "through space" and stop (when they heard the whistle from the aliens) and throw the Frisbee to the other side of the room, run and get the Frisbee, and continue.

Nutritional Activity

Children made vegetable aliens using toothpicks and vegetables. They ate their aliens and tried vegetable chips. Children discussed how they could add vegetables to their diet and each child chose a favorite vegetable.

Take-Home Incentives

Frisbee, carrot sticks with peanut butter packet, celery stick packet, vegetable drink.

Children were encouraged to eat more vegetables and play outside with the Frisbee.

SUMMARY

The Centennial Vision provides a vision for the OT profession that includes a powerful, science-based profession that meets society's needs. The vision involves developing emerging areas of practice while strengthening the evidence and support for practice. This chapter provides an overview of the vision and some examples of how to explore the emerging areas of practice. It provides practical and applicable information for creating and implementing innovative group protocols in emerging practice areas. Two unique groups in less traditional practice areas are described.

REVIEW QUESTIONS

1. What is the purpose of AOTA's Centennial Vision?
2. List the four adjectives used to describe the profession of occupational therapy and give examples of how practitioners can participate such that the vision is met by the year 2017.
3. List and describe the role of the OT practitioner in the identified practice areas.
4. List and give examples of the components of developing and designing a creative group protocol.

REFERENCES

1. American Occupational Therapy Association: *Centennial vision*, 2008, Retrieved 4/15/2012 from http://www.aota.org/News/Centennial/Background/36516.aspx?FT=.pdf.
2. Brickel CM: The clinical use of pets with the aged, *Clin Gerontol* 2(4):72-75.
3. Freedman C: Personal communication, 9/20/2011.
4. Hesketh K, Waters E, Green J, Salmon L, Williams J: Healthy eating, activity and obesity prevention: a qualitative study of parent and child perceptions in Australia, *Health Promot Int* 20(1):19-26, 2005.
5. Katcher A, Friedmann E, Beck A, Lynch J: Looking, talking, and blood pressure: the physiological consequences of interaction with the living environment. In Katcher A, Beck A, editors: *New perspectives on our lives*

with companion animals, Philadelphia, 1983, University of Pennsylvania Press.
6. Kielhofner G: *Model of human occupation: theory and application*, ed 4, Baltimore, 2008, Lippincott, Williams & Wilkins.
7. Martin F: Animal-assisted therapy for children with pervasive developmental disorders, *West J Nurs Res* 24(6):657-670, 2002.
8. Mayo Clinic: *Childhood obesity*. Retrieved 10/3/2007 from http://www.mayoclinic.com/health/childhood-obesity/DS00698/DSECTION=risk.
9. National Institute of Health: *Can pets keep you healthy? Exploring the human-animal bond*, 2009, Retrieved 4/15/2012 from http://newsinhealth.nih.gov/pdf/NIHNiH%20Feb09.pdf.

10. Proctor KL, Clarke GP, Ransley JK, Cade J: Micro-level analysis of childhood obesity, diet, physical activity, residential socioeconomic and social capital variables, *Area* 40(3):323-340, 2008.
11. Rathsam S: Puppy uppers, *Parks & Recreation* 37(11):58-62, Nov 2002.
12. Salotto: *Pet assisted therapy: a loving intervention and an emerging profession: leading to a friendlier, healthier, and more peaceful world*, Norton, MA, 2001, DJ Publications.
13. Speroni KG, Earley C, Atherton M: Evaluating the effectiveness of the kids living fit program: a comparative study, *J School Nurs* 26(6):329-337, 2007.

Ethical Practice

Michelle Parolise, Deborah Hyman

KEY TERMS

autonomy	fidelity
beneficence	locus of authority
confidentiality	morals
conflict resolution	nonmaleficence
deontologic theories	procedural justice
divine command	social justice
ethical dilemma	teleologic theories
ethical distress	veracity
ethics	virtue ethics

CHAPTER OBJECTIVES

1. Outline the steps to ethical decision making.
2. Identify the seven ethical principles as outlined in the American Occupational Therapy Association Code of Ethics.
3. Discuss ethical considerations that may occur specific to groups.
4. Describe the ethical principles found in ethical scenarios specific to occupational therapy practice.
5. Outline the resolution and enforcement process for the code of ethics.
6. Understand the importance of following a professional code of ethics.

The American Occupational Therapy Association (AOTA) Code of Ethics is a "statement of principles used to promote and maintain high standards of conduct" in all occupational therapy (OT) practice. It serves as a "guide to professional conduct when ethical issues arise."[4] Inevitably, ethical issues and the need to establish the best outcome to a dilemma arise in practice, because OT practitioners have intimate contact with and a profound influence on the lives of the individuals, groups, and populations they serve. Although each OT practitioner has a personal set of values, he or she represents the profession as a whole when interacting with clients, caregivers, colleagues, authority figures, and subordinates. An understanding of the AOTA Code of Ethics[4] is essential for carrying out one's professional responsibilities.

After providing a brief description of ethical theory, the chapter outlines the ethical decision-making process and clearly presents the principles of the AOTA Code of Ethics.[4] Providing case scenarios specific to OT practice helps to reinforce the concepts. The chapter concludes with a discussion of the enforcement and resolution process.

ETHICAL THEORY

Morals are the personal values, principles, and beliefs that determine what is right and wrong for the individual.[13] Many theories of moral development exist. Freud proposed that the child's relationship with his or her parents affects moral development. Kohlberg, Piaget, and Gilligan link moral development to cognitive and physical development. They hypothesize that the child moves through stages of value acquisition as he or she develops. Gilligan theorizes that males and females differ in this respect.[6] Massey attributes the development of morals to events that take place during childhood and adolescence that result in a group or generation that subscribes to a similar morality.[6] Social learning theorists like Bandura view moral behavior as learned through modeling and reinforced by rewards and punishments.[9]

Ethics are a "system for decision making in the arena of moral values."[6] Both morals and ethics are culture based and influenced by factors such as age, ethnicity and race, religion, gender, gender identification, environment, social milieu, personality, emotional makeup, intelligence, physical health, economic status. The degree of control that an individual perceives himself or herself as having influences the ethical position.[10] Ethical theories provide the framework for decision making and help define ways to solve professional dilemmas. These theories can be categorized as follows:

Virtue ethics examine the characteristics of the individual and theorize that the individual with certain traits (such as compassion) behave in an appropriate way.[8]

Divine command ethics postulate that there is a set of rules created by a divine source for directing of moral behavior.[13]

Teleologic theories hold that an action is ethical or unethical depending on its consequence. In practice, teleologic theories look for a solution to a dilemma that will achieve the best outcome for the most number of people.[8]

Deontologic theories hold that an action itself is either ethical or unethical with no regard for its consequence. When applied, deontologic theories hold that there is a universal duty to obey rules and follow principles.[8]

Professional organizations such as AOTA provide its members with guidance in dealing with ethical dilemmas.[3,4,13] The establishment and enforcement of the code of ethics ensure maintenance of the standards of the profession. Practitioners rely on professional ethics as opposed to moral beliefs. The ethical decision-making process involves a systematic reasoning structure to enable practitioners to make professional decisions.

ETHICAL DECISION MAKING

OT practitioners facing potential ethical dilemmas use a process to guide their analysis and subsequent actions. Purtilo[11] lists six steps to assist OT practitioners to arrive at a "caring response" (Box 13-1). The "caring response" includes meeting client needs and performing professional responsibilities.

These steps provide a method to thoughtfully act on ethical issues as they arise, staying in agreement with the AOTA Code of Ethics. Some situations cross legal boundaries. Thus, when gathering data and considering alternative courses of action, practitioners examine laws or regulations for practice.[8]

The OT practitioner should reflect on the outcome using the following questions as guides[5,8,11]:

1. Is it the truth?
2. Is it fair to all concerned?
3. Will it build goodwill and better friendships?
4. Will it be beneficial to all concerned?

Reflection facilitates professional growth and provides the practitioner with tools for resolving subsequent situations.

AOTA CODE OF ETHICS—PRINCIPLES

The AOTA Ethics Commission (EC) informs and educates OT personnel regarding ethical matters and ensures compliance with the ethical standards.[2,3] The ethical standards of OT can be found in three documents: Occupational Therapy Code of Ethics[4], Guidelines to the Occupational Therapy Code of Ethics[2], and Core Values and Attitudes of Occupational Therapy

Practice.[1] The procedures to enforce the Code of Ethics are described in "Enforcement Procedures for the Occupational Therapy Code of Ethics and Ethics Standards."[3] The Code of Ethics is based on the core values of the OT profession (Box 13-2). Table 13-1 presents the principles of the AOTA Code of Ethics.

Ethical dilemmas occur when there is a struggle to decide what course of action to take in a difficult situation. The "Occupational Therapy Code of Ethics and Ethics Standard"[4] provides standards to guide practitioners in making the right choice to protect the public and the profession. The following scenarios are based on real-life situations that we have encountered and serve to illustrate a range of ethical dilemmas presented in OT practice. OT practitioners rely on knowledge of

---

BOX 13-1   Steps to Ethical Decision Making[11]

Step 1: Gather relevant information.
- What is the context of the dilemma?
- What is the situation?
- What are the associated facts?
- Who are the involved players?

Step 2: Identify the type of ethical problem.
- **Ethical distress** is the discomfort experienced when the OT practitioner is prevented from doing what is believed to be right.
- An **ethical dilemma** occurs when the practitioner is required to choose between conflicting alternatives.
- The **locus of authority** problem questions who should resolve ethical issues.

Step 3: Use ethical theories or approaches to analyze the problems.
- Examine the AOTA Code of Ethics, Standards of Practice, and laws and regulations.
- Define the principles involved according to the Code of Ethics.

Step 4: Explore the alternatives.
- Who will benefit?
- Will anyone be hurt?

Step 5: Complete the action.
Step 6: Evaluate the process and outcome.

AOTA, American Occupational Therapy Association; *OT*, occupational therapy.
Adapted from Purtilo R. (2005). Ethical Dimensions in the Health Professions, ed. 5, St. Louis, Saunders.

BOX 13-2   Core Values and Attitudes of Occupational Therapy Practice[1]

Altruism: caring, an unselfish concern for and desire to help others
Equality: fairness in all interactions and seeing all people as having equal rights
Freedom: respect for the client's personal choice and self-direction
Justice: being impartial in all interactions and adhering to laws and standards
Dignity: treating all clients with respect and assisting them to participate in meaningful occupations
Truth: honesty in all written and verbal communication
Prudence: self-discipline; moderation; and the use of reasoning, judgment, and reflection in making decisions

ethical decision making and the Code of Ethics when deciding the best course of action.

BENEFICENCE

Principle 1: "Occupational therapy personnel shall demonstrate a concern for the well-being and safety of the recipients of their services."[4]

The term **beneficence** refers to the act of producing good, as in an act of charity.[10] Beneficence is consistent with the OT core value of altruism. AOTA interprets this principle as meaning that OT personnel need to take action to not only provide service that is for the good of their clients but to also protect their clients from harm.[4] Working in a service profession such as OT does not automatically make a person altruistic. Being altruistic involves an attitude of doing good for every client. Beneficence requires OT personnel to put the needs of the client above personal needs or the needs of the facility.

To carry out this principle, OT personnel must have an understanding of the scope of OT practice and remain competent. Thus, practitioners use current equipment and provide evidence-based intervention. Responses to referral, completion of evaluations, and periodic reassessment should be completed in a timely manner to ensure that the client is receiving the best possible care and that services are terminated when the client is no longer able to benefit from them. The OT practitioner must be able to determine when the client could benefit from the services of another discipline and make necessary referrals. Finally, OT personnel must report behavior that is unethical when it is observed.[3,4]

TABLE 13-1	Ethical Principles[4]
Principle 1: Beneficence	Occupational therapy personnel shall demonstrate a concern for the well being and safety of the recipients of their services.
Principle 2: Nonmaleficence	Occupational therapy personnel shall intentionally refrain from actions that cause harm.
Principle 3: Autonomy and Confidentiality	Occupational therapy personnel shall respect the right of the individual to self-determination.
Principle 4: Social Justice	Occupational therapy personnel shall provide services in a fair and equitable manner.
Principle 5: Procedural Justice	Occupational therapy personnel shall comply with institutional rules; local, state, federal, and international laws; and AOTA documents applicable to the profession of occupational therapy.
Principle 6: Veracity	Occupational therapy personnel shall provide comprehensive, accurate, and objective information when representing the profession.
Principle 7: Fidelity	Occupational therapy personnel shall treat colleagues and other professionals with respect, fairness, discretion, and integrity.

AOTA, American Occupational Therapy Association.
Data from American Occupational Therapy Association: Enforcement procedures for the Occupational Therapy Code of Ethics and Ethics Standards, *Am J Occup Ther* 64(Suppl.):S4-S16, 2010.

CASE SCENARIO

Adam, a new OT graduate, accepts his job in a hand clinic where he is promised mentoring during his first year of employment. In his first week, the clinic receives more than the normal number of referrals and one of the practitioners is out sick. The supervisor asks Adam to complete an evaluation on his own, stating that someone will review it with him during the next week. Adam feels unsure of his ability to complete the evaluation effectively, but he does not want to disappoint the supervisor and he wants to demonstrate a helping attitude. What should Adam do?

Application: *The principle of beneficence suggests that Adam should not do the evaluation if he does not have the competency to complete it independently because he could make an error that would cause harm to the client. However, Adam may demonstrate his helpful attitude in other ways. One suggestion may be that he could pair up with a more experienced OT to help with the evaluation. He could then independently complete the parts of the evaluation in which he is competent; the experienced OT could complete the rest of it. He could also offer to cover client interventions, allowing the experienced OT time to do the evaluations.*

NONMALEFICENCE

Principle 2: "Occupational therapy personnel shall intentionally refrain from actions that cause harm."[4]

Nonmaleficence is an "ethical principle of doing no harm."[16] On the surface, this may seem like a simple principle because it seems obvious that an OT practitioner would not want to harm any client. However, there are inherent risks in some aspects of OT intervention that can cause harm regardless of the intent to do good. Before starting treatment, the OT practitioner must identify the risk of the intervention and proceed only if the benefits outweighs the potential risks.[11] For example, the practitioner may consider taking a risk with a client to increase his or her independence, or the practitioner may decide to limit the client's independence because of safety concerns.

AOTA outlines circumstances that have the potential to cause harm and cautions OT practitioners to avoid any relationship or activity that could exploit the recipient of services; compromise the therapeutic relationship; or inhibit making clear, objective decisions.[2,4] These activities include conflicts of interest, sexual relationships, personal problems, or anything that blurs the boundaries of the relationship between the client and OT practitioner. It is important to understand the differences between a friendship and a therapeutic relationship. Friendships are give-and-take relationships that are beneficial to both parties involved. A therapeutic relationship is intentional and the client is always the focus.[14] Having a friendship with a client can cloud judgment and result in a violation of this principle. This concept suggests that practitioners resolve their own personal problems so they are equipped to work with a variety of clients. Personal problems can result in the practitioner being intolerant, mentally unavailable, or treating the client as a sounding board, all of which can be potentially harmful.

Nonmaleficence includes the practitioner's duty to avoid abandoning the client when the OT services can no longer be provided by helping the client transition to appropriate services.[4] This may be especially difficult when working with a client who has limited financial or human resources available. The OT practitioner needs to be aware of resources offered in the community and work closely with other disciplines to arrange for the best possible outcome.

CASE SCENARIO

Dena is a certified occupational therapy assistant (COTA) working in a school-based practice. During an individualized education plan (IEP) meeting, the team decides that the child will not be afforded treatment over the summer. The mother is hesitant but eventually agrees to the plan. (Figure 13-1A) After the meeting, the mother speaks to Dena privately and offers to pay Dena $100 per week to provide OT services in their home (Figure 13-1B, 13-1C). Dena explains that she cannot provide services without an OT supervisor. The mother states that it does not need to be called "OT" and

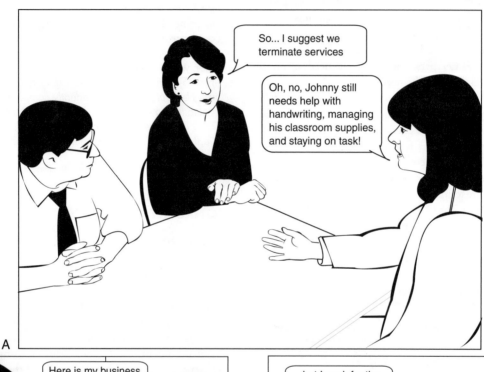

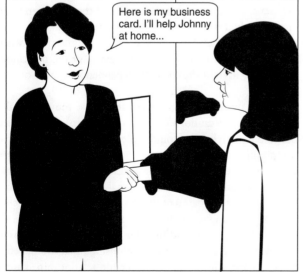

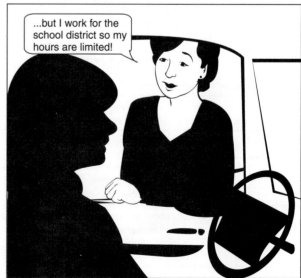

Figure 13-1 *Nonmaleficence:* Occupational therapy practitioners are expected to advocate for clients and engage in therapeutic relationships that allow clients to make objective decisions. In this example, the practitioner should be advocating in the individualized education plan meeting and not arranging outside services. **A,** The practitioner agrees with team members that the child should not receive services. **B,** Following the meeting, the practitioner suggests to the mother that the child would benefit from services. **C,** The practitioner suggests that she can provide the services but not through the school.

that no paperwork will be required. Dena feels uncertain but she really needs the money. What should she do?

Application: *Although this may sound tempting, this situation represents a conflict of interest. Although the mother is not calling it "OT," the COTA is being asked to attend to the child because of her professional role. If Dena accepts the work, it implies that the child really does need treatment over the summer. This could put the school district in a bad light with the parents and open up some potential legal problems. If Dena and the supervising OT feel strongly that the child needs treatment over the summer, they should have advocated for the child during the IEP meeting. Dena should not accept this private work.*

AUTONOMY AND CONFIDENTIALITY

Principle 3: "Occupational therapy personnel shall respect the right of the individual to self-determination."[4]

Confidentiality is essential in all areas of health care. OT personnel have access to privileged personal health information and they are responsible for protecting this information during verbal, written, and electronic communication.[11] They must understand and follow the Health Insurance Portability and Accountability Act of 1996.

Personal rights, freedom, and autonomy are highly valued concepts and are consistent with client-centered care. The term *self-determination* refers to the client making decisions regarding personal health care. To make an informed decision, the client must be aware of the purpose of the intervention, including the possible risks and benefits. Practitioners are responsible for informing clients fully. Collaboration between the practitioner, the client, and family members is key. Collaboration is more than just choosing goals; it includes updates on progress, selection of intervention activities, and changes in goals as needed. Collaboration is more difficult when working with a client who has impaired judgment, cognitive skills, or speech skills. **Autonomy** refers to the client's right to make choices about his or her intervention, including the right to refuse intervention. The OT practitioner is responsible for making every attempt to communicate with the client, family, or conservator of the client. Once a client is informed, the practitioner must respect the client's decisions regarding intervention.

CASE SCENARIO

Anna is an OT working in an outpatient day treatment program for adults with brain injuries. Eve, one of her clients, is a 32-year-old woman who has good receptive speech but moderate expressive aphasia. One day, Eve compliments Anna's hair and asks her what product she uses to color it. Anna tells her that she can purchase the product from her hairdresser, who works locally. Later that day Anna calls the hairdresser, telling him that one of her clients is going to come in to buy hair color. She does not provide Eve's name or specific information but does say that Eve has difficulty with speech. She does not tell Eve that she did this because she wants her to feel good about her ability to communicate in the community. Is Anna in violation of the code of ethics?

Application: *Anna has good intentions; however, calling the hairdresser is a breach of confidentiality. The fact that she does not provide Eve's name or diagnostic information does not make it less of a violation of confidentiality. Although the hairdresser would be able to ascertain that Eve had a speech problem, he would have no right to know that she was one of Anna's clients. Anna is not being truthful with Eve (Principle 6, veracity) regarding her community skills. If Eve was unable to do this task on her own, then Anna should have suggested that she have a family member or friend assist her with it.*

SOCIAL JUSTICE

Principle 4: "Occupational therapy personnel shall provide services in a fair and equitable manner."[4]

Social justice is also called *distributive justice* and this refers to "normative principles designed to guide the allocation of the benefits and burdens of economic activity."[6] Social justice ensures a fair distribution of resources so that individuals and groups receive fair treatment and the opportunity to participate in society.[4]

The need to reform the system for health care in the United States is a topic of significant debate. One of the major problems is the high number of people who do not have health insurance. It is estimated that more than 41 million Americans are uninsured.[12] Many of these people need OT services. Government-sponsored health insurance is available for certain groups. For example, Medicare is a federal program that provides insurance for people who are older than 65 or who have certain disabilities. Medicaid is administered by states to provide insurance to certain people who have low income and fit into recognized eligibility groups.[15]

Social justice refers to fairly distributing services and supplies. Social justice is considered when deciding who receives attention in the case of a disaster during which numerous people require medical attention at the same time. For example, there are times when the amount of medical supplies available is inadequate, such as during the H1N1 flu vaccine shortage in 2010. Available cadaver organ donation is another example of a shortage of a needed resource.[7] A shortage of trained OT personnel can cause difficulty in meeting community needs.

OT practitioners advocate for fair treatment of their clients and help clients obtain needed services and resources. Subsequently, practitioners consider how age, gender, culture, or economic status may affect OT services.

CASE SCENARIO

An outpatient pediatric facility provides services for children who have Medicaid. Evaluations at this facility include standardized testing. The standardized evaluation process takes approximately three hours to complete. Medicaid pays approximately one third less than private insurance and does not cover the therapist's time to complete the long evaluation. The team decides to use a checklist to streamline the evaluations for children receiving Medicaid so that they can be completed within one hour. Should the OT practitioners provide different evaluations based on insurance coverage?

Application: *OT evaluation and intervention should be based on the client's needs and not the amount that insurance pays for services. OT practitioners should do everything possible to advocate that the child receive the type of evaluation needed. This could include accepting less pay for the evaluations of children covered by Medicaid.*

PROCEDURAL JUSTICE

Principle 5: "Occupational therapy personnel shall comply with institutional rules, local, state, federal, and international laws, and AOTA documents applicable to the profession of occupational therapy."[4]

The intent of **procedural justice** is to provide fair processes for sound decision making. It implies that policies, regulations, and laws are formulated fairly, applied consistently, and result in reasonable decisions. It is the ethical duty of OT practitioners to be familiar with and follow policies, procedures, guidelines, and rules.

OT personnel need to ensure that their duties are consistent with ethics, standards, and regulations irrespective of their role (such as owner, partner, or employee) in the organization. Practitioners must follow standards for supervising others. Professionals are responsible for educating employers, employees, colleagues, and students regarding current legal and ethical compliance and for maintaining current credentials. They are required to participate in continuing education programs to keep their knowledge and skills current. All OT personnel are responsible for preventing discrimination and advocating for disabled workers in the workplace. This means that fees are commensurate with services and independent of the payment process. All compensation, including gifts, need to be declared to stakeholders and all monies received allocated in accordance with the directions of the contributor. OT personnel need to cooperate with ethical committees and comply with decisions.

CASE SCENARIO

Bart is a recent COTA graduate with a moderate hearing loss. He was encouraged to apply for a job at a transitional living center by Gary, who is an occupational therapist registered (OTR) and will be his supervisor if he gets the job. The rehabilitation director respects Gary's work and opinion and is excited that Bart has been recommended because the position has been difficult to fill. After the interview, the director calls Gary to tell him that, although Bart has good academic skills and the interview went well, he is not "what they are looking for." What should Gary do?

Application: *Gary is required to uphold Principle 5, procedural justice, by following the facility procedures that support a fair and equitable opportunity. Bart should not be denied a position because of his hearing impairment. If Gary believes Bart was declined employment because of his disability (hearing loss) alone, the workplace may be discriminating and Gary should report this.*

VERACITY

Principle 6: "Occupational therapy personnel shall provide comprehensive, accurate, and objective information when representing the profession."[4]

Veracity refers to "a duty to tell the truth" and "avoid deception."[15] Within working relationships, veracity is assumed and information conveyed is accepted as truthful. OT practitioners are obligated to communicate accurately and to make certain that the recipient clearly understands the message so he or she can make an informed decision. Veracity is an integral part of practice, research, and education leading to the development of trusting and productive relationships.

Upholding the principle of veracity means that OT practitioners accurately represent themselves and, when appropriate, acknowledge their part in causing mistrust in the profession. They must be unambiguous, comprehensive, and timely in their communication, irrespective of the audience. This includes crediting sources of information and avoiding plagiarism. Practitioners must always be truthful in communication, including explaining and documenting services, marketing and advertising, commenting on the performance of others, and presenting in writing or orally. The OT practitioner is truthful when communicating to persons, groups and organizations such as service recipients, supervisors, subordinates, colleagues, payers, research subjects, students, and the public (Figure 13-2).

CASE SCENARIO

Wendy is an OTR who works at a private hand clinic. She overhears Nadia, the COTA, introduce herself to a new client as an occupational therapist. When asked why she uses that title rather than the designation COTA, Nadia explains that the intervention is the same and that the patient cannot tell the difference. Furthermore, she elaborates that she likes the title of occupational therapist better and she has more experience than the OTR. What action, if any, should Wendy (the OTR) take?

Application: *Nadia has violated Principle 6, veracity, by misrepresenting her credentials and using misleading verbiage. The OTR may report this to Nadia's supervisor or to the appropriate authorities.*

FIDELITY

Principle 7: "Occupational therapy personnel shall treat colleagues and other professionals with respect, fairness, discretion, and integrity."[4]

Fidelity is defined as "the quality or state of being faithful."[8] In a broad sense, it is the commitment to follow through on proposals and keep promises. *Fidelity* refers in particular to the relationships that OT practitioners have with other service providers and organizations.[1] This includes other health care professionals, administrators, caregivers, and support staff. Fidelity guides OT practitioners, educators, and researchers in fulfilling their responsibilities in a fair and respectable way to the organization, students, research subjects, and colleagues while meeting the client's reasonable expectations.[11]

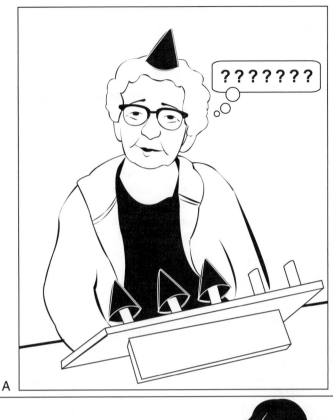

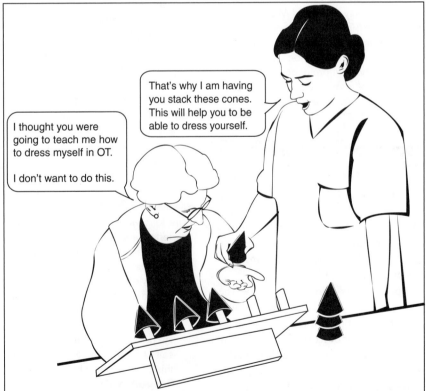

Figure 13-2 *Veracity* refers to providing comprehensive and accurate information when representing the profession. In this example, the client does not understand the connection between stacking cones and dressing. The practitioner does not clearly provide the client information and is not representing the profession accurately. **A,** The practitioner is not clear about why the client needs to stack cones. **B,** The client is left confused and unable to see the connection.

Adhering to the principle of fidelity involves respecting others in the workplace and maintaining their privacy. OT practitioners cannot use their profession or information from their role as an occupational therapist to create conflict or for personal gain and they are obligated to encourage OT practitioners to follow the Code of Ethics. If breaches in the Code of Ethics occur, OT personnel first use internal resources before reporting to external bodies.[2] If OT personnel are involved in a disagreement with other people or an organization, they need to use **conflict resolution**. Fidelity includes providing accurate feedback regarding the performance of others (including students), in a considerate manner and without prejudice or derision. OT practitioners treat others with respect, avoid exploitation of others in the workplace, prevent misappropriate of resources, and show integrity in behaviors.

CASE SCENARIO

David works as an OT practitioner in a skilled-nursing facility in a small, rural community. He is scheduled to work on activities of daily living (ADLs) with Mrs. Roberts at 10 a.m. When he enters her room, he sees that Mrs. Roberts' bed is empty and the certified nursing assistant (CNA) is pocketing candy from the gift basket on Mrs. Roberts' nightstand. What action, if any, should David take?

Application: *David has a duty to protect Mrs. Roberts and this extends to her possessions. In accordance with Principle 7, fidelity, he needs to demonstrate respect for the CNA and maintain her privacy. His best action would be to approach her tactfully to get more information. He should try to resolve this with internal organizational resources before reporting to authorities outside the facility.*

COMPLIANT RESOLUTION PROCESS AND ENFORCEMENT

The purpose of the AOTA Code of Ethics is to "protect the public and to reinforce its confidence in the occupational therapy profession rather than to resolve disputes."[4] The EC outlines the process for a just resolution of an ethics complaint in the *Enforcement Procedures for the Occupational Therapy Code of Ethics and Ethics Standards*[3] (Figure 13-3).

Any individual, group, or entity within or outside the AOTA can lodge an ethics complaint, including state regulatory boards (SRBs), the National Board for Certification in Occupational Therapy (NBCOT), or other professionals.[3] The EC recommends that the complainant discuss the alleged ethical violation with the respondent first. If an acceptable resolution is not achieved, the complainant may submit a formal statement of complaint to the EC.

The EC, Disciplinary Council, or the Appeal Panel evaluates the complaint and disciplines the respondent if necessary by instituting the following sanctions:

- Reprimand: a private, official notification of disapproval
- Censure: A public, official notification of disapproval
- Probation of membership (with terms): Conditions need to be met to avoid further sanctions.

- Suspension: Temporary prohibiting of AOTA membership
- Revocation: Permanent barring from AOTA membership

AOTA publishes the outcome of the process (except reprimands) and notifies relevant parties (e.g., SRBs, the NBCOT).

ETHICAL PRACTICE IN GROUP SCENARIOS

Group sessions pose unique ethical dilemmas and thus practitioners benefit from thoughtfully considering the possibilities. Clients in groups may sometimes ask questions about others. The OT practitioner must maintain confidentiality (Principle 3, autonomy and confidentiality). Although members can reveal information about themselves, the practitioner must not elicit the information and coerce members to reveal private information. The practitioner considers the individual's needs within the group activity. Designing activities that are beneficial to all members can be challenging. Practitioners demonstrate a concern for the client's well being and safety (Principle 1, beneficence) when designing groups to help them achieve their stated goals. When designing group activities, practitioners consider how the individual will respond to the activity, making sure it will not do them any harm (Principle 2, nonmaleficence). For example, the practitioner considers the client's psychological state and course of intervention. Pushing a client to complete an activity when he or she is not ready may harm his or her progress.

All group members are entitled to benefit from the activities (Principle 4, social justice). While engaging in activities, practitioners follow policies, procedures, and state and federal laws (Principle 5, procedural justice). Practitioners are truthful about their qualifications and intervention strategies (Principle 6, veracity). Following the Code of Ethics provides a foundation for OT practice. Practitioners adhere to these principals to provide fair and equitable therapy to a variety of clients. Finally, practitioners are respectful, fair, and discrete when dealing with colleagues (Principle 7, fidelity).

CASE SCENARIOS

The following case scenarios based on our actual clinical experience illustrate ethical principles of the OT profession. A brief description follows each scenario.

1. Michael is a pediatric OT who is starting a Mommy and Me early intervention group for 2-year-old children who are either at risk for or have developmental delays. In planning for the group, Michael decides that there should be introductions for the initial treatment session. He asks each parent to introduce both the child and himself or herself and to tell the group why they are there. Is this an ethical problem?

   Response: *At first glance, this may appear to be a violation of Principle 3, autonomy and confidentiality, because the group members will be divulging private information. However, because each parent can share what he or she wants the group to know about them, this is not a violation of the Code of Ethics. This is a common practice in therapeutic groups in that the sharing enhances the cohesiveness of the members.*

2. Erin is an OT who works in the school and leads a handwriting group with second graders who have problems with praxis. She leads a variety of activities in the group

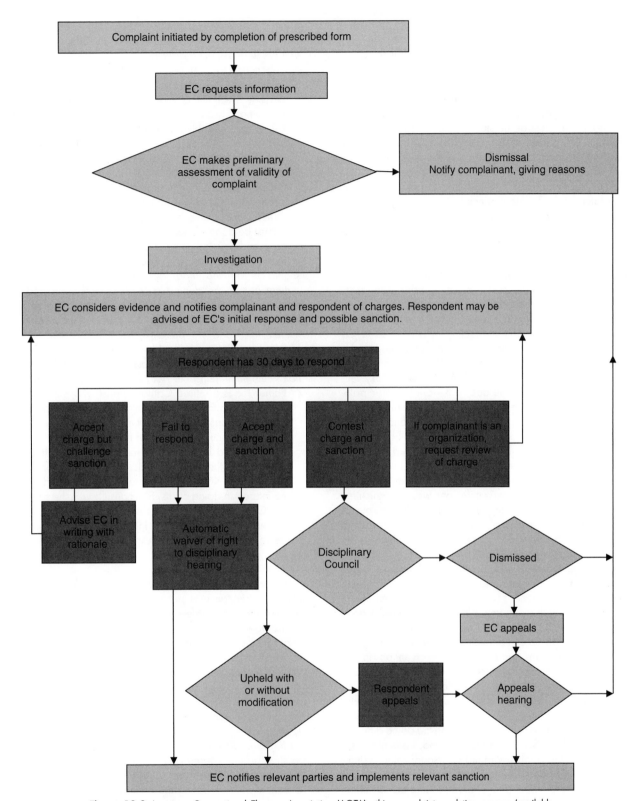

Figure 13-3 American Occupational Therapy Association (AOTA) ethics complaint resolution process (available through there AOTA).

that include writing practice but also fun activities for hand and finger strengthening, tactile discrimination, coordination, and increasing proprioceptive input to hands. One day the teacher asks Erin to have the children complete their reading assignment during OT time. Should Erin do this?

Response: *Erin should not comply with this request. Although Principle 7, fidelity, states that OT practitioners should maintain "collegial and organizational relationships," Erin should explain to the teacher that she cannot assist with the reading skills. Doing so would violate Principle 1, beneficence, because Erin does not have* expertise in teaching reading. Furthermore, providing intervention that is out of her scope of practice is a violation of Principle 6, veracity, because she is billing, documenting, and intervening toward the goal of improving handwriting skills.

3. Logan is a COTA who works in an outpatient facility with at-risk youth. One of his clients, Amy, has been defiant with most of the staff but has been cooperative during OT groups. She appears to have a "crush" on Logan. He interacts with Amy in a friendly manner and teases her light-heartedly to coax her to cooperate. He considers this effective therapeutic use of self. Has he violated any OT ethical principles?

Response: Logan's light-hearted teasing may be interpreted as flirting by Amy, who already has inappropriate feelings for him. This is not good therapeutic use of self and is a violation of Principle 2, nonmaleficence. The flirtatious nature of the relationship may interfere with Amy's progress. Logan should find a more appropriate way to encourage Amy to cooperate with treatment.

4. Sue is a COTA working in a skilled-nursing facility. Mary, a long-term resident of the facility, was referred to OT after a 5-day stay in the acute hospital for pneumonia. The intervention plan prescribed ADL training for two weeks. During the second OT intervention, Mary tells the COTA, Sue, that she does not want to participate. Sue explains that the intervention is necessary if Mary wants to do things for herself. Mary responds by saying, "Honey, I am 93 years old and tired. I have been taking care of myself all my life and now I just want someone to take care of me." According to Medicare diagnosis-related group guidelines, Mary must receive 150 minutes of OT intervention per week for the next two weeks or the facility will receive a lower rate of reimbursement. Sue is afraid that if she suggests that Mary be discharged for OT services, the administration will be angry with her. What should Sue do?

Response: Sue should recommend discharge to the supervising OTR. According to Principle 3, autonomy and confidentiality, the patient has the right to refuse treatment. This has to do with autonomy. Although the administration may not like this, Sue's ethical responsibility is to respect her patient's right to self-determination. It is possible that the OTR may require Sue to continue intervention. In this case, Sue should ask for direct supervision to determine meaningful goals and activities for Mary.

5. Virginia is an OT working in a hospital with Scott, who is recovering from a stroke. Scott's wife visits him every night in the hospital. However, during the day a different woman, whom Scott calls his girlfriend, visits him. This behavior goes against Virginia's personal value system; she feels that Scott's wife should know about the girlfriend. One day, the girlfriend comes into the OT clinic while Scott is receiving intervention. Virginia observes that his wife is standing at the clinic door watching them talk. After the session, Scott's wife questions Virginia about the identity of the woman talking to her husband. Considering the OT ethical principles, how should Virginia handle this?

Response: According to Principle 3, autonomy and confidentiality, Virginia must maintain Scott's right to privacy. She should explain to the wife that she is ethically bound to maintaining confidentiality and cannot provide any information without Scott's consent. She can suggest that the wife ask Scott directly.

6. Rebecca is an OT who is part of a dysphagia team in an acute hospital. She receives a referral do to a bedside swallowing evaluation on an adolescent with a traumatic brain injury who is functioning at a Rancho Los Amigos cognitive level 4 (agitation). The patient also has human immunodeficiency virus (HIV). The bedside evaluation includes an oral evaluation in which the therapist must put her gloved finger into the patient's mouth. Because the patient is confused and easily agitated, Rebecca is afraid of being bitten and contracting HIV. When she explains this to the supervisor, she is told that it must be done. Describe the issues associated with this case and develop some solutions.

Response: Principle 4, social justice, states that there should be fair and impartial treatment of all patients. This patient cannot be denied a feeding evaluation and the right to eat safely based on having a diagnosis of HIV. However, it is reasonable that the therapist wants to keep herself safe, and the patient's agitation presents a risk. In this case, Rebecca should work with her supervisor to develop a way to perform the essential parts of the evaluation while minimizing her risk of contracting the virus.

7. Father Joe is a retired Catholic priest who was referred to a day treatment program following a hospitalization for depression. This is the first episode of depression for him and it occurred soon after retirement at age 75. The OT evaluated him and assigned him to a craft group that Karen, the COTA, leads. Although Father Joe is cooperative, Karen can see that he is bored and he has no interest in doing crafts. She consults with the supervising OT and they do not believe that any group would appeal to Father Joe's prior interests. The supervisor suggests that he continue attending the craft group because he is cooperating. What ethical principles are illustrated by this scenario?

Response: In this case, Karen should advocate for her client. Father Joe was put into the craft group because it is what was available on the OT schedule, not because of therapeutic value to him based on the OT evaluation. That fact that he is cooperating with the craft group is not relevant to this scenario. This is a clear violation of Principle 1, beneficence, which states that the evaluation and intervention should be specific to the client's needs. This could also lead to a violation of Principle 6, veracity, if the documentation of the treatment provided reports that Father Joe is making progress based on his participation in the craft group. Because Father Joe does not fit into any of the existing groups offered by OT, he should be provided with individual treatment or be set up to work independently on a meaningful task during the craft group.

8. Emily is an OT working in a skilled-nursing facility. In the morning she completes bedside ADL training. One day, while she is doing a bedside intervention, a CNA is feeding breakfast to the patient in the next bed. Because the patient was previously on the OT caseload for feeding, Emily is familiar with her. The patient requires a pureed diet and eats slowly; she occasionally needs cues to tuck her chin down to prevent choking. Emily observes the CNA turning on the patient's television

and watching a talk show while feeding the patient. She pays more attention to the television than to the patient and only talks to the patient to tell her to "hurry up and eat." What ethical principles are presented in this scenario? Describe the decision-making process and possible solutions.

Response: *Based on Principle 1, beneficence, Emily should "remove conditions that will cause harm to others."[1] Feeding can cause harm to the patient because she is at risk for choking and should be watched and cued as needed. Therefore, Emily needs to address this situation. In doing so, Emily needs to keep Principle 7, fidelity in mind, which calls for her to treat colleagues with respect and maintain good relationships with them. To address this issue Emily should first ask to speak with the CNA in private and explain her concerns to her. If the conflict cannot be resolved this way, then Emily should go to the CNA's supervisor.*

9. Jessica is an OT assistant (OTA) student at a skilled-nursing facility. At this facility, the intervention is done bedside and consists primarily of therapeutic exercise. After her second week, she was asked to write a progress note on one of the patients. When her supervisor, Dan, reviewed the note, he told her that she needed to include progress on the patient's ADL status. Jessica said that she did not know what to write because she did not observe the patient doing self-care. Dan told her that she should be able to make inferences regarding ADL status based on how she was doing in the exercise program. The next day, Dan called Jessica's academic fieldwork counselor, Beth, and told her that he was having difficulty with the student because she did not understand functional documentation. He told Beth that he expected the students to be able to write notes about ADLs based on observations of them in exercise. Describe the ethical principles from the student and academic fieldwork coordinator's point of view.

Response: *There are several possible violations of the code of ethics in this scenario. Principle 1, beneficence, requires OT treatment to be up to date and geared to the individual needs of the patient. Principle 6, veracity is based on OT practitioners being truthful and accurate. Having adequate strength and endurance does not automatically mean that a person can self-dress. Finally, Principle 7, fidelity calls for Beth to be collegial in handling this situation. She should initially ask for a meeting with Dan at the facility to assess how treatment and documentation are being done. She should ensure that Dan understands the school's expectations and AOTA's requirements for the fieldwork experience. If Beth feels that the treatment at the facility is unethical and her meeting with Dan does not go well, she should contact the OT supervisor of the facility.*

10. Barbara is the lead OT in a school district in a rural area where she provides one-on-one service delivery. There is a shortage of therapists in the district. Barbara decides to assign therapists to the children in elementary school because they are fun to work with and generally make more progress than the adolescents in the transition program who have many challenging behaviors. Describe the ethical principles and Barbara's actions.

Response: *In accordance with Principle 4, social justice, Barbara needs to advocate for services for all recipients. She needs to make an effort to provide necessary services either by offering pro bono services with the consent of her employer or by finding equitable solutions such as considering group treatment.*

11. Alisha, an OTR with advanced sensory integration training, has been working with Olivia, a 5-year-old with sensory processing disorder at a private pediatric clinic. Olivia wants to be able to keep up with her peers on the climbing frame and monkey bars. Alisha documented that Olivia is not progressing to meet these goals and that her lack of progress may be due in part to the fact that she is overweight. Alisha recommends to Olivia's mother that she restrict Olivia's calorie intake. Does Alisha's recommendation conform to the Code of Ethics?

Response: *Alisha is violating Principle 1, beneficence. OT personnel must stay within their scope of practice and personal expertise within that scope. Alisha is making a recommendation outside of her scope of practice. A physician or dietitian should make the recommendation for a restricted-calorie diet.*

12. Gideon is an OTR in a large county hospital. He observes one of the staff therapists, Melissa, demonstrating the use of magnets to a patient for the purpose of pain control. She shows the patient the magnets and spends half of the 45-minute treatment session helping the patient to position them. At the end of the day, when he and Melissa complete their documentation, he notices that Melissa bills for the intervention using standard OT treatment codes. Describe the ethics involved and solutions. How should Gideon proceed?

Response: *Melissa is violating Principle 5, procedural justice, as she is using standard billing for an alternative therapy. This means that fees are not commensurate with services. In addition, Melissa is not accurately describing the types of services and so has violated Principle 6, veracity. In accordance with Principle 7, fidelity, Gideon is required to expose any breach of the Code of Ethics. He must first attempt to resolve the issue with Melissa. If this fails, he needs to report the breach to the appropriate authorities.*

13. Mrs. Barlow is a resident of a senior assisted-living facility with moderate to middle-stage Alzheimer's disease. She has marked loss of memory for recent events, gets lost easily, and is aphasic. The OTR suggested that they pin a note on her back with her name, room number, and a request to "return if found." The COTA working at the adjacent skilled-nursing facility has observed Mrs. Barlow wandering around the facility. Describe the ethical issues. How should the COTA proceed?

Response: *The OTR has violated Principle 3, autonomy and confidentiality. The note contains private information. Additionally, it goes against the core value of dignity to have an adult wearing a note pinned to her back. Principle 1, beneficence, instructs OT personnel to report any unethical actions. The COTA should therefore request that the note be removed from Mrs. Barlow's back. If the OTR refuses, the COTA should report it to the proper authorities.*

14. Mina is an OTR working with young adult substance abusers. She is leading a group aimed at developing positive recreational activities in the community. The group elects to participate in ceramic painting at a specialty store. One group member, Chris, chooses to decorate a mug with the slogan: "Reality is for people who can't handle drugs." Chris responds to Mina's

concerns regarding the appropriateness of the slogan by saying that it is a joke. What is Mina's ethical duty?

Response: *Although it seems that Mina has a duty to uphold Principle 3, autonomy and confidentiality, by respecting Chris's right to self-determination, this is not applicable. Mina's responsibility is to ensure a therapeutic experience for Chris by following the program rules and regulations. A program serving clients with substance abuse problems would not allow him to make this reference to drugs on his project. Because they are in a group setting, Mina should take him aside when giving feedback in adherence to Principle 3, autonomy and confidentiality.*

15. An OT student, Leila, is assigned to do level II fieldwork under the supervision of Brandon. He is the lead OTR and the director of rehabilitation. During the second week of the rotation, Leila receives a "friend request" on a social network site from Brandon. She rejects the request because she wants to safeguard her personal information. Brandon explains to her that he prefers to communicate this way and that networking is approved by the facility. He adds that he is "friends" with all the staff. Leila confirms his request and later finds out that his site has pictures of Brandon and the other therapists in social situations that make her uncomfortable. Describe the ethical issues presented.

Response: *Brandon has contravened Principle 2, nonmaleficence, by inflicting harm on a student because he pressured Leila to accept his request after her initial refusal. He also violated Principle 7, fidelity, by using his position as Leila's fieldwork educator to allow himself access to her personal information.*

SUMMARY

Ethics is the branch of philosophy that deals with the distinction between right and wrong.[16] Ethical principles can be applied to an individual or to a group. Whereas individuals develop morals based on culture, religion, and family values that provide them with direction of how to act, a code of ethics informs a group of professionals how to act. Therefore, the AOTA Code of Ethics is a set of standards for how OT practitioners behave. As such, practitioners apply these ethical principles to practice.

This chapter clearly defines the ethical principles of the OT profession by illustrating the application through case scenarios. Practitioners use the ethical decision-making process to clearly identify and analyze solutions to ethical dilemmas faced in practice.

REVIEW QUESTIONS

1. What are the 6 steps to ethical decision making as outlined by Purtillo?
2. What are the 7 principles outlined in the OT Code of Ethics?
3. What are some ethical issues that might arise in occupational therapy practice?
4. What is the importance of following a code of ethics?
5. What is the process for enforcing the OT code of ethics?
6. How are the OT core values and attitudes illustrated in the OT Code of ethics?

REFERENCES

1. American Occupational Therapy Association. (1993). Core values and attitudes of occupational therapy practice. *American Journal of Occupational Therapy*, 47: 1085–1086.
2. American Occupational Therapy Association, Guidelines to the occupational therapy code of ethics. *American Journal of Occupational Therapy*, 60:652–658, 2006.
3. American Occupational Therapy Association: Enforcement procedures for the Occupational Therapy Code of Ethics and Ethics Standards, *Am J Occup Ther* 64(Suppl): S4-S16, 2010.
4. American Occupational Therapy Association. (2010a). Occupational therapy code of ethics and ethics standards (Suppl): S17–S26, 2010.
5. Bailey DM, Schwartzberg SL: *Ethical and legal dilemmas in occupational therapy*, Philadelphia, 1995, FA Davis.
6. Edge RS, Groves JR: *Ethics of health care: a guide for clinical practice*, ed 2, Albany, 1999, Delmar.
7. Jonson AR, Edwards KA: *Resource allocation, ethics in medicine*, Seattle, 2010, University of Washington School of Medicine. Retrieved from http://depts.washington.edu/bioethx/topics/resall.html.
8. Kornblau BL, Starling SP: *Ethics in rehabilitation: a clinical perspective*, Thorofare, NJ, 2000, Slack.
9. Levine LE, Munsch J: *Child development: an active learning approach*, Los Angeles, 2011, SAGE.
10. *Merriam-Webster's pocket dictionary new edition*, Springfield, MA, 2006, Merriam-Webster.
11. Purtilo R: *Ethical dimensions in the health professions*, ed 4, Bethesda, MD, 2005, American Occupational Therapy Association.
12. Ruger JP: Ethics in American health 1: ethical approaches to health policy, *Am J Pub Health* 98(10):1751-1756, 2008.
13. Scott R: *Professional ethics: a guide for rehabilitation professionals*, St Louis, 1998, Mosby.
14. Taylor R: *The intentional relationship: OT and therapeutic use of self*, Philadelphia, 2008, FA Davis.
15. U.S. Department of Health Services Centers for Medicare and Medicaid Services. Retrieved from http://www.cms.gov/.

Managing Difficult Groups

Lisa Mahaffey

KEY TERMS

aggressor	harmonizer
blocker	information-seeker
compromiser	initiator-contributor
dominator	observer
encourager	opinion seeker

CHAPTER OBJECTIVES

1. Identify the stages of groups and roles of members.
2. Identify common group management issues.
3. Discuss how to manage difficult group behavior.
4. Describe a problem solving mode for working in groups.
5. Describe the four-step intervention model to address group members' needs and specific member issues.

Most everyone is involved in the group process at some time or another. Occupational therapy (OT) students spend many hours working together on projects and classroom activities. Children are grouped in gym class, on the playground, or in the classroom working on experiments or other tasks. Workers might convene to develop a new project or to discuss the plan for a client or student. When groups of people work well together, they can accomplish goals and often learn something about themselves. Occasionally, that group experience is less than optimal. Most of us have sat in a group where a member takes over and leads the discussion somewhere uninteresting or uncomfortable. Sometimes a member simply does not get involved, leaving the work to others. There are any number of reasons why a group may

struggle with completing the established tasks. The goal of this chapter is to identify some of the more common reasons why groups break down and to introduce a model for pinpointing the problem and implementing a solution.

COMMON MANAGEMENT ISSUES

Regardless of the time and energy put into planning, groups fall short because there are many opportunities for things to go wrong. Sometimes the problem is simply one of planning—not having the right activity for that mix of people. Other times, problems can be seasonal or a result of things that happened that day or time of year. Many problems occur during the group's initial formation or when new members join an already established group. A shortened length of stay in acute-care settings means membership can change daily. Groups can be large or small, depending on the number of clients invited to join the program. Both large and small groups have their challenges. Small groups provide opportunity for individual attention, but fewer opportunities to learn from peers. The smaller groups do not encourage people to engage in rich social interaction and they provide little opportunity to explore social behaviors.

CASE STUDY

Julie is an OT practitioner running groups in an inpatient pediatric unit for children with mental health issues. Julie notes that when there is a group of six or eight, there are moments when the children can explore their own behavior and learn from the feedback of others. Cole, a 7-year-old child with a diagnosis of bipolar disorder, comes into the hospital and joins five children who have already been working for three days on managing behavior, on fine motor and calibration skills, and, as a team, doing a gardening task. Cole immediately has trouble with speaking out of turn and acting impulsively. On the first day he proclaims the task "dumb" and pulls a recently planted flower from a pot. Cole demands a lot of attention from Julie by doing what he wants and avoiding the tasks assigned to him. He disregards Julie's redirection and becomes verbally aggressive when the other children express frustration with his behavior. He makes no connection between their anger and his behavior. Julie and the staff work with Cole to help him understand the responses of the other children and by day two he is able to make a friend on the unit and attend a group without incident. For the next few days, Cole struggles with impulsiveness, but with empathic feedback, becomes increasingly more aware of the effect his actions have on the rest of the group, and he begins to try new ways of interacting. On Cole's fourth day in the hospital, all but one of the other children are discharged. Because there are now only two group members, Cole's demands for attention are easily met and the therapist sees no interpersonal problems. Although she is able to work on other goals with Cole, the opportunity to learn more effective interpersonal skills is diminished significantly. This case illustrates how management in a group must change. A child may show different behaviors in different groups. Larger groups may challenges members in new ways.

Large groups require different teaching styles. There are few hands-on tasks that lend themselves to large groups. Lecture and discussion are the most common forms of provision for large groups. In large groups, there is more opportunity for members to sit back and not participate and they also provide more opportunity for members who have a tendency to monopolize. Because of shortened lengths of stay, it can be challenging for a group leader to remember everyone's name or keep track of the therapeutic needs of each member. This lends an impersonal feeling to the group. In acute care, membership changes daily and each new member alters the group dynamics. Sometimes the shifts are subtle and have a minimal effect and other times the atmosphere changes completely. The OT practitioner must develop strategies to engage all members including those that may disrupt the group process.

CASE STUDY

Tanya is running an OT group in a drug and alcohol rehabilitation program. Length of stay is, on average, two to three weeks. Groups have between 10 and 20 members. Tanya has been running a group with approximately 12 members, exploring the effect of alcohol on the responsibilities of daily life roles. Everyone in the group has children and they agree that they were not managing their responsibilities as well as they had led themselves to believe. After working on this task for two sessions, the members are actively exchanging ideas for resuming parenting roles and engaging their children as part of their recovery. A new patient, Rick, is admitted to the program. He and his wife, both cocaine users, have lost their children to the state foster care system. Rick is angry because, despite the fact that he has been sober for six weeks, the state is refusing to give them back. On his first day with the group, he directs this anger toward Tanya. Some members side with Rick, but others challenge Rick's assertion that the state should give them back so soon. These members become loud and animated. Other members sit quietly, adding little. One member leaves the room crying. Tanya attempts to sort through all the responses of members and several times tries to redirect the group to the task planned for the day. In the end, Rick's issue takes up the bulk of the time and many group members express disappointment that the group got out of hand. In large groups, members may monopolize the discussion or try to promote individual agenda. Leading large groups requires practitioners identify group goals and help

members work towards them. Larger groups need direction, structure and clear goals. Leaders must be aware of how members interact and keep the group moving forward.

GROUP ROLES

OT practitioners work in assisted-living programs, schools, long-term care facilities, and community mental health settings. In these settings, long-term groups are effective for many OT goals. Regardless of the population, there is a period of time for group members to develop their roles, understand the norms of the group, and begin to work together efficiently. Yalom and Leszcz[11] state that there are three stages to group formation. The first stage is characterized by getting to know each other; hesitant participation; searching for a meaning to the group and participation; and a dependency on the leader and other members for structure, for approval, and for an understanding of their role within the group. The third stage is cohesiveness and a willingness to work within the group, but on their own issues. The group is more concerned about helping each other and maintaining a safe environment for growth.[11]

The second stage is the most challenging for a leader. During this stage, members begin to let their guards down, become more familiar with their peers, and try to establish their position within the group structure. Some members feel a need to dominate in the group or to impress others. Some show little empathy and want to tell people what to do to change. No matter the age of the participants, a pecking order emerges that may include some contempt toward the leader, the group, or even individual members. In an attempt to resist self-examination, self-disclosure, and change, some members become ambivalent to the group and leader or attempt to control the direction of the group. Others may conclude they will not be the leader's favorite member and decrease participation.[11] For the leader, the management of this dynamic process determines the future working ability of the group. The leader must be prepared to handle the interpersonal challenges of this stage by working with members to help them understand their responses to the situation. This means allowing members to express their feelings, even if they are unflattering, and then helping them explore those feelings without a negative emotional response. If successful, members are left feeling emotionally safe and will trust the leader and the group process. Sometimes when there are negative emotions in a group, one member may become a scapegoat. Allowing this to happen may lead the group to believe that, if it were not for that member, the group would be fine. Pushing out a member rarely solves all the issues unless that member is truly disruptive and unable to benefit from the experience.[11]

Therapists in school and other pediatric settings have time to assess children and match them according to goals. Although the goals for pediatric groups are wide ranging, the children are matched within the group to help them develop interpersonal skills. This presents the greatest challenge, but also, under effective leadership, the greatest opportunity for members to learn.

CASE STUDY

Clare is an OT practitioner in an elementary school that provides services for children on the autism spectrum (Figure 14-1). She has put together a group of four children, age 10, diagnosed with Asperger's syndrome who need to improve interpersonal skills. Clare has decided that for the fall quarter she will work on playground skills. All four children express a desire to have friends, but when they are observed on the playground, she notes that they tend to move off by themselves. Clare organizes a game in which they must work together, using equipment to gather foam circles in a particular order. They need to plan a strategy to move quickly, but the first time through they gather only 3 of the 12 circles. One child becomes distracted, two fight over who will climb to get the circles, and one just quits when no one listens to her ideas. In the discussion with Clare afterward, they blame each other and one child "melts down," lying on the floor sobbing while the others continue to yell at each other. After regrouping, they identify a plan to split up the tasks and agree to take turns. On the second run, they collect 7 of the 12 circles before the interaction breaks down. This time, Clare films the entire process, and the children watch the video and are able to assess their actions in the game and what they would do differently the next time.[10]

Clare knows that she needs to set up a situation in which the children are bound to clash if she is to teach them how to handle things differently. By using video, the children can see their behavior and perhaps find new ways of interacting. It is easy to forget that some of the best lessons are learned when there is tension in a group, or a failure by a group or members of a group. It is the leader's responsibility to help members see their responsibility in the group situation and identify more effective actions.

REVIEW OF GROUP DYNAMICS

As mentioned earlier, sometimes the difficulty in the group is simply the result of poor planning. One example is doing a project that involves short-term memory, like current events, with a group of adults with early dementia. Although some members will respond well, those who shut down or become anxious will negatively affect the dynamics of the group. As leaders develop a stronger understanding of their client population, planning activities that fit their needs becomes second nature. Group dynamics is defined as the "interacting forces within a small human group."[8] Those interacting forces make up the relationships between members and there are a number of variables within these relationships.[4]

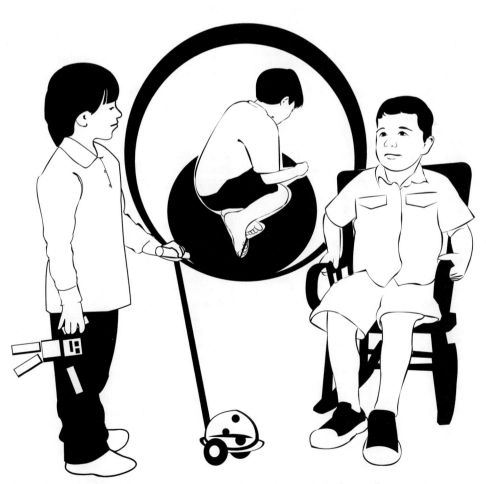

Figure 14-1 Children with Asperger's syndrome frequently work in groups to develop socially appropriate responses.

Consider the relationship between the group leader and its members. Leadership can take on a direct approach, in which the leader decides what the activity is, what the discussion will be about, who speaks first and second, and so on. This may work well with a group of people who need that structure, such as a group of adults with an exacerbation of severe mental illness, or children with attention-deficit/hyperactivity disorder. This structure helps the leader manage the action and influence the dynamics of the group with the potential effect of decreasing creativity and free thought. A more "hands-off" style of leadership allows for more group interaction. Long-standing groups with a fairly constant membership get to a point at which the leader spends much of the time observing. However, if the leader starts out using this style for newer groups, it can lead to tangential discussions, long silences, or a takeover by more powerful group members. In such a group there can be a tendency for the leader to engage in an interaction with a single member, leaving the others to observe. Early on the leader must work harder to establish the norms and manage conflicts so that members feel they can trust the leader and benefit from the group process.[9,11,5]

The other dynamic variables lie within the relationships of the members. Members can take on a variety of roles in the group. These roles can either be productive, supporting the work of the group and enhancing the therapeutic relationships, or unproductive, distracting the group and leading to dissatisfying results. Benne and Sheats[2] identify three sets of roles for group members. Two sets are focused on bringing the group members together and moving the group toward its end goal, and one set describes the roles individuals take on primarily to meet their own needs. The group task roles include the **initiator-contributor**, the **information seeker**, and the **opinion seeker**. (See Box 14-1 for all 12 roles and their definitions.) The group building and maintenance roles include the **encourager**, the **harmonizer**, the **compromiser**, and the **observer** (Box 14-2). Individual roles include the **aggressor**, the **blocker**, and the **dominator** (Box 14-3).[2] One member often fills more than one role and members take on different roles on different days, depending on the tasks and individual skills or interests. Not every role is filled or even needed in some groups. However, a group lacking members willing to take on important tasks or harmonizing roles or the existence of members engaging in behaviors consistent with individual roles are the crux of most group challenges[2,9,11] (Figures 14-2, 14-3, and 14-4).

All of the individual roles are used to meet the needs of those engaging in them. They include narcissistic needs such as constant attention or a need to feel superior. Other times the person acts in an attempt to overcome feelings of insecurity or poor self-esteem, or to avoid making life changes or taking responsibility for his or her problems. It is important to keep in mind that the "problem member" really is not solely responsible. It is their interaction, combined with the others in the group, that challenge the leader. It also is not the leader's job to "fix" the problem but rather to help that person, and the group, recognize what is happening and make the needed changes.[11]

BOX 14-1   Group Task Roles 2, 5

Initiator-Contributor: This person suggests new ideas or goals or new ways to accomplish specific tasks or solve problems.

Information Seeker: This person is most concerned with establishing the facts that surround or affect the tasks and goals of the group. He or she does this by asking for clarification and seeking out authoritative resources for information related to the task.

Opinion Seeker: This person is less concerned with the facts and more concerned with what people think—the general values of the group related to the task.

Coordinator: The person taking on this role will try to coordinate the various subtasks, pull together groups of members working on different pieces of the task, and work to clarify the relationship between the ideas and suggestions made by others.

Information Giver: The person who takes on this role offers information or opinions related to the task of the group.

Opinion Giver: This person provides statements related to his or her beliefs about a particular task or the group process as a whole.

Elaborator: The person taking on this role will consider suggestions and ideas, and then will provide specific examples, develop a rationale for that suggestion, or explain why it won't work for the task at hand.

Orienteer: This person periodically evaluates and summarizes the progress of the group related to its defined goal.

Energizer: The person taking on this role works to stimulate the group to a "better" activity. They also encourage decision making and forward movement.

Evaluator-Critic: This person tends to look at the expectations or standards of the group and compare current progress with that expectation.

Procedural Technician: This person takes care of details, small tasks that can be overlooked, to keep the group moving forward in its goal.

Recorder: This person keeps a record of the group's progress in the form of written notation, minutes for meetings, or simply recalling verbally past decisions and suggestions.[2]

BOX 14-2   Group Building and Maintenance Roles 2

Encourager: This person agrees with, praises, and supports the suggestions, opinions, beliefs, and overall contributions of other group members.

Compromiser: This person gives up some component of his or her idea or suggestion to allow for coordination with other group members' ideas or suggestions.

Harmonizer: This person attempts to decrease tension in the group by serving as a mediator, helping members in conflict negotiate an acceptable solution.

Gatekeeper: This person works to make sure there is a flow of communication by encouraging and facilitating participation between members.

Standard Setter: The person who takes on this role works to set the standards for what the group will achieve, then applies norms while measuring the groups ability to meet those standards.

Group Observer or Commentator: This person keeps a mental or written record of the group process and provides comments related to the group's progress, history, or situations within the group.

Follower: This person simply goes along with the group decisions and process. He or she listens to others during discussions and does what is asked.[2]

BOX 14-3   Individual Roles 2

Aggressor: This person tends to verbally attack others through disapproval of their statements, values, and beliefs. He or she might also attack the group as a whole and any issues it might be working on. This person gains much power, primarily through fear, by making it unsafe for others to speak or participate in a meaningful way.

Dominator or Monopolist: This person tends to fill large amounts of the group's time, often asserting authority over individual members or the group as a whole, or attempting to establish superiority in some way. Like the aggressor, the dominator can work to lower the status of other members, making participation uncomfortable.

Blocker: This person blocks any forward movement through negativity, resistance, and oppositional behavior. Often the blocker is doing this to mitigate discomfort related to self-disclosure or some action the group is taking.

Self-Confessor: This person uses the group as an audience and often has a goal to reveal personal information intended to shock or affect the group in some way. It is not unusual for the self-confessor to wait until there are only a few minutes of group time left to reveal this information, affecting the closure of the group session.

Recognition Seeker: This person's primary goal is to draw attention to himself or herself. This can be done any number of ways (e.g., telling gossip, engaging his or her neighbor in private conversation, focusing and fidgeting with something, or "one-upping" others in the group when they share information).

Playboy: This person lacks involvement in the group process and instead looks to engage others in activities that are often playful or flirtatious. Although rarely negative, this person causes the group to remain superficial and unable to make progress on goals.

Help-Seeker: This person uses self-deprecation and expressions of insecurity to get members of the group to feel sympathy for him or her. He or she then often rejects the help provided by the group because he or she is convinced it won't help. This person is also referred to as the *help-rejecting complainer.*[11]

Special Interest Pleader: This person brings individual special interests to the group and attempts to convince others of the value and need to focus on those interests, rather than on the issues of the group.[2]

FIGURING OUT THE PROBLEM

The most effective technique for improving group outcomes and strengthening group leadership is to review the group and discuss all the variables immediately after it ends.[3] Some leaders begin this process in the actual group, asking members how it went, what they learned, and what they did not like. Afterward leaders might consider such things as the flow of the group, the strongest members, the membership roles, the compatibility between the group activity and the functional status of members, and the desired outcomes.[5,9] This could be done in a written format if there is one group leader or as a discussion between co-leaders. Box 14-4 lists a set of questions that may be useful in assessing the dynamics and outcome of the group.[9]

Although doing this process every day may avert problems or make the group and group leadership more effective, a different process is needed when a situation negatively affects members or therapeutic progress. The leaders must assess the situation and use their observation skills along with their knowledge of group dynamics and theory to determine the factors that are negatively affecting the group.

CASE STUDY

One of Jack's responsibilities as an OT practitioner in the cardiac rehabilitation program is to run a group that specifically focuses on role balance and healthy lifestyle choices. This program is designed to be ten weeks long and Jack has structured his group to meet three times a week for the last six weeks. Meetings last up to 90 minutes and are interactive, with projects and homework related to developing a more balanced lifestyle. Jack has built in activities focused on developing cohesiveness. On the third day of week one, 47-year-old Rob proclaims the entire process a waste of time. Having had a heart attack and surgery for multiple blocked arteries, he believes he should be using his rehabilitation hours to exercise and get in shape. During the first two meetings Rob asks Jack questions about

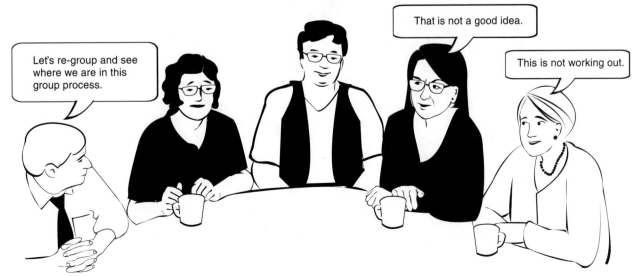

Figure 14-2 The role of *harmonizer* may develop to help members get along. Some roles, such as those of the *blocker* and *aggressor*, can disrupt group process.

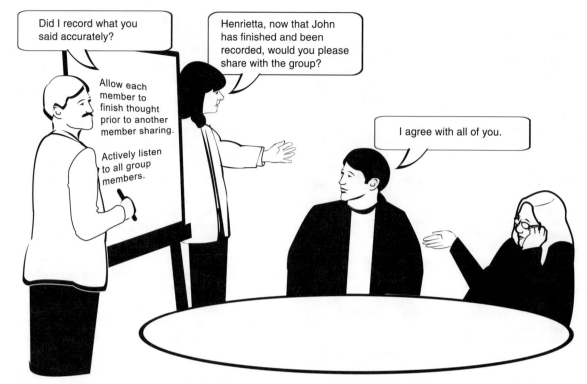

Figure 14-3 The *recorder* keeps track of the decisions, whereas the *coordinator* keeps the group on task and assigns functions if needed. The *follower* does little to assert his or her needs.

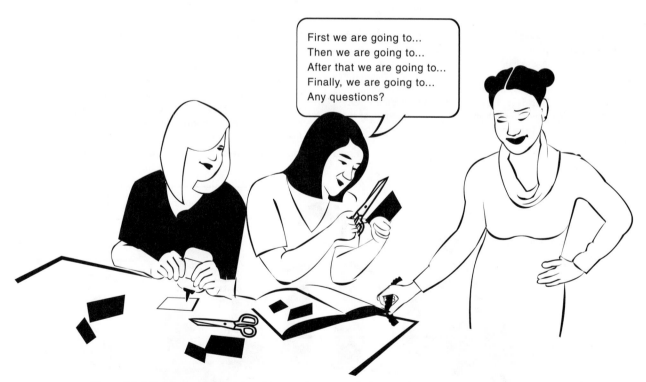

Figure 14-4 The *dominator* monopolizes the group discussion and takes over the project. *Recognition seekers* strive to be acknowledged and praised. They may not be interested in the group project, but rather want to be recognized as essential members.

BOX 14-4	Guiding Questions for Assessing Group Dynamics and Outcomes

- **Were the goals accomplished?** State the outcome and identify your rationale.
- **Was the group successful in helping individuals accomplish their short- or long-term goals?**
- **Was the group content and structure adequate for accomplishing the goals?** Leadership; time and length of meeting; format; sequence, methods, and procedures; media, modalities, and techniques employed; norms and behaviors reinforced implicitly or explicitly; methods of reinforcement; and stage of the group
- **Did the structure provide for an "optimal experience" or a "flow state?"**
- **Did the structure allow for new learning or reinforcement of the current level of role functioning or occupational performance, or did it reinforce functioning below current level of ability?**
- **Did the structure provide an opportunity for evaluation and feedback regarding the group procedures, process, and member progress?**
- **What changes would you make regarding group goals and structure for the next group or the next time this group is led?**
- **Were you as leaders adequately prepared for the group?** Consider time, place, materials, personal knowledge, and physical and emotional environments.
- **How did you function within that role?** Consider how your behavior and position affected the group, what you did that was effective, leadership opportunities missed, and what you think you learned from this group session.
- **Was the group interaction as you anticipated?** What can you identify as a basis for understanding the problems?
- **In the future, what might you do differently as the group leader?** Give rationale.

(Adapted from Schwartsberg SL, Howe MC, Barnes MA: *Groups: applying the functional group model*, Philadelphia, PA, 2008, FA Davis.)

BOX 14-5	A Four-Step Intervention Model

1. **Problem:** Identify the specific issues in the group. Who is involved, what are the behaviors, and how is it affecting other group members and the group process? Be as specific as possible; identify the group roles. In addition to identifying any individual roles that group members are taking on, look to see if any members have taken on the task roles or the building and maintenance roles that support the group process. Pay attention to the basic dynamics of the group: Who is talking? Who is quiet? Who has formed alliances? And so on.
2. **Interpretation**: What are possible explanations for the behaviors? Given what you are observing, what do you think is really going on with the members at the center of the issue? What is your understanding of the response of the remaining group members?
3. **Intervention**: Consider the identified problem and the proposed theory and the desired outcome of the intervention. Identify two or three possible approaches. Use the various group members' roles and the group's dynamics to intervene whenever possible.
4. **Outcome and Reassessment:** What was the effect of the intervention? Using the specific details from question 1, assess any changes resulting from the intervention process. Is there any new information about the group or its members gleaned from the intervention process? Determine if there needs to be further action, or ongoing action, to move toward the identified goal.

heart attacks and treatment. If Jack's answer does not contain details, Rob supplies them to the group. For Jack this appears to be an attempt on Rob's part to show that he, Rob, is more knowledgeable. During group discussions, Rob often asks questions to his peers as if he were running the discussion. He responds to the questions posed by Jack and also to the questions other members ask Jack. When someone shares a concern, Rob provides them with advice—often without empathy for the person's situation or feelings. Jack notices that by the end of the second session, the few members still engaged direct their questions to Rob. Although Rob was an active member, he shares almost no information about his own lifestyle. By the third session, Rob's behavior has effectively shut down participation of all the others. Unless encouraged by Jack, the other seven members simply sit quietly and let Rob do the talking. When Rob comments again that the group is a waste, a couple people shake their heads in frustration, but several others nod in agreement. Consider Jack's cardiac rehabilitation group on lifestyle balance. After reviewing the three groups and thinking about the different dynamics related to Rob, Jack decides that Rob feels a need to appear knowledgeable and maybe superior to Jack and the others in the group (dominator role). Rob also avoids any talk about himself, which might indicate a desire to

avoid the discomfort related to admitting his responsibility for his disease and the need to change his life (blocker). Rob also insists that he should be using his time to work out. Jack considers that many of the younger men in this program drive themselves hard in work or "leisure" activities, taking little time to care for their health. Any one of the theories could be accurate, completely faulty, or one part of the problem. Identifying several potential causes allows the therapists to create a multifaceted intervention plan. If one part of the plan fails, the therapist has other options and the information gleaned from the failed intervention process will help the therapist determine the next step. It is helpful to have a model to use to identify the issues affecting the group, and a plan for intervening (Box 14-5).[3]

In Jack's case, he had already determined that Rob was a challenge. Although Jack had been running these groups for more than one year, he admits his experience with members like Rob is limited. When Jack starts to look at the group dynamics, it occurs to him that the group has deferred to Rob, that there are no members taking on productive task roles, and that everyone has adopted a follower role. Jack was undecided as to whether Rob's chosen role is dominator, blocker, or aggressor.[2] He decides, as part of the intervention plan, to attempt to engage the other group members in supportive roles. The next group involves exploring leisure using a detailed list of leisure values. Jack creates a question sheet that will help his group review their assigned leisure activity. He sends this out by e-mail, asking each person to come on Monday prepared to present an activity. Jack's hope is that everyone will come expecting to take a turn talking about the activity, and that this will not only encourage them to participate more but will discourage Rob from taking over. In addition, he plans to challenge Rob when he interrupts or makes negative statements by asking his peers if they agree and how they would change the group. Jack also plans to model "challenging" Rob when he interrupts by saying, "I really would like to hear what Ann has to say. When you interrupt, Ann cannot finish and the group does not benefit from her research or from hearing her thoughts on the matter." Jack hopes to give the other members permission to respond to Rob's behavior and assert their own positions. An intervention is often more effective when it comes from peers rather than the leader, so Jack decides if Rob interrupts someone and they appear frustrated, he will ask that person to state how that behavior affects him or her. One last plan Jack has is to unemotionally "observe" the dynamics of the group: "I noticed that by the end of last week Rob was doing all the talking and the rest of you sat quietly. I was hoping we could have some good discussions and work together to learn about lifestyle balance. What do you think is happening?" Jack knows Rob will jump in, so he has planned to point out how much Rob has "contributed" to the group, and then ask him to give the others a chance to speak first.

Jack's assessment of both Rob and the group, based on the membership roles and dynamics, helps him identify an intervention plan that is focused more on the group. Jack's plan is to empower the other group members to assert their position and stand up to Rob's need to dominate. In addition to empowering other members, this also mitigates the chance that the group makes Rob a scapegoat. By facilitating a group intervention, Jack maintains a position of leader and teacher rather than disciplinarian and Rob may learn the effect he has on others. Were Jack to "set rules" in the group, for instance telling Rob he can only speak when asked, the entire group could end up feeling like it is unsafe to talk. If Jack chooses not to intervene, the group members will lose confidence in his ability to lead the group or even help them

ADDRESSING MEMBERS' NEEDS

CASE STUDY

Rhonda decides to start a group for the people who come to the outpatient clinic with rheumatoid arthritis (RA). Initially, when she began the group she thought this would be for people who were newly diagnosed. She planned on providing education about RA as well as joint protection, energy conservation, and the power of engagement in meaningful activity. A month into the program, she realizes that her membership will be a mix of people—many newly diagnosed, some having lived with the disease for many years, and a number of older adults with clear joint disfigurement. One particular day she has three newly diagnosed women in a group of seven. Her plan includes teaching about joint protection using written handouts and a didactic model of teaching. One group member is older and has difficulty hearing. She is irritable and complains that it was too late for her because her hands were useless. Rhonda attempts to empathize and move on, but the woman insists on complaining about her situation. Rhonda gives the group a break with the intention of removing the

woman from the group. After considering the dynamics of the group, the membership, and the fact that there are people in three different stages of the illness, Rhonda decides to open the group to questions and answers. Rather than standing in front, she pulls them into a tight circle and sits next to the women with impaired hearing. She then points out to those who have had the disease for a time how frightened the new members are. This sparks a discussion about living with the illness. Rhonda uses her teaching points to formulate questions and model the behavior of asking the older woman questions. The women began to talk among themselves with Rhonda, either asking a question or clarifying a response when necessary. After the session, Rhonda reassesses the effect of her intervention and is grateful she did not remove the woman. She also realizes that by having the older women become the experts, she has learned more about RA than she had reading books.

Varied Membership

Groups with members who are at different ages, stages of recovery, or, stages of the disease process can present a major challenge for a group leader. By presenting material to those who are further along in recovery, you leave behind those who have not learned or developed the requisite skills. By catering to those who are newer, you tend to go over material learned and mastered by the first group. Rhonda's solution to engage those with experience to teach those with less can be effective as long as the leader creates an environment in which interaction is comfortable and meets the goals of the members. The older woman did seem to want to talk and complain about her disease and her affected hands, so Rhonda asked her to share what she might have done differently for the younger women who were at risk of the same situation. The younger women in the group were able to see the importance of joint protection. Those in between could bridge that by talking about how they did not take it seriously, but could now see its importance. Rhonda's knowledge of group dynamics helped her overcome a difficult situation and create an opportunity for all members to learn and feel empowered.

Life Stage

Another challenge is life stage.[7] The needs of adolescents can be very different from those of adults. Sheila is working in an inpatient mental health unit that admits both teens and adults. She has been asked to develop a group that addresses the life skill of money management. In her needs assessment, the life stage issues she must address become clear. Most of the teens have no income and few expenses because they live with an adult who has that role. Some of the young people on the unit have never held a job. The adults vary more. Most have some income and some expenses and some hold good-paying jobs and pay the mortgage regularly. Sheila also notes that in both age groups there is huge variation in competency with money. Sheila needs to find the common ground and come up with activities that improve or support success for everyone. In the end, she puts together a set of activities that address every aspect of money management. That way she can choose one based on the needs of those who come to the group that day.

She finds several activities that consider the value of money and attitudes toward money and money management that seem to cross all levels of ability. She also finds that tapping into the money skills of those members who manage well, within the context of the group, gives them a feeling of success.

Cognitive Functioning

Another challenge for the group leader is running a group in which there are different levels of cognitive functioning. Examples include the older adult population in which one or more members may have dementia, groups of children on the autism spectrum, or adults diagnosed with severe mental illness. When this happens, the leader must consider the needs of the group first, but finding a possible solution by using the intervention model could mean the person remains in the group and benefits from the interaction with the others. Sitting near that person, or getting a willing peer to work with him or her, are a couple ways to keep the person engaged and the disruption to the group at a minimum.

Group Experience

Most older adults have not experienced therapy groups. Those with persistent mental illness have difficulty may find group activities overwhelming. If the therapist believes that group intervention is important, he or she may have to begin with educating the members on how to be in a group.

Lana is working in a school that has classrooms for children on the autism spectrum (Figure 14-5). She decides to create small groups that focus on developing basic skills to teach them to work and play together. One group consists of three 10-year-old boys. After several failed sessions during which she has asked them to work together to accomplish a task, Lana uses the intervention model and identifies specific issues with each of the boys. None of the three has ever needed to rely on others. They all avoid group situations, although all three expressed interest in having friendships and holding jobs. One child is easily over stimulated by the number of items in the OT space. Another is interested in insects and talks about little else. Eventually, the other two boys simply disengage, refusing to listen or work with him. Lana decides to begin with activities that are more parallel. One such activity includes observing a large group of "typical" kids on a playground. The boys are to write down things they see the others do that seem good to them and then things that appear not so desirable. This task leads to the exploration of effective friendships and play. Lana also figures out how to engage the kids by using their passions. Although insect day was a challenge for her, it was on that day that the boys began to work together, in part because they agreed that Lana's fear of insects was funny. Lana recognizes that when they joined together to frighten her, they were finally working as a team. In this example, all

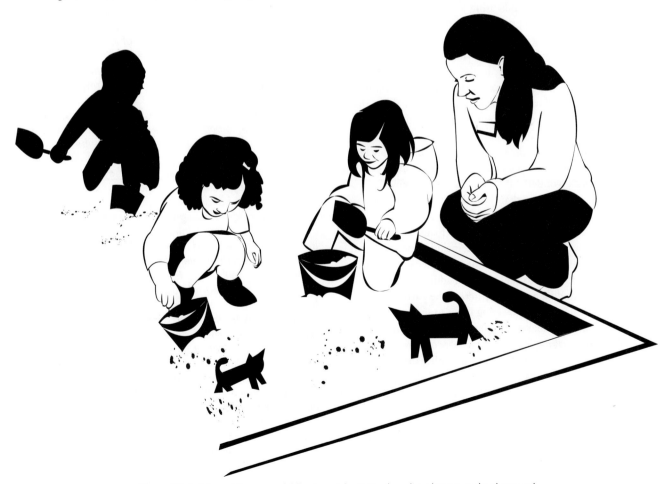

Figure 14-5 A therapist engages children in social activities through exploration on the playground.

three boys have a similar condition, age, and life stage. This allows the practitioner to develop group sessions to support each child's goals. All of the members of this group have difficulty being a group member and this becomes one of their goals.

PROBLEM GROUP MEMBERS

This chapter identifies a number of individual roles[2] taken on by members who are specifically focused on getting their own personal needs met—needs that are at odds with the social interaction required in the group process. The behaviors common to those roles are sometimes the biggest challenges in the group process and for the group leader. It is impossible to cover all the potential problems and solutions in this chapter, so in this section the most common individual member group challenges are addressed using the intervention model proposed. The hope is that the reader will be able to use the steps to identify his or her own creative solutions for group member challenges.

Monopolist

Probably the most common challenge is the person who dominates. Yalom refers to this person as the *monopolist*.[11] This person is often compelled to respond to the questions asked, offer information and solutions, and relate to personal situations in great detail. He or she may not tolerate even the briefest silence and work to join conversations using a variety of techniques, taking up large amounts of group time with a crisis or personal upheaval. The remaining members have little opportunity to participate and may be left thinking what they have to offer is not of interest or concern, or, as in the case of Jack and Rob, wondering if the leader is really capable. There are a number of possible interpretations for this action. The first thing that comes to mind is a need for attention. This could either be attention from the group or a desire to have the favor and attention of the leader.[11] Other times, the excessive talking may be a way to avoid certain topics or control the direction of the group. In Rob's case, Jack wondered if Rob felt a need to prove he was smarter or somehow better than Jack. Many times this person is not aware of how monopolizing affects fellow members, so any solution in this situation would likely focus on increasing the person's awareness. Jack's solution included pointing out the dynamic and letting Rob know he was interested in hearing what the others had to say. Jack also addressed the resulting dynamic by finding a way to structure the participation of other members, thereby empowering them to speak up.

At one point, Jack makes a statement to the group that he feels Rob has been taking more than his share of time. Several of the members agree, but two defend Rob, stating they were fine with it. Jack points out that they have not had an opportunity to participate and they both respond by saying they learn more from listening. When Jack asks the group if they thought that just listening was as effective as total participation, Rob responds by saying that he thinks people would benefit more from participating actively. Jack agrees and asks Rob to help him keep other members more accountable for their participation. In the end, this solution works the best. Rob takes on a role of record keeper

and works hard to keep track of each member's participation as well as the progress of the group. He receives positive attention from Jack regarding his desire to have everyone participate equally and begins to take pride in his ability to engage the two members who were quiet. As he listens to others share and take responsibility for their lifestyle choices, he also becomes more comfortable talking about his diet and lifestyle.

Jack's group illustrates the importance of considering several possible interpretations before identifying interventions. Multiple interpretations lead to multiple intervention strategies, which in turn gives the leader more flexibility during the actual group situation.[3] Another common challenge is the group member who remains quiet.

Passive Members

CASE STUDY

Christine is running a group for teens with eating disorders. This is a small group of three to six members who are working on exploring and developing skills in a variety of leisure occupations.[7] On the first day, Christine notices that Jill is sitting sideways on the couch with her head down on her knees. When encouraged to respond, Jill answers with one or two words and little more. After the group, Christine approaches her to ask if there was a reason why she was so quiet in the group. Jill states that she is tired and dealing with a lot. In the next session, Jill repeats this behavior and Christine notes that several members who were active in the first session have also gotten quiet. Christine notes in her observation of the behaviors that even though Jill has said and done little in the group, she seems to draw the attention of the other members. They watch her when they do respond and their responses have gotten shorter. In the third group, Christine finds that Jill is the only one answering the questions she poses, so she points that out, along with how much more active they were in the first session. The members, with the exception of Jill who remains turned away, respond by saying that because the group falls after lunch, they are uncomfortable and sleepy from their medications. Christine notes that Jill looks at handouts and group materials and then tosses them aside. Although Jill is always pleasant when approached, her body language and lack of response indicate disinterest and occasionally disdain. Christine thinks about possible interpretations to identify an intervention. Clearly, the time is challenging. Christine thinks that the methods used, discussion or worksheets, may not be conducive to keeping the group alert and engaged. She is also aware that the reason she is doing this group is that many of her clients do not value balance and leisure activity.[1] She wonders if Jill is having difficulty identifying the relevance. She notes that Jill's continued silence has affected the others and wonders if they, too, are questioning the value of the group. She wonders if they feel unsafe talking, fearing someone will think they are wrong or foolish. Christine also wonders if there is fear that talking about allowing themselves to have fun will be looked down on by the members. The last things she considers are general lack of confidence and possibly anger toward her or toward some aspect of the program.

Given these explanations, Christine begins to develop an intervention that covers multiple possibilities. Addressing the fact that after lunch they have difficulty staying alert, Christine decides that her group needs to be more interactive and task oriented. She begins to develop a resource of activities that require working together to reach a solution and others that require use of their hands and bodies. Because the group is focused primarily on leisure engagement, Christine collects supplies for activities they can explore and hopefully continue when they leave. All of her tasks have an end goal of helping the clients to see the value of occupation in developing their identity.[7] Because all the tasks are goal oriented and active, Christine figures they will be more likely to stay alert and engaged. To address the power that Jill has within the group, Christine decides she will approach Jill before the next session and talk to her about these observations. Specifically, she will point out how others look toward her and how her silence is affecting the group. Because she suspects Jill's silence is more about resistance, she will allow Jill to respond, and then point this out to her as an observation. "I am wondering if you are uncomfortable with the activities we are doing. Sometimes I wonder if you feel these activities are silly or worthless?" Christine hopes her statements will give Jill permission to be honest, and with that admission, she can determine the next step. She will also ask Jill to take a leadership role in the task activities because the others seem to defer to her. Christine thinks maybe this will encourage everyone to participate. Last, because Christine wants the group to develop new interests, she must have a better way to help them figure out what to explore first. This process will also help her narrow down the task activities and supplies. She spends the next session helping them break down previously enjoyed tasks into the component parts—for instance "being outdoors," "having a product to give others," or "learning a new skill." The teens use the results to narrow down their exploration of activities to those that share the same characteristics. The results also empower them to assert themselves when they don't want to do something.

In her evaluation of the outcome, Christine notes several things. Her discussion with Jill was very beneficial. Jill explained that she had been quiet because she was dealing with a difficult and sometimes frightening situation at home and it seemed to her that leisure activities were silly. With help from Christine, she was able to see the value in finding things she loved and the importance of developing her sense of competence and identity separate from her family situation. She also was able to see the value in shutting down worry and sadness for 45 minutes and allowing her brain a break. She did not recognize how her actions affected others and she agreed that she might be a different and more effective influence. She was able to find value in taking the lead and learning to encourage others in a positive way. With Jill's change, the rest of the group members felt more comfortable being active. They identified a list of things they wanted to try and began to encourage each other in the exploratory process. Christine's example of honestly sharing her concerns about the group dynamics encouraged them to be more direct and honest with her. With that sense of safety, they felt able to tell her when they liked something and, more importantly, when they didn't. When a new member joined the group, they reviewed the rules. "Be honest and direct," "be willing to try things (take risks)," and "allow yourself to have fun."

Sidetracking

Occasionally, a group member will take great interest in a topic that is of little interest to other members and he or she lacks the ability to notice this fact. OT practitioners see this often in groups with people on the autism spectrum. Simply setting limits on the person rarely helps that person see the interpersonal problems that result from this behavior. The solutions for this can vary from getting peers to give feedback, videotaping a group session and encouraging the person to look for social cues, or role playing interactions with peers taking the role of the obsessive focus on a topic of little interest. The end goal is to help the individual increase his or her awareness of this tendency as well as allowing the group to move forward on developing goals.

Occasionally, a group will have a member who poses a personal problem, yet when suggestions are offered by the members or the leader, the person points out why they won't work. Although most members come to the group situation looking for help, they also want to be helpful to others. This member, often referred to as the "help-rejecting complainer,"[11] creates a great deal of frustration among group members who are left feeling helpless when all of their suggestions are rejected. They eventually give up and reject the individual by ignoring him or becoming harsh and confrontational. The leader often notes any help offered to this member is immediately rejected. The first solution is to encourage the group not to offer any. This can be modeled by the group leader or suggested as an explicit rule. Teaching the group to listen and empathize with the person can decrease the sense of rejection felt by the group and increase the member's sense of connection to fellow members. After a while, the member may feel safe enough to accept feedback regarding the tendency to reject the solicited help.[11]

Children and adults on the autism spectrum; adults with closed head injury; people with more severe, persistent mental illness; and people coming to terms with traumatic injury are examples of populations who, because of underlying body dysfunction, might experience moments of emotional over-responsiveness or impulsive tendencies. When someone has one of these moments in the group, the leader must consider the needs of the larger group. In the observation and interpretation parts of the intervention model, the leader needs to determine if the person has the capacity to regain control in a short period. The leader must also pay close attention to the responses of the other members in the group. Sometimes, especially if the group has been together for a while, the members will respond with compassion and will work together to help the member remain a part of the group. Other times, the other group members are afraid or become extremely anxious when they are forced to face their fears of losing control. In the end, the decision to have that member remain in the group must take into account the needs of all members. Many times, the member who is exhibiting this behavior is not able to benefit from the group process, so having him or her step out for a while is the best option. If the group is a long-term group, it is important for the leader to use the intervention model and create a plan to reintroduce that member in a way that minimizes bias and fear for everyone, once he or she is ready to return.[11]

Challenging

Gerard Egan, in the book *The Skilled Helper*,[6] describes the concept of *challenging*. Challenging is used when the group is experiencing difficulties with one or more members, or is stalled or moving in a less than therapeutic direction. In Egan's helping model, part of the job of the skilled helper is to develop opportunities to learn and change that fit well with the OT intervention concept of enabling participation in occupation. When the leader challenges someone, or the group, he or she provides relevant, helpful, supportive feedback that is inconsistent with the individual's current thinking process.[6] The intention is to increase awareness, encourage risk taking, or provide assistance in exploring more effective ways of doing things. Challenging is used in many of the earlier scenarios, particularly when the intervention is designed to increase awareness of the effect on others. Group members can learn to challenge each other by observing the modeling of the leader. In the example of Jack and Rob, Jack uses several techniques to change the dynamics, including helping Rob see how his dominating is affecting the participation of others. Pointing out to Rob that his tendency to take over might be the reason for the silence of his peers is likely to be inconsistent with his belief. Jack then challenges Rob to take on a role of encouraging others to participate, something he would not have considered.

These challenges lead Rob to explore his actions and move forward in his therapy.

CASE STUDY

Scott is running a group in a senior center with community-dwelling older adults who are in their late 60s and early 70s. These people have been referred to Scott's group by area physicians. The group's focus is on losing weight and getting fit. Scott works with a dietitian who designs an eating plan for each member. Scott's role is to help them incorporate activities into their day that decrease their sedentary tendencies. Scott also works on fear of falling, fall avoidance, improving self-efficacy, and creating a balanced lifestyle. The group has agreed to form a team for an upcoming walk to raise money for a cure for cancer. They begin to identify some ways they might raise money and promote awareness in the community. They all agree they will need to train for the walk. Out of concern for the varied levels of physical fitness, the group creates a training schedule that is, in Scott's opinion, not progressive enough to affect their physical fitness. One day he asks the group to spend time exploring the benefits of different forms of exercise. They also discuss how much exercise is needed to increase fitness and decrease weight. By doing this, he challenges some of their fears about working too hard, and encourages them to push themselves and each other a little more. He helps them explore the problems they identify to determine what is of real concern and what is unnecessary worry. In the end, the group develops a much more challenging plan for training that will change their thinking and improve their health.

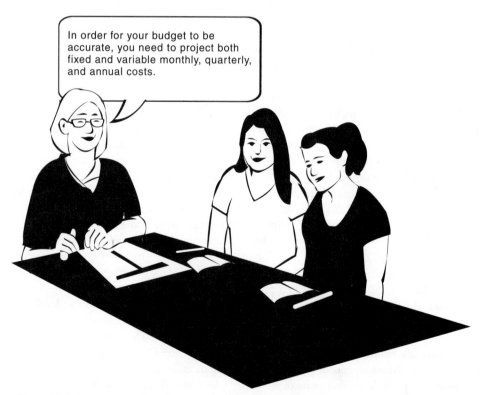

Figure 14-6 A practitioner works with women who are preparing to live in an apartment on preparing a budget.

LEARNING TASK

You have developed a group in a community homeless shelter for women with young children who are preparing to move into their own apartments under a supported living situation (Figure 14-6). The organization that provides these programs has identified money and household mismanagement as the primary reasons for people losing their apartments.

CASE STUDY

You have developed a six-week group program in which members meet twice a week for 90 minutes to learn bud-geting skills, systems to manage bills, cleaning and home repair, and safety in the home. At least two sessions will be offered on parenting skills that you have identified as an issue. You have five women who have been in the shelter for about a year and a half. Alexis, a 32-year-old woman with three small children and a diagnosis of schizo-affective disorder, is quiet but attentive during the first two sessions. Jackie, the only women who could be described as Alexis' friend, is talkative and open to feedback. She also has three small children. Other group members include Sha-niqua who is 19 and has a 17-month-old, and Lisa and Janelle, both in their late 20s and each with one toddler. In the third session, Alexis appears distracted and irritable with her peers and the group in general. Jackie attempts to talk with Alexis but Alexis asks her to leave her alone. After that, the group becomes much quieter than during the two previous sessions and you are having a difficult time get-ting them to complete the money management task for the day. The task is one that requires them to work together to research and solve a problem related to money. The three younger women start working on the task but then begin to talk among themselves about an unrelated topic. Jackie

continues to try and engage Alexis, who just becomes more agitated.

The intervention model described in this chapter provides a structure for how to intervene in this group.

1. **Identify the problem:** What are the specific behaviors, interactions or facts related to the problem? Include any roles members have taken on and the effects they have on the group. What are the basic dynamics of the group? Who interacts with whom and so on?
2. **Interpretation:** Identify three or four possible causes for the current group dysfunction. Is it something to do with member interaction, the group tasks, or the size or context of the group?
3. **Intervention:** Based on your interpretation, what interventions would you try to get this group back on track to learn what they need to know?
4. **Outcome and reassessment:** What would you hope would be the outcome of the interventions? What might go wrong with your interventions and how could you tweak them to change the response?

SUMMARY

Understanding group dynamics and members' roles helps OT practitioners manage difficult behaviors in groups. This chapter describes some of the common reasons why groups break down and introduces a four-step model for identifying the problem and implementing a solution. The chapter provides clear examples of how practitioners can be more effective in leading groups. This final chapter provides a pragmatic approach to group work that is important for any practitioner.

REVIEW QUESTIONS

1. Some groups fall short of the goals because of poor planning. Identify three or four things you must consider when planning for a large group, a small group, and groups in which the membership changes daily because of short hospital stays.
2. OT practitioners run groups in facilities where people stay involved for a long period. In this case, group challenges often come during the second stage of group development according to Yalom and Leszcz.[11] What would you do as a leader to manage the issues common to the second stage of group development?
3. Most of what goes wrong in a group is tied into group dynamics. Having a good understanding of the roles people take in a group can help a leader identify the problematic dynamics and implement a solution. Using three or four of the group building roles and one individual role, create a scenario in which the interplay of these dynamics can cause challenges to the group.
4. Using a case study from the chapter, identify two or three different ways the leader could address the problems.
5. Egan, in his book *The Skilled Helper,* identifies the concept of "challenging." Consider the scenario you created in question 3. How might the leader of this group go about challenging the person who has taken on the individual role?

REFERENCES

1. Abeydeera K, Willis S, Forsyth K: Occupation focused assessment and intervention for clients with anorexia, *Int J Ther Rehabil* 13:296, 2006.
2. Benne KD, Sheats P: Functional roles of group members. In Bradford LP, editor: *Group development*, ed 2, La Jolla, CA, 1978, University Associates, pp 52-61.
3. Bradford LP: *Group development*, La Jolla, CA, 1978, University Associates.
4. Cartwright DP, Lippitt R: Group dynamics and the individual. In Bradford LP, editor: *Group development*, ed 2, La Jolla, CA, 1978, University Associates, pp 36-51.
5. Cole MB: *Group dynamics in occupational therapy*, ed 3, Thorofare, NJ, 2005, Slack Incorporated.
6. Egan G: *The skilled helper: a problem-manage-ment and opportunity-development approach to helping*, ed 9, Belmont, CA, 2010, Brooks/Cole, Cengage Learning.

7. Kielhofner G: *Model of human occupation: theory and application*, ed 4, Philadelphia, PA, 2008, Lippincott Williams & Wilkins.

8. *Merriam-Webster Dictionary Online*. Retrieved 6/2011 from http://www.merriam-webster.com/dictionary/group%20dynamics.

9. Schwartsberg SL, Howe MC, Barnes MA: *Groups: applying the functional group model*, Philadelphia, PA, 2008, FA Davis.

10. Skog K, Virnig E, Castaneda C, Deitz J: Promoting participation and success on the playground, OT Practice Online. Retrieved from www.aota.org/Pubs/OTP/1997-2007/Features/2006. (log-in required).

11. Yalom ID, Leszcz M: *The theory and practice of group psychotherapy*, ed 5, New York, NY, 2005, Basic Books.

Glossary

Kate McLean Hanrahan

acquisition the learning or developing of a skill, habit, or quality

active engagement teaching clients through "doing" by using visual, auditory, and movement to reinforce learning.

active listening a communication technique in which the listener feeds back what he or she heard from the speaker; a way of restating what was heard to confirm.

activities of daily living activities that are oriented toward taking care of one's own body that are "fundamental to living in a social world; they enable basic survival and well-being" (Rogers & Holm, 1994, pp. 181-202; Christiansen & Hammecker, 2001, p. 156).

activity purposeful and meaningful tasks or actions that results in an end product.

activity analysis analyzing the typical demands of an activity, the range of skills involved in its performance, and the various cultural meanings that might be ascribed to it (Crepeau, 2003, p. 192).

activity group engage clients in meaningful activity, but may not necessarily occur within the context of the actual occupation.

activity match the process of identifying an activity that will interest the client and serve to motivate the client to achieve goals.

activity synthesis combining separate elements of an activity to form a coherent whole specific to the person (*American Heritage*).

adaptation changing how an activity is completed by changing the steps, often using equipment to change the activity requirements.

adjourn to suspend the group indefinitely or until a later stated time.

aggressor role a person who tends to verbally attack others, or the group as a whole through disapproval of their statements, values, and beliefs. Gaining much power, primarily through fear, by making it unsafe for others to speak or participate in a meaningful way.

agnosia a condition typically caused by neurologic damage resulting in the loss of ability to recognize objects, persons, sounds, shapes, or smells, although the specific sense is not defective nor is there any significant memory loss.

altruism selfless concern for the well being of others.

applied behavioral analysis design, implementation, and evaluation of environmental modifications to produce socially significant improvement in human behavior.

area of occupation Various kinds of life activities in which people, populations, or organizations engage, including activities of daily living, instrumental activities of daily living, rest and sleep, education, work, play, leisure, and social participation.

anosmia the absence of olfactory or smell sensation.

aural perceptual mode listening to verbal instructions to learn a new task or follow directions.

authoritarian style leaders who employ a high level of control in the decision making of the group.

autonomy the client's right to make choices about his or her intervention, including the right to refuse intervention.

beliefs any cognitive content held as true by the client (Moyers & Dale, 2007).

beneficence providing service that is for the good of clients and to also protect clients from harm.

biomechanical the application of the principles and physics of human movement and postures with respect to gravity.

blocker roles activities that disrupt the group. May dominate discussions, verbally attacking other group members, and distract the group with trivial information or unnecessary humor.

body functions the physiologic functions of body systems, including psychological functions

body structures anatomic parts of the body such as organs, limbs, and their components that support body function.

case method of instruction using a case study to provide an opportunity for a learner to brainstorm and apply knowledge being learned, with a facilitator available for answering questions.

categorical fluency skill of naming items in a category, such as naming as many animals or as many words beginning with a certain letter as possible in 1 minute.

catharsis the purging of emotions or relieving emotional tensions.

Centennial Vision a statement by the American Occupational Therapy Association describing the future of the occupational therapy profession as powerful, widely recognized, science driven, and evidence based.

children and youth the American Occupational Therapy Association has stated that more practitioners are needed to work with school-aged children and youth, especially in using assistive technology.

client-centered care emphasize the readjustment of power within the therapeutic relationship and support client control over decision making and problem solving.

client factors factors residing within the client that may affect performance in areas of occupation. Client factors include values, beliefs, and spirituality; body functions; and body structures (see Table 1-2).

closed group a group no new members join in which membership remains the same over time.

cognitive aspects actions or behaviors that a client uses to plan and manage the performance of an activity.

cognitive-behavioral therapy psychotherapeutic approach that addresses dysfunctional emotions, behaviors, and cognitions through a goal-oriented, systematic process.

cohesiveness when a group feels a sense of belonging, validation, and acceptance.

collaborative group members share materials and supplies while working on a single project as the final group outcome. An example is a group of adolescents making a poster board collage sharing magazines, scissors, glue, and other materials and supplies to make one collage that represents the group's thoughts and feelings.

communication style a client's ability to communicate in a clear, well-paced, and detailed yet succinct manner that is appropriate to his or her developmental level and cognitive ability.

compromiser roles this person gives up some component of his or her idea or suggestion to allow for coordination with other group members' ideas or suggestions.

condition the demands or aspects of a goal that is modified by altering the demands of the setting, the behavior, or the frequency.

conductive hearing loss hearing loss involving damages to structures of the outer or middle ear or tympanic membrane.

confidentiality the act of being responsible for protecting private health information during verbal, written, and electronic communication.

configuration designing, arranging, or shaping with a view for use.

conflict resolution the methods and processes involved in facilitating the peaceful ending of a disagreement.

context a variety of interrelated conditions within and surrounding the client that influence performance. Contexts include cultural, personal, temporal, and virtual (see Table 1-5).

cooperative group group members share materials and supplies while working on individual projects as the outcome. For example, children making bird seed pine cones share the peanut butter, spreading utensils, and other media, but each child completes an individual end product.

copying a term used when teaching prewriting strokes, which refers to drawing a stroke from a picture.

corrective recapitulation of the primary family experience occurs when group members identify the therapist with members of their own family. The therapist can help the group members in identifying these patterns and in developing healthy interactions.

creative group protocol outline of an innovative group developed by a therapist that includes needs assessment, group design, how to implement, and evaluation.

democratic style allows for a higher level of involvement from group members in achieving the outcomes of the group; the group leader delegates responsibility for group tasks to group members as appropriate.

deontologic theories theories that hold that an action itself is either ethical or unethical with no regard for its consequence and that there is a universal duty to obey rules and follow principles.

developmental group focus on teaching group-interaction skills that are considered developmental stage–specific, working from parallel to mature groups.

developmental levels the physical, psychological, social, moral, and spiritual aspects one experiences during the various ages and stages in life.

development of socialization skills working with the other group members during the activity process and group discussion, improving and developing appropriate social skills.

developmental tasks age-related norms that reflect social expectations for normal development.

direct teaching teaching that involves instructing or demonstrating each step of an activity.

direct service (pull out) the occupational therapist provides services in the school environment outside of the special education classroom.

disability physical or mental condition that limits a person's movements, senses, or participation in activities.

divine command ethics that postulate that there is a set of rules created by a divine source for directing of moral behavior.

dominator roles this person tends to fill large amounts of the group's time, often asserting authority over individual members or the group as a whole, or attempting to establish superiority in some way.

dress-up group a type of group that teaches basic self-care skills such as ability to dress, undress, and use fasteners.

early adolescence encompasses the middle school years (11 to 13 years old); the majority of young people in this age group are experiencing puberty.

emerging occupational therapy practice areas fields of work within the occupational therapy profession that will become more prominent in the future. They include mental health; productive aging; children and youth; health and wellness; work and industry; and rehabilitation, disability, and participation.

empathy the ability to share and understand feelings of another.

empowerment the act of promoting self-actualization and understanding one's influence over a situation.

encourager role this person agrees with, praises, and supports the suggestions, opinions, beliefs, and overall contributions of other group members

endurance the ability to sustain engagement in an activity that involves physical strength.

environment the external physical and social environment that surrounds the client and in which the client's daily life occupations occur (see Table 1-5).

episodic memory type of long-term, declarative memory in which we store memories of personal experiences that are tied to particular times and places.

ergonomics the evaluation and design of effective work environments that promote optimal productivity.

ethical dilemmas a challenge practitioners face when there is a struggle to decide what course of action to take in a difficult situation.

ethical distress the discomfort experienced when the occupational therapy practitioner is prevented from doing what is believed to be right.

ethics a "system for decision making in the arena of moral values."

evaluation The process of obtaining and interpreting data necessary for intervention.

evaluation group groups that allow for assessment of both interpersonal and activity skills.

existential factors attributes of life addressing the meaning of life, acceptance of mortality, and recognition of personal responsibility.

fidelity "The quality or state of being faithful; the commitment to follow through on proposals and keep promises to all those with whom you have professional relationships, including clients, co-workers, and organizations."

Fitness, yoU, and Nutrition (FUN) program a program that uses a multilevel approach to improve health and wellness in children and families. Based on the Model of Human Occupation, children with a variety of physical and nutritional activities explore and discover, which they find motivating, interesting, and valuable.

fluid intelligence the speed and accuracy with which one can reason abstractly and problem solve.

frame of reference system of compatible concepts from theory that guides a plan of action within a specific occupational therapy domain of concern (Mosey, 1986).

formal instructional environment characterized by individual work, emphasis on assessment, and use of external motivators with the result typically being academic achievement.

forming the first stage of group development as defined by Tuckman (1965). This stage encompasses the transition from a group of individuals to a functioning team; members build confidence and trust in each other as well as their leader.

functional group groups that result in end products or help members achieve desired skills and abilities.

generalization expanding learning or the transfer of skills.

global mental functions basic cognitive skills and emotional stability, deemed to be more fixed, and are not altered significantly through the typical aging process.

goals and objectives the individual objectives each child is trying to achieve that guide the activities planned by the therapist to address these needs.

grading conditions that make goals achievable within the time frame or context of therapy by outlining the circumstances under which the client is expected to exhibit the behavior, resulting in conditions that make the goal more demanding or increase the support for desired behavior

group climate emotional atmosphere the group members experience, indicative of the level of comfort members feel with each other, their leader, and their environment.

group cohesiveness how the members bond or interact.

group design and protocol the specifics of the group, including such things as group membership, time, duration, location, purpose, goals, costs, and specific activities and often budget, supplies, equipment, and supervision

group-facilitation techniques techniques that group leaders use to monitor and observe members' behaviors, interactions, and relationships to ensure that the group is a supportive, safe, nonjudgmental setting for learning, taking risks, and gaining skills for all members.

group length the time duration of each group session.

group norms established guidelines and expectations for behaviors within a group.

group projects a means of facilitating learning within a group of people that allows members to assist each other, gain a sense of camaraderie and contribute to the final project without the burden of completing all aspects alone.

group protocol structured set of guidelines to promote meaningful and efficient communication and task participation within a group.

group setting the environment in which the group is conducted.

group size the number of participant individuals that make up the group.

group time of day the time of day at which the group is held; this can effect participation.

habituation repeated performance of a task or occupation that results in the formation of habits and roles.

handwriting group groups designed by occupational therapists to build a solid foundation of skills required for efficient and legible handwriting.

haptic perceptual mode using manipulation of objects (hands on) to learn or to complete a task.

harmonizer role this person attempts to decrease tension in the group by serving as a mediator, helping members in conflict negotiate an acceptable solution.

health and wellness an emerging practice area that examines habits and routines and designs individualized plans while considering the unique health needs of clients.

hyposmia decrease in sense of smell.

imitation the physical or motor modeling or demonstration of the desired stroke to be drawn in a prewriting group.

imitative behavior by observing the group leader and other group members interacting in an appropriate, socially acceptable manner, others are able to mimic the actions of their peers.

implementation involves leading the groups and documenting the session results.

inclusive ("push-in") therapeutic model that requires the occupational therapy practitioner to provide direct services in the special education classroom.

indirect teaching helps individuals gain ability and feel empowered by encouraging self-initiation and problem-solving to learn a new skill in an environment that allows the learner to make choices.

inevitable personal event naturally occurring communication, reaction, process, task, or general circumstance that occurs during therapy and that has the potential to detract from or strengthen the therapeutic relationship.

informal instructional environment characterized by freedom in choosing activities and minimal emphasis on assessment or the use of external motivators, fostering thoughtful and creative learners who learn to develop solutions through problem solving.

initiator-contributor roles this person suggests new ideas or goals or new ways to accomplish specific tasks or solve problems.

instrumental groups groups that focus on clients' maintaining their current level of function and meeting health needs.

intentional relationship model focuses on four main components of the therapist-client relationship: (1) the client, (2) the interpersonal events that occur during therapy, (3) the therapist, and (4) the occupation.

interactive perceptual mode a means of learning through group discussions

interest groups informal groups formed around common interests.

interpersonal characteristics relevant aspects that the client brings into a therapeutic relationship that differ when the client is in different situations.

interpersonal learning when group members become more aware of their behavior and their interaction skills and how their behavior affects other people.

involuntary group participation participation in a group at the advisement of a physician, because of pressure from family and friends, is court ordered, or required for obtaining other services.

judging determining the appropriateness or importance of an activity or object.

"just-right" challenge challenge that is not so easy as to bore clients or so difficult as to make clients frustrated.

kinesthetic perceptual mode engaging in movements or learning through doing.

laissez-faire style leader allows the group to control all decision making and problem solving.

late adolescence between 17 to 25 years. A time of consolidation of values, self-identity, and self-efficacy in performance skills required to meet the choices and demands of the roles of early adulthood such as work and forming a stable intimate relationship.

learning gaining awareness and understanding by active participation in activities that lead to skills.

locus of authority an ethical dilemma that involves determining who should have the authority to make an important moral decision.

locus of control the extent to which individuals believe that they can control events that affect them.

long-term goals goals that delineate what group members will achieve over the life of the group program.

maintenance roles social-emotional activities that help members maintain their involvement in the group and raise their personal commitment to the group.

maladaptive dynamics serve the needs of at least one individual within the system but are inefficient and involve negative feelings or outcomes for at least one of the involved individuals.

materials, supplies, and equipment the media and items used in therapy that therapists choose and becoming familiar with to facilitate success for the group members when participating in an activity.

meaningful repetition practice needed to fully integrate the movements or sequence of steps.

media items used during the intervention process.

memory a great number of constructs related to remembering.

mental health an emerging area of occupational therapy practice calling for increased involvement of practitioners with people diagnosed with mental health conditions throughout the lifespan, especially in community and school settings.

methods means of accomplishing a task.

middle adolescence the high school years between the ages of 14 and 17. This is the period of the most intense psychosocial development when the salient relations with friends and other peer-mediated influences displace parental relationships and opinions.

mode shift within the intentional relationship model, this occurs when there is a conscious change in one's way of relating to a client.

model of human occupation a conceptual practice model based on open systems theory that attempts to explain how occupations are motivated, patterned, and performed.

morals the personal values, principles, and beliefs that determine what is right and wrong for the individual.

multimodal the ability of a therapist to use all six of the modes identified in the intentional relationship model flexibly and comfortably and to match those modes to the client and the situation.

narrative reasoning used to learn about the client's life story.

needs assessment includes the reasons for the group and often includes a description of the gap that the group is addressing, the rationale for the group, and cost effectiveness of the proposed group.

nonmaleficence the ethical principle of doing no harm, including taking risks in some aspects of occupational therapy intervention that can cause harm regardless of the intent to do good.

nonverbal communication communication that does not involve the exchange of words but includes gestures, facial expressions, and eye contact.

norming the third stage of group development as defined by Tuckman (1965). This stage is characterized by the recognition of individual differences and shared expectations.

objectives: short-term goals that contribute to the accomplishment of the long-term goal.

objects tools, materials, and equipment used in the process of carrying out the activity.

observer roles this person keeps a mental or written record of the group process and provides comments related to the group's progress, history, or situations within the group.

occupation-based group groups that engage children in the natural context while focusing on areas of occupation, such as activities of daily living, instrumental activities of daily living, education, rest and sleep, work, and play.

occupations "Daily activities that reflect cultural values, provide structure to living, and meaning to individuals; these activities meet human needs for self-care, enjoyment, and participation in society" (Crepeau et al., 2003, p. 1031).

occupational or activity analysis process of describing an occupation or activity in terms of several characteristics, including the purposes, task characteristics, task duties, necessary skills, and abilities required to perform the activity.

occupational identity a subjective construct made up of an individual's volition, habituation, and performance capacity in daily occupations.

occupational performance analysis tool used by practitioners to determine necessity for modification of adaptation to tasks by evaluating a client's performance capacity and analyzing activity requirements.

occupational profile interview tool used to understand the client's history, roles, and motivations.

occupational therapy practice framework official document of the American Occupational Therapy Association, intended for internal and external audiences, to present a summary of interrelated constructs that define and guide occupational therapy practice. It outlines occupational therapy's contribution to promoting the health and participation of people, organizations, and populations through engagement in occupation.

olfactory perceptual mode incorporating scents into an activity.

open group a group that allows for new participants to join the group, so membership is always changing.

opinion seeker roles this person is less concerned with the facts and more concerned with what people think and the general values of the group related to the task.

parallel group members work in close proximity to each other, but do not share materials or interact with each other.

paternalistic style closely regulates the behavior of group members to assist in achieving individual and group goals.

participation engagement in activities.

participative style more flexible approach in which the leader adapts the amount of direction and feedback to the specific needs and abilities of the group members.

perceived efficacy (self-efficacy) one's belief in one's ability to succeed in specific situations, playing a large role in how a person approaches goals, tasks, and challenges.

perception the ability to make sense of and interpret incoming sensory information.

perceptual modes of learning pathways for processing sensory information from the environment for use during learning process.

perceptual pathways for learning neuronal networks interact during the process of learning that include the patterns of sensory information; what is being learned determines how learning is planned, executed, and monitored and the importance of what is learned and the emotions associated with learning (Rose & Meyer, 2002).

performing the final stage of group development as defined by Tuckman (1965). The group begins to accomplish a significant amount of work. Everyone is participating and problems and challenges arise.

performance capacity the physical and mental abilities that underlie skilled occupational performance.

performance patterns patterns of behavior related to daily life activities that are habitual or routine. They can include habits, routines, rituals, and roles (see Table 1-4).

performance skills observable, concrete, goal-directed actions clients use to engage in daily life occupations (Fisher, 2006).

personal causation one's sense of competence and effectiveness, and awareness of his or her abilities

personal disclosure when a leader contributes personal information, it is done with the intention to be therapeutic, enhance the group process, and contribute to a group member or members collectively meeting the group goals.

pet-assisted therapy (PAT) uses trained animals and handlers to achieve specific physical, social, cognitive, and emotional goals with patients.

physical environment the environment, and all of its related characteristics in which group activities are conducted.

physical, social, and personality traits characteristics of group members that influence the success of the group and individual.

plain language clear and concise language (at a sixth-grade level) that highlights key aspects and helps an individual learn.

playfulness an integral part of learning that allows the exploration of interests, development of skills, and learning of social rules while enjoying an activity and taking pleasure in the moment.

postgroup analysis following completion of a group session a practitioner must assess the group and his or her leadership from his or her perspective and the perspectives of the individual members.

postural control voluntary movement that allows control of the position of the body in space for the purpose of stability and orientation during occupational mobility.

praxis ability to carry out skilled, purposeful, sequential motor acts as part of an overall plan.

preparatory methods methods and techniques that prepare the client for occupational performance. Used in preparation for or concurrently with purposeful and occupation-based activities.

presbycusis age-related decrease in the sense of hearing.

presbyopia condition in which, with age, the eye exhibits a progressively diminished ability to focus on near objects (farsightedness).

present functional levels determine the fit of each member to the group or activity or decide if additional personnel are needed for the group to convene.

prewriting group groups designed by occupational therapists to develop prewriting skills such as scribbling, hand strength, fine motor control, and grip pattern.

prewriting strokes strokes used to form the uppercase and lowercase letters and numbers, which are combined to draw simple and complex geometric shapes.

print perceptual mode incorporating reading and written material into a learning opportunity.

procedural justice to provide fair processes for sound decision making related to policies, regulations, and laws being formulated fairly, applied consistently, and resulting in reasonable decisions.

procedural memory memory for motor performance skills, which is deeply ingrained, often automatic, and is less affected by the aging process.

process group groups that work on the members' interpersonal abilities.

productive aging helping older adults remain safely in their homes or on their own.

projective activities therapeutic activities that use a variety of media such as art, music, movement, or sociodrama as vehicles for self-exploration and self-expression.

prospective memory the ability to remember to do a task or planned action in the future.

psychiatric rehabilitation model process of restoration of community functioning and well-being of an individual who has a psychiatric disability through seeking changes in a person's environment and in a person's ability to deal with his or her environment

psychoeducational groups closed and time-limited groups that are designed to educate participants and assist them in skill development while learning and applying their new knowledge by practicing skills in life situations.

psychodynamic therapy focuses on unconscious processes as they are manifested in a person's present behavior, with the goals being self-awareness and understanding of the influence of the past on present behavior.

psychosocial aspects pertaining to intrapersonal, interpersonal, and social experiences and interactions that influence occupational behavior (Mosey, 1996).

purposeful activity specifically selected, goal-directed activities that allow the client to develop skills that enhance occupational engagement.

quality of life the general well-being of individuals across all contexts of life.

recognition recognizing and identifying items and other aspects of the world.

rehabilitation to restore to good health or useful life, as through therapy and education.

required actions and performance skills the usual skills that would be required by any performer to carry out the activity. Sensory, perceptual, motor, praxis, emotional, cognitive, communication, and social performance skills should each be considered. The performance skills demanded by an activity will be correlated with the demands of the other activity aspects (e.g., objects, space).

resiliency the ability to successfully cope with change.

role playing engaging in a pretend scenario to try out new skills and abilities in a safe environment to prepare for participation in new activities.

sarcopenia the loss of strength in skeletal muscle as one ages, starting in middle age.

self-actualization a healthy self-concept, self-esteem, and sense of one's identity as an autonomous individual allowing one to understand his or her full potential.

self-determinism, hope, and empowerment characteristics gained through participation in psychoeducational group therapy as one develops a greater understanding of oneself and his or her actions.

self-understanding the insight one has into one's problems and the understanding of how one's behavior positively or negatively influences the problems one is dealing with in life.

semantic memory the portion of long-term memory concerned with ideas, meanings, and concepts that are not related to personal experiences.

sequence and timing process used to carry out the activity (e.g., specific steps, sequence, timing requirements).

short-term goals goals that define the desired outcomes of a single session and do not always depend on all members having attended previous sessions.

social demands social environment and cultural contexts that may be required by the activity.

social justice ensures a fair distribution of resources so that individuals and groups receive fair treatment and the opportunity to participate in society; provides normative principles designed to guide the allocation of the benefits and burdens of economic activity.

social learning theory (SLT) theory used to develop groups that aim to decrease behavioral problems, improve social behaviors and social skills, and to improve feelings of self-efficacy in performance.

social systems perspective applied when therapists understand the interpersonal aspects of their interactions with each client in the group as well as the interpersonal aspects of the mutual interactions between members.

social participation organized patterns of behavior that are characteristic and expected of an individual or given position within a social system.

social skills the interpersonal and communication skills necessary for successful social participation, relationships, and community engagement.

space demands physical environmental requirements of the activity (e.g., size, arrangement, surface, lighting, temperature, noise, humidity, ventilation).

special occasion group groups designed to work on a specific skill such as handwriting that is designed around a special occasion such as holidays or seasons.

spirituality "The personal quest for understanding answers to ultimate questions about life, about meaning, and about relationship with the sacred or transcendent, which may (or may not) lead to or arise from the development of religious rituals and the formation of community" (Moreira-Almeida & Koenig, 2006, p. 844).

storming the second stage of group development as defined by Tuckman (1965). The group is likely to see the highest level of disagreement and conflict. The leader must take on a negotiator and supporting role.

talk-based therapy therapeutic groups that use self-disclosure and sharing of experiences and feelings to promote insight and self-understanding.

tasks basic actions required to complete activities or occupations.

task-focused analysis focuses on and describes the basic actions required to perform each step of the skill being assessed.

task group groups that have specific outcomes and tasks to be accomplished.

task-focused group groups designed to address specific client factors and performance skills such as sensory processing, fine motor skills, strength, endurance, and range of motion.

task-oriented group group that allows for focus on both self-awareness and interactions with other group members during a structured activity.

teaching imparting knowledge or a skill.

thematic groups groups that focus on the clients learning the knowledge, skills, and activities for a specific activity.

teleologic theories state that an action is ethical or unethical depending on its consequence, and that the solutions to a dilemma should achieve the best outcome for the most number of people.

therapeutic factors qualities or traits that allow the facilitator to establish rapport with members and facilitate the group process.

therapeutic media items used in therapy during the intervention process.

topical groups similar to thematic groups with the difference being the focus of implementing the group activity in the community.

universal design for learning curricular flexibility to reduce barriers to provide appropriate supports and challenges and to maintain high academic achievement standards for all students enrolled in primary and secondary public education programs.

universality the realization that other members of a group have similar concerns and feelings and may have very similar experiences.

values principles, standards, or qualities considered worthwhile or desirable by the client who holds them (Moyers & Dale, 2007).

veracity practitioners are obligated to communicate accurately and truthfully and to make certain that the recipient clearly understands the message so he or she can make an informed decision.

verbal communication communication that includes both written and spoken words.

virtue ethics examine the characteristics of the individual and theorize that an individual with certain traits behave in an appropriate way.

visual aids items that provides cues to remind clients of key points, sequences, and directions.

visual perceptual mode incorporating demonstrations or models when teaching a new skill to a group of learners.

volition a person's values, interests, and self-efficacy about personal performance.

voluntary group participation members attend based solely on their personal desire to attend the group.

work and industry an emerging area of occupational therapy practice in which practitioners help clients achieve the most functional and optimal engagement in employment or volunteer activities.

worker roles task-oriented activities that involve accomplishing the group's goals.

REFERENCES:

American Occupational Therapy Association: Occupational therapy practice framework: domain and process, *Am J Occup Ther* 62:625–683, 2008.

Christiansen CH, Hammecker CL: Self care. In Bonder BR, Wagner MB, editors: *Functional performance in older adults*, Philadelphia, 2001, FA Davis, pp 155–175.

Crepeau E: Analyzing occupation and activity: A way of thinking about occupational performance. In Crepeau E, Cohn E, Schell B, editors: *Willard and Spackman's occupational therapy*, ed 10, Philadelphia, 2003, Lippincott Williams & Wilkins, pp 189–198.

Crepeau E, Cohn E, Schell B, editors: *Willard and Spackman's occupational therapy*, Philadelphia, 2003, Lippincott Williams & Wilkins.

Fisher A: Overview of performance skills and client factors. In Pendleton, Schultz-Krohn W, editors: *Pedretti's occupational therapy: practice skills for physical dysfunction*, St Louis, 2006, Mosby/Elsevier, pp 372–402.

Mosey AC: *Psychosocial components of occupational therapy*, New York, 1986, Raven Press.

Mosey A: *Psychosocial components of occupational therapy*, Philadelphia, 1996, Lippincott-Raven.

Moyers PA, Dale LM: *The guide to occupational therapy practice*, ed 2, Bethesda, MD, 2007, AOTA Press.

Moreira-Almeida A, Koenig HG: Retaining the meaning of the words religiousness and spirituality: a commentary on the WHOQOL SRPB group's "A cross-cultural study of spirituality, religion, and personal beliefs as components of quality of life" (62:6, 2005, pp. 1486-1497). Social Sci Med 63:843-845.

Rogers JC, Holm MB: Assessment of selfcare. In Bonder BR, Wagner MB, editors: *Functional performance in older adults*, Philadelphia, 1994, FA Davis, pp 181–202.

World Health Organization: *International classification of functioning, disability, and health (ICF)*, Geneva, 2001, Author.

Exercises and Forms for Practice

CHAPTER 1

IMPORTANT QUESTIONS TO CONSIDER WHEN DETERMINING OCCUPATIONAL GOALS

- What things give you meaning?
- How do you spend your days?
- What type of activities do you enjoy?
- What type of things make you excited?
- How would you describe yourself?
- What would you like to get back to doing?
- What would you like to accomplish in therapy?

FACTORS TO CONSIDER WHEN FORMING A GROUP

- Group and individual goals
- Age
- Gender
- Characteristics of members
- Setting

- Contexts (cultural, personal, temporal, physical, social, virtual)
- Needs of members
- Strengths and weaknesses
- Size of group
- Types of possible activities
- Duration
- Associated costs
- Personnel
- Length of membership and how it is established

BOX 1-2   **General Group Activity Analysis**

Name:
Group Activity:
Goal:
Steps (include sequence):
Preparation needed:
Client factors:
- Cognitive
- Social
- Motor
- Physical and environmental contexts
Precautions

TABLE 1-1   Values, Belief, and Spirituality

Name:

Activity:

Group:

Category and Definition	Examples	Example for This Activity
Values: Principles, standards, or qualities considered worthwhile or desirable by the client who holds them	**PERSON** Practice honesty with self and with others. Adhere to personal religious convictions. Practice commitment to family. **ORGANIZATION** Fulfill obligation to serve the community. Practice fairness. **POPULATION** Practice freedom of speech. Ensure equal opportunities for all. Practice tolerance toward others.	
Beliefs: Cognitive content held as true	**PERSON** He or she is powerless to influence others. Hard work pays off. **ORGANIZATION** Profits are more important than people. Achieving the mission of providing service can effect positive change in the world. **POPULATION** People can influence government by voting. Accessibility is a right, not a privilege.	
Spirituality: The "personal quest for understanding answers to ultimate questions about life, about meaning, and the sacred"[3] (p. 28)	**PERSON** Daily search for purpose and meaning in one's life. Guiding actions from a sense of value beyond the personal acquisition of wealth or fame. **ORGANIZATION AND POPULATION** (see "Person" examples related to individuals within an organization and population).	

From American Occupational Therapy Association: Occupational therapy practice framework: domain and process, *Am J Occup Ther* 62:634, 2008.

TABLE 1-2	**Client Factors: Body Functions and Structures**

Name:

Activity:

Group:

Body Functions		**Application to the Activity**
Categories	**Body Commonly Considered by Occupational Therapy Practitioners (not intended to be all-inclusive list)**	
Mental functions (affective, cognitive, perceptual		
■ Specific mental functions	Specific mental functions	
■ Higher-level cognitive	Judgment, concept formation, metacognition, cognitive flexibility, insight, attention, awareness	
■ Attention	Sustained, selective, and divided attention	
■ Memory	Short-term, long-term, and working memory	
■ Perception	Discrimination of sensations (e.g., auditory, tactile, visual, olfactory, gustatory, vestibular-proprioception), including multisensory processing, sensory memory, spatial, and temporal relationships (Calvert, Spence, & Stein, 2004)	
■ Thought	Recognition, categorization, generalization, awareness of reality, logical and coherent thought, and appropriate thought content	
■ Mental functions of sequencing complex movement	Execution of learned movement patters	
■ Emotional	Coping and behavioral regulation (Schell, Cohn, & Crepeau, 2008)	
■ Experience of self and time	Body image, self-concept, self-esteem	
GLOBAL MENTAL FUNCTIONS	**GLOBAL MENTAL FUNCTIONS**	
■ Consciousness	Level of arousal, level of consciousness	
■ Orientation	Orientation to person, place, time, self, and others	
■ Temperament and personality	Emotional stability	
■ Energy and drive	Motivation, impulse control, and appetite	
■ Sleep (physiological process)		
SENSORY FUNCTIONS AND PAIN	**SENSORY FUNCTIONS AND PAIN**	
■ Seeing and related functions, including visual acuity, visual stability, visual field functions	Detection and registration, modulation, and integration of sensations from the body and environment	
	Visual awareness of environment at various distances	
■ Hearing functions	Tolerance of ambient sounds; awareness of location and distance of sounds such as an approaching car	
■ Vestibular functions	Sensation of securely moving against gravity	
■ Taste functions	Association of taste	
■ Smell functions	Association of smell	

Continued

TABLE 1-2 Client Factors: Body Functions and Structures—Cont'd

SENSORY FUNCTIONS AND PAIN	SENSORY FUNCTIONS AND PAIN
■ Proprioceptive functions	Awareness of body position and space
■ Touch functions	Comfort with the feeling of being touched by others or touching various textures such as food
■ Pain (e.g., diffuse, dull, sharp, phantom)	Localized pain
■ Temperature and pressure	Thermal awareness
Neuromusculoskeletal and movement-related functions	**Neuromusculoskeletal and movement-related functions**
■ Functions of joints and bones	
■ Joint mobility	Joint range of motion
■ Joint stability	Postural alignment (this refers to the physiologic stability of the joint related to its structural integrity as compared to the motor skill of aligning the body while moving in relation to task objects)
■ Muscle power	Strength
■ Muscle tone	Degree of muscle tone (e.g., flaccidity, spasticity, fluctuating)
■ Muscle endurance	Endurance
■ Motor reflexes	Stretch, asymmetrical tonic neck, symmetrical tonic neck
■ Involuntary movement reactions	Righting and supporting
■ Control of voluntary movement	Eye—hand-foot coordination, bilateral integration, crossing the midline, fine- and gross-motor control, and oculomotor (e.g., saccades, pursuits, accommodation, binocularity)
■ Gait patterns	Walking patterns and impairments such as asymmetric gait, stiff gait. (Note: Gait patterns are considered in relation to how they affect ability to engage in occupations in daily life activities.)
CARDIOVASCULAR, HEMATOLOGIC, IMMUNOLOGIC, AND RESPIRATORY SYSTEM FUNCTION	**CARDIOVASCULAR, HEMATOLOGIC, IMMUNOLOGIC, AND RESPIRATORY SYSTEM FUNCTION**
■ Cardiovascular system function	Blood pressure functions (hypertension, hypotension, postural hypotension), and heart rate
■ Hematologic and immunologic system function	
■ Respiratory system function	
■ Additional functions and sensations of the cardiovascular and respiratory systems	Rate, rhythm, and depth of respiration
	Physical endurance, aerobic capacity, stamina, and fatigability

TABLE 1-2	Client Factors: Body Functions and Structures—Cont'd	
VOICE AND SPEECH FUNCTIONS	(Note: Occupational therapy practitioners have knowledge of these body functions and understand broadly the interaction that occurs between these functions to support health and participation in life through engagement in occupation. Some therapists may specialize in evaluating and intervening with a specific function, such as incontinence and pelvic floor disorders, as it is related to supporting performance and engagement in occupations and activities targeted for intervention.	
■ Voice functions		
■ Fluency and rhythm		
■ Alternative vocalization functions		
DIGESTIVE, METABOLIC, AND ENDOCRINE SYSTEM FUNCTION		
■ Digestive system function		
■ Metabolic system and endocrine system function		
GENITOURINARY AND REPRODUCTIVE FUNCTIONS		
■ Urinary functions		
■ Genital and reproductive functions		
SKIN AND RELATED-STRUCTURE FUNCTIONS	**SKIN AND RELATED-STRUCTURE FUNCTIONS**	
■ Skin functions	Protective functions of the skin—presence or absence of wounds, cuts, or abrasions	
■ Hair and nail functions	Repair function of the skin—wound healing	
BODY STRUCTURES		
Categories	**Examples are note delineated in the "Body structure" section of this table.**	
Structure of the nervous system Eyes, ear, and related structures Structures involved in voice and speech Structures of the cardiovascular, immunologic, and respiratory systems Structures related to the digestive, metabolic, and endocrine systems Structure related to the genitourinary and reproductive systems Structures related to movement Skin and related structures		

From data adapted from the International Classification of Functioning (World Health Organization, 2001) in Table 2 from American Occupational Therapy Association: Occupational therapy practice framework: domain and process, *Am J Occup Ther* 62:635-637, 2008.

TABLE 1-3   Activity Demands

Name:

Activity:

Group:

Activity Demand Aspects	Definition	Examples for this Activity
Objects and their properties	Tools, materials, and equipment used in the process of carrying out the activity, including inherent properties	
Space demands (relates to physical context	Physical environmental requirements of the activity (e.g., size, arrangement, surface, lighting, temperature, noise, humidity, ventilation)	
Social demands (relates to social environment and cultural contexts)	Social environment and cultural contexts that may be required by the activity, including rules of conduct, expectations of others	
Sequence and timing	Process used to carry out the activity (e.g., specific steps, sequence, timing requirements)	
Required actions and performance skills	The usual skills that would be required by any performer to carry out the activity, including sensory, perceptual, motor, praxis, emotional, cognitive, communication, and social performance skills Performance skills demanded by an activity correlated with the demands of the other activity aspects (e.g., objects, space)	
Required body functions	"[P]hysiological functions of body systems (including psychological functions)" (WHO, 2001, p. 10) that are required to support the actions used to perform the activity	
Required body structures	"Anatomical parts of the body such as organs, limbs, and their components" that support body function (WHO, 2001, p. 10) that are required to perform the activity	

Table 3 from American Occupational Therapy Association: Occupational therapy practice framework: domain and process, *Am J Occup Ther* 62:638, 2008.
WHO, World Health Organization.

TABLE 1-4 Performance Skills

Name:

Activity:

Group:

Skill	Examples
Motor and praxis skills	
Sensory-perceptual skills	
Emotional regulation skills	
Cognitive skills	
Communication and social skills	

TABLE 1-5 Contexts

Name:

Activity:

Group:

Context and Environment	Application to Activity
Cultural	
Personal	
Temporal	
Virtual	
Physical	
Social	

CHAPTER 2

BOX 2-1 Analysis of Cognitive Skills

Name:
Activity:
Group:

Skill	Example
Judging	
Selecting	
Organizing	
Problem Solving	
Sequencing	
Prioritizing	
Understanding	
Being aware	

BOX 2-2 Psychosocial Skills Considered for Activity

Skill	Example
Responding	
Reading	
Persisting	
Controlling	
Displaying	
Coping	
Problem Solving	
Recovering	
Listening and responding	
Engaging	
Relaxing	
Responding	

BOX 2-3 Occupational Profile

Name of Client:
Reason for seeking services:
Concerns related to occupational therapy:
Client's goals:
Describe client's life experiences:
How would client define self?
Where does client live and with whom does he or she interact?

BOX 2-4 Activity Configuration

Name:
Occupational Profile summary
Goals:
Objectives:
Suggested activities:
Rationale:
   The activities promote the goals and objectives (use of the right arm and hand) while considering the individual profile of client.

BOX 2-5 Activity Analysis

Activity:
Materials:
Equipment:
Group members:
Precautions:
Sequence:
Requirements:
Contexts:
Activity demands:

BOX 2-6 | Understanding Occupation, Activity, and Task

Name:
Describe what makes something an occupation, activity or task.
    Provide an example.
Occupation:
Activity:
Task:

BOX 2-7 | Properties of Media

Name:
Activity:
Describe the media used in an activity using the following terms:
Texture
Consistency
Size
Purpose
Shape
Color
Sensory properties

TABLE 2-1 | Adapting and Grading Tasks

Name:
Activity:
Group:
Describe the task required to complete the activity and provide
examples of how to make the task easier or more difficult.

Task	Easier	Harder

CHAPTER 3

BOX 3-1 | Group Protocol

Name:
Topic:
Members:
Setting:
Rationale:
Goals:
    Long Term:
    Short Term:
Outcome Measures:
Meeting Schedule:
Materials:
    List all materials needed—type, number, etc.
    Include cost of each item.
    Include method of acquiring each item.
Session Plan:
1. Introduction (10 minutes)
■ Introduce leaders and set the tone.
■ Introduce members.
■ Review purpose and expectations.
■ Provide outline of session.
2. Activity
■ Describe the activity step by step in detail.
■ Identify the physical, cognitive, and psychosocial skills needed
    for participation.
    ■ Physical:
    ■ Cognitive:
    ■ Psychosocial:
■ Describe how the activity can be adapted if needed.
■ State the therapeutic goals.
3. Closure
■ Review application to daily life.
■ Assess goal achievement.
4. End Group
Additional Information.

BOX 3-2 | Model for Group Leadership

Name:
Activity:
Group:
1. Introduction

Application to this Activity

Warm-Up and Setting the Mood: Includes lighting, room arrangement, materials, and
  position of the leader. Is the group formal or informal?
Expectation of the Group and Explaining the Purpose: Describe the behavioral expectations
  and purpose of the group. For example, members are expected to remain in the
  group and participate. Everyone should support each other. If anyone is having
  difficulty remaining in the group or following the expectations, let the leader
  know.
Brief Outline of the Session: Give an overview and show a completed project if applicable. Be sure to include time for clean up and remind group members to help.

2. Activity

Application to this Activity

Timing and Therapeutic Goals: Carefully review the therapeutic goals and time each part
  of the activity. Being aware of time is essential.
Physical and Mental Capacities of the Members: Understanding the physical and mental
  capacities of members helps practitioners design group activities. Monitor the
  members' capacities as they work to be sure they can complete the activities.
  Guide members or adapt activities as needed so all can participate.
Knowledge and Skill of the Leader: Be knowledgeable about the activity and skill level
  required prior to leading the group. Complete the activity and note the areas that
  may be difficult. Allow extra time for those areas and preplan how to adapt the
  activity if the group needs it.
Adaptation of an Activity: Examine each step and determine what changes can be
  made to the activity if needed. Have additional materials (that are already
  adapted) available. For example, have directions in large print or precut
  materials.

3. Sharing
Clients Share Experiences: Provide opportunities for each client to share his or her experience in the activity. Relate this experience to others.
Leader Acknowledge Each Member: Leaders should acknowledge each member positively,
  using the person's name and emphasizing improvement.

4. Processing
Members Express Feelings about Experience and Others: Allow members to express their
  feelings about the experience and how the group performed. The leader must ask
  questions and be open to the feedback.

5. Generalizing
Address Cognitive Learning Aspects of the Group: Reflect on the cognitive aspects of the
  group and determine how the group went.

6. Application
How Does This Apply to Everyday Life? Ask members how they might use skills from the
  group in other settings and in their daily life. Discuss different scenarios with the
  group.

7. Summary
Review Goals, Content, Process: Emphasize to members how the group addressed their
  goals. Did they feel challenged? Would they be able to use skills learned in other
  settings? Are there any areas on which they need to continue to work? What did
  they like or dislike about the process or content?

Cole MB: *Group dynamics in occupational therapy*, 3rd ed, Thorofare, NJ, 2005, Slack.

CHAPTER 4

TABLE 4-1 Client Interpersonal Characteristics

Name:
Activity:
Provide an example for a group that you observed that describes the interpersonal characteristic.

Interpersonal Characteristic	Group Therapy Example
Communication style	
Capacity for trust	
Need for control	
Capacity to assert needs	
Response to change and challenge	
Affect	
Predisposition to giving feedback	
Capacity to receive feedback	
Response to human diversity	
Orientation toward relating	
Preference for touch	
Capacity for reciprocity	

TABLE 4-2 The Inevitable Interpersonal Events of Occupational Therapy

Name:
Activity:
Group:
Provide an example for groups you observed of an interpersonal event.

Interpersonal Event	Definition	Group Therapy Example
Expression of Strong Emotion	External displays of internal feelings are shown with a high level of intensity beyond usual cultural norms for interaction. Can be positive or negative expressions.	
Intimate Self-Disclosures	Statements or stories reveal something unobservable, private, or sensitive about the person making a disclosure. These can be stories about oneself or about close others.	
Power Dilemmas	Tensions arise in the therapeutic relationship because of clients' innate feelings about issues of power, the inherent situation of therapy, the therapist's behavior, or other circumstances that underscore clients' lack or loss of power over aspects of their lives.	
Nonverbal Cues	Communications do not involve the use of formal language. Some examples of these are facial expressions, movement patterns, body posture, and eye contact.	
Crisis Points	Unanticipated, stressful events cause clients to become distracted or temporarily interfere with clients' ability for occupational engagement.	
Resistance and Reluctance	Resistance is a client's passive or active refusal to participate in some or all aspects of therapy for reasons linked to the therapeutic relationship. Reluctance is disinclination toward some aspect of therapy for reasons outside the therapeutic relationship.	
Boundary Testing	Client behavior violates or asks the therapist to act in ways that is outside the defined therapeutic relationship.	
Empathic Breaks	Therapist fails to notice or understand a communication from a client, or communication or behavior initiated by the therapist is perceived by the client as hurtful or insensitive.	
Emotionally Charged Therapy Tasks and Situations	Activities or circumstances can lead clients to become overwhelmed or experience uncomfortable emotional reactions such as embarrassment, humiliation, or shame.	
Limitations of Therapy	The available or possible services, time, resources, or therapist actions are restricted.	
Contextual Inconsistencies	Refers to any aspect of a client's interpersonal or physical environment that changes during the course of therapy.	

TABLE 4-3 The Six Therapeutic Modes

Name:
Activity:
Group:
Provide an example of each mode.

Mode	Definition	Group Therapy Example
Advocating	Ensure that the client's rights are enforced and resources are secured. May require the therapist to serve as a mediator, facilitator, negotiator, enforcer, or other type of advocate with external persons and agencies.	
Collaborating	Expect the client to be an active and equal participant in therapy. Ensure choice, freedom, and autonomy to the greatest extent possible.	
Empathizing	Ongoing striving to understand the client's thoughts, feelings, and behaviors while suspending any judgment. Ensure that the client verifies and experiences the therapist's understanding as truthful and validating.	
Encouraging	Seize the opportunity to instill hope in a client. Celebrate a client's thinking or behavior through positive reinforcement. Convey an attitude of joyfulness, playfulness, and confidence.	
Instructing	Carefully structure therapy activities and be explicit with clients about the plan, sequence, and events of therapy. Provide clear instruction and feedback about performance. Set limits on a client's requests or behavior.	
Problem Solving	Facilitate pragmatic thinking and solving dilemmas by outlining choices, posing strategic questions, and providing opportunities for comparative or analytical thinking.	

TABLE 4-4   The Six Steps of the Interpersonal Reasoning Process

Name:
Activity:
Group:
Provide an example of each step of interpersonal reasoning from a group that you lead.

Step of Interpersonal Reasoning	Definition	Example
Anticipate.	Use observational skills, information from others who have interacted with the client, and your direct experience interacting with the client to anticipate the likely interpersonal events that may occur during therapy, given your knowledge of the client's interpersonal characteristics.	
Identify and cope.	Use IRM language to label a difficult client characteristic or interpersonal event when it occurs. Do what it takes to collect yourself and get emotional perspective on the situation. Remind yourself not to take it personally.	
Determine if a mode shift is required.	Ask yourself the following questions to determine whether a mode shift is required: What mode am I currently using with this client, if any? What are the effects of the mode on the client? Would another mode better serve the interpersonal needs of this client at this moment?	
Choose a response mode or mode sequence.	Interact within the mode or modes that you think the client prefers or needs at this moment. Think about a sequence of modes that you might use to accommodate changes in what the client might need from moment to moment.	
Draw on any relevant interpersonal skills associated with the modes.	Think about other communication, rapport-building, and conflict resolution skills that you might draw on in association with your mode use.	
Gather feedback.	Gather nonverbal or verbal feedback from the client as to whether he or she feels comfortable with the way you approached the event or difficulty.	

IRM, Intentional relationship model.

TABLE 4-5 Examples of Dynamics that Have the Potential to Interfere with the Process or Desired Outcome of Therapy

Name:
Activity:
Group:
Provide examples of the dynamics observed in a group that you observed or led.

Dynamic	Example
Help-Seeking/Help-Rejecting	
Competitive	
Enabling Negative Behavior	
Dominance/Submission	
Enmeshment	
Disengagement	
Approach/Avoidance	
Idealizing/Devaluing	
Reluctance/Reassurance	
Demonstrative/Voyeuristic	
Helpless/Rescuing	
Chaotic/Organizing	
Manipulating/Conceding	
Scapegoating	

CHAPTER 5

TABLE 5-1 Using Tools for Teaching

Name:
Activity:
Group:
Describe how you would use each tool with group members in the activity.

Tool	Example
Meaningful repetition	
Plain language	
Just right challenge	
Objects to stimulate learning	
Colorful handout	
Active engagement	

TABLE 5-2 Perceptual Learning Styles and Characteristics

Name:
Activity:
Group:
Describe how each of the learning styles could be used in the desired activity.

Perceptual Learning Style	Characteristics	Examples
Print	Takes notes. Learns best by seeing. Reads often.	
Aural	Remembers and repeats ideas. Excellent listener. Enjoys drama, music, dialogues.	
Interactive	Enjoys small-group discussions. Prefers to discuss things. Learns best through verbalization.	
Visual	Learns through watching demonstrations. Drifts when extensive listening is required. Likes picture graphs and other visual aids.	
Haptic	Learns through touching. Likes to trace words and pictures. Likes tasks that require manipulating objects.	
Kinesthetic	Learns by doing and moving. Gestures while speaking. Finds reasons to move, which increases concentration.	
Olfactory	Learns best by smelling and tasting. Associates smell with past experiences. Scents increases learning.	

TABLE 5-3 Perceptual Pathways

Name:
Activity:
Group:
Provide an example of each pathway.

Pathway	Example
Print: reading	
Aural: listening	
Interactive: discussing	
Visual: watching demonstrations	
Haptic: manipulating	
Kinesthetic: moving	
Olfactory: smelling	

TABLE 5-4   Checklist for Teaching Process

Name:
Activity:
Group:
Complete the form as related to the group activity.

Preparation		Description of Activities
	Space	
	Supplies and materials	
	Completed project	
	Handouts	
	Time needed	
	Costs	
	Travel	
	Precautions (allergies, sunscreen)	
	Activity plan (introduction, activity, conclusion)	
Activity	Group members' needs	
	Special considerations	
	Directions	
	Wrap up, reminders	
	Clean up	
Follow up		
Suggestions for next time		

BOX 5-6 Williams Motor Learning Principles

Name:

Activity:

Group:

Provide examples of how you might use these principles in a group session.

Area	Principle	Application in Group
TRANSFER OF LEARNING	Skill experiences need to be presented in logical progression.	
	Simple, foundational skills should be practiced before more complex skills.	
	Skill practice should include "real" life and simulated settings.	
	Skills with similar components are more likely to show transfer effect.	
FEEDBACK		
Modeling or Demonstration		
	Demonstration is best if it is given to the individual prior to practicing the skill and the early stages of skill acquisition.	
	Demonstration should be given throughout practice and as frequently as deemed helpful.	
	Demonstrations should not be accompanied by verbal commentary as this can reduce attention paid to important aspects of the skill being demonstrated.	
	It is important to direct the individual's attention to the critical cues immediately before the skill is demonstrated.	
Verbal Instructions		
	Verbal cues should be brief, to the point, and involve 1-3 words.	
	Verbal cues should be limited in terms of numbers of cues given during or after performance.	
	Only the major aspect of the skill that is being concentrated on should be cued.	
	Verbal cues should be carefully timed, so they do not interfere with performance.	
	Verbal cues can and should be initially repeated by the performer.	
Knowledge of Results and Knowledge of Performance		
	A variety of different combinations of both KR and KP typically helps to facilitate learning.	
	KP error information may help performer change important performance characteristics and thus may help facilitate skill acquisition.	
	Information about "appropriate" or "correct" aspects of performance helps to motivate the person to continue practicing.	
	It is important to balance between feedback that is error-based and that based on "appropriate" or "correct" characteristics of the performance.	
	KP feedback can also be descriptive or prescriptive; prescriptive KP is more helpful than just descriptive KP in early or beginning stages of learning.	
	KP and KR should be given close in time to but after completion of the task.	
	KP and KR typically should not necessarily be given 100% of the time.	
	Learning is enhanced if KP and KR are given at least 50% of the time.	
	A frequently used procedure for KR and KP is to practice a skill several times and then provide the appropriated feedback.	

Continued

BOX 5-6   Williams Motor Learning Principles—cont'd

Area	Principle	Application in Group
DISTRIBUTION AND VARIABILITY OF SKILL PRACTICE		

Shorter, more frequent practice sessions are preferable to longer, less frequent practice.

If a skill or task is complex, requires a relatively long time to perform, or requires repetitive movements, relatively short practice trials or sessions with frequent rest periods are preferable.

If the skill is relatively simple and takes only a brief time to complete, longer practice trials or sessions with less frequent rest periods are preferable.

It can enhance skill acquisition to practice several tasks in the same session.

If several tasks are to be practiced, divide the time spent on each and either randomly repeat practice on each or use a sequence that aids the overall practice.

Providing a number of different environmental contexts in which the skill is practiced appears to facilitate learning.

With regard to the amount of practice, more is not necessarily always better.

Clinical judgment should be used to recognize when practice is no longer producing changes; at this time a new or different task could and probably should be introduced.

WHOLE VERSUS PART PRACTICE

Whole practice is better when the skill or task to be performed is simple.

Part practice may be preferable when the skill is more complex.

If part practice is used, be sure that the parts practiced are "natural units" or "go together," so to speak.

To simplify a task, reduce the nature or complexity of the objects to be manipulated (e.g., use a balloon for catching instead of a ball, etc.)

To simplify a task, provide assistance to the learner that helps to reduce attention demands (e.g., provide trunk support during practice of different eye-hand coordination tasks).

To simplify a task, provide auditory or rhythmic accompaniment; this may help to facilitate learning through assisting the learner in getting the appropriate "rhythm" of the movement.

MENTAL PRACTICE

Mental practice can help to facilitate acquisition of new skills as well as the relearning of old skills.

Mental practice can help the person to prepare to perform a task.

Mental practice combined with physical practice works best.

For mental practice to be effective, the individual should have some basic imagery ability.

Mental practice should be relatively short, not prolonged.

KP, Knowledge of performance; *KR,* knowledge of results.

WORKSHEET 5-1   Understanding Pathways of Learning

Name:

Activity:

Group:

Use the following worksheet to identify how an activity can help clients learn.

Process	Questions	Examples
Recognition	What is required for this activity? What must the client process? What is the sensory input?	
Strategic	What must the client "figure out"? What steps in the activity require problem solving? Must the client arrange things in relationship to others?	
Affective	What does the learner feel about the activity? What is the importance of the activity? Was the activity pleasurable? How did the learner assess his or her performance? What did the learner gain from the activity?	

CHAPTER 6

BOX 6-1   Development of a Group Intervention

Preplanning a Group Program
List the characteristics of the target population (age, diagnosis, status such as inpatient, outpatient, community-based, socioeconomic status;, health insurance, etc.).

_____

_____

_____

_____

List the occupational therapy needs of the target population.

_____

_____

_____

_____

Are the needs of the target population most effectively met by a group intervention? Justify the answer with empirical evidence that supports a group intervention as the optimal mode of therapy.

_____

_____

_____

_____

Identify the type of group intervention (frame of reference) that is supported by the empirical evidence for these clients' needs (e.g., psycho-education, cognitive-behavioral therapy, motor-relearning theory, sensory integration theory, social learning theory, gestalt therapy, illness management and recovery).

_____

_____

_____

_____

Identify the type of group structure (open, closed; time limited; directive; problem-, diagnosis-, or population-specific).

_____

_____

_____

_____

Identify the schedule of group and time frame (number of sessions; whether they are daily, weekly, or biweekly; and duration such as 8 weeks, permanent program, or as needed).

_____

_____

_____

Identify criteria for admission: Define the gate-keeping process (e.g., all inpatients admitted to unit, all presurgical total hip patients, self- or physician-referral, children currently enrolled in occupational therapy).

_____

_____

_____

_____

Identify list of resources required to implement program and costs: Practitioner expertise to deliver program (does it require specialized skills such as cognitive behavioral therapy training, or sensory integration certification to implement group), space, equipment, materials. How will these resources be provided? Create a budget if necessary.

_____

_____

_____

_____

Identify source of reimbursement.

_____

_____

Identify how the group intervention's effectiveness will be measured and reported to clients and payment providers. Measurement and communication of group outcomes is often overlooked in the planning phase. Pretesting is fundamental in demonstrating the effectiveness of occupational therapy services and the communication of outcomes is crucial to sustaining services.

_____

_____

_____

_____

BOX 6-2   Planning a Group Program

When program will be implemented: date_____

Where program will be implement: room_____

Number of sessions_____

Staff_____

Number of groups members to be enrolled_____

Identify purpose of group:

Outline frame of reference and core assumptions of this approach:

Identify long-term goals:

Identify screening, and pre- and postest evaluation:

Outline the sessions:

List all materials, personnel, and resources needed to implement program:

BOX 6-3   Reviewing Goal Structure

Until you are proficient in writing goals, check off that you have included all the elements within each of your goals. I have below identified the components of the earlier example:

Group members will **identify six fears** that **interfere with their ability to talk in social settings**
    [Actors]   [Behavior]   [Condition]
demonstrated by **verbally sharing these fears** by **end of the communications skills group session.**
    [Measurement or Criteria]   [Timeframe]

Actor
Behavior
Condition
Measurement or Criteria
Timeframe

BOX 6-4   Guidelines for Individual Session

This template provides instructions for an individual session. Write this outline so another occupational therapy practitioner could follow it and run the session. Once these instructions are developed, they can be reused for future groups.

Purpose of Group Session
Briefly state the purpose of the session. This will be used in the introduction of the session.

_____
_____
_____
_____
_____

Goals for Group Session
Write the specific goals to be achieved in this group. The relationship to the long- term goals need to be clear as these short-term goals are the steps to achieving them.
1. _____
2. _____
3. _____

Materials Needed

_____
_____
_____
_____
_____

Introduction
Outline the key points for the introduction that state the purpose of the session; expectations of the session, including goals; and reiterate group norms as applicable to an individual sessions. Describe what will happen in the session and the time frame.

_____
_____
_____
_____
_____

Warm-up: Describe the Warm-up (Icebreaker)
A warm-up is short (5-10 minutes of a hour session). It energizes and focuses on bringing group members together around a common purpose expressed by the short-term goals of the group. Therefore the warm-up is not a random activity. It is carefully chosen to orient the members to the theme or topic of the group activity and its demands are consistent with the stage of group development. For example, when a group is new, warm-up activities are likely to

emphasize common themes or shared problems to reinforce members' sense of belonging and similarities. At the productive stage of group development, the warm-up may require disclosure of more personal information or be more emotionally demanding.

_____
_____
_____
_____
_____

Activity or Intervention
Outline the steps of the activity. This might be a discussion group, in which case the talking points are outlined, or it might be a task group in which the directions for a specific activity are documented.

_____
_____
_____
_____
_____

Conclusion of Group
In the conclusion phase of the group a number of tasks need to be completed, so it is important to make sure there is adequate time to address them. These are (1) summation of the group by either members or group leader, (2) application and generalization to occupational performance in everyday life, and (3) homework to reinforce transfer of learning and generalization of skills or behaviors.

_____
_____

Postgroup Evaluation
Document immediately following a group session. Critique the group and write comments and recommendations for the next time this group session is run. In a busy schedule, it is difficult to recall the details of a specific group. Taking 5 minutes to document an evaluation of the group will significantly reduce time planning this session in the future and continue to improve occupational therapy services. This feedback could include changes to the activity, points about structuring the activity, time management, or points for facilitating this group.

_____
_____
_____
_____
_____

BOX 6-5   **A Postgroup Observation Checklist**

POSTGROUP EVALUATION

AREA OF OBSERVATION COMMENTS AND ACTIONS

Group Climate
- ☐ Space—room
- ☐ Lighting, heating, ventilation, seating suitability
- ☐ No interruptions of distractions
- ☐ Organization and materials supported group goals
- ☐ Openness and appropriate level of trust among members
- ☐ Sense of cohesion among members

Group Norms
- ☐ Therapeutic group norms maintained
- ☐ Lateness, absences
- ☐ Members listened to each other
- ☐ Members were respectful of others
- ☐ Decisions made collectively and accepted

Group Goals—Productivity
- ☐ Goals were clear and stated
- ☐ Goals understood by members
- ☐ Goals relevant to members
- ☐ Goals for group met

Group Activity
- ☐ Occupation based
- ☐ Facilitated members' goal attainment
- ☐ Activities supported group goals
- ☐ Activities presented clearly and understood
- ☐ Activity demands appropriate and relevant

Participation—Interaction
- ☐ Cooperation encouraged participation
- ☐ Member-to-member interaction
- ☐ Members interested and involved
- ☐ Members restless and disengaged
- ☐ Balanced participation (no member dominated or withdrawn)
- ☐ Members listened and built on each others' ideas and actions

Leadership
- ☐ Directions and introduction clear
- ☐ Positively facilitated members' participation
- ☐ Encouraged group interaction
- ☐ Constructively set limits
- ☐ Elicited members' feelings and ideas
- ☐ Time management ensured completion of activities with full member participation
- ☐ Concluded group with summary
- ☐ Reinforced generalization of learning beyond group session

General Comments

Box developed using
Dimock H G : *How to observe your groups*, ed 3, North York, Ontario, 1993, Captus Press.

CHAPTER 7

TABLE 7-1 Suggestions for Changing Activities

Activity:

Be specific on how you will change the requirements for this activity.

Activity Requirement	Easy	Difficult
Time		
Strength		
Repetitions		
Speed		
Accuracy		
Variety		
Cognitive		
Materials		
Attention		
Other:		

TABLE 7-2 Goals for Selected Groups

Complete the following table using a variety of groups.

Group Name	Member characteristics	Goal	Purpose

BOX 7-1 Group Guidelines

Name of Group: _____

Group Goal: _____

Leaders: _____

Number of Members in Group: _____

Length of sessions: _____ Number of sessions: _____

Location: _____

Cost per week: _____

Equipment: _____

Types of sessions: _____

_____

_____

_____

_____

_____

_____

_____

Comments: _____

_____

_____

_____

_____

BOX 7-2 Considerations When Planning a Group Session

Comment on each consideration in regard to your group.

- Age: Will some members serve to mentor others? Would their pairings help facilitate progression toward goals?
- Gender: Are there members who will work better with the same or opposite gender?
- Personality characteristics: Consider the extrovert, introvert, passive, aggressive, manipulative, blocking, caring, empathetic characteristics of clients when requiring group members to interact.
- Goals: How do group members' goals relate?
- Physical: Are there certain members who need help with physical tasks? Consider how you will encourage success for all members in the group.
- Cognitive: Consider how each member can handle the cognitive tasks of the group.
- Social: What are the social requirements of the group? How can you facilitate social participation?
- Emotional level: What are the psychosocial characteristics of members? What is the purpose of the group and what type of intensity of emotions may be displayed? Are members able to support each other? Are group members safe to disclose personal information if needed?

Writing Individual Goals

Practice writing goals defining each required element.
Who: Who is the Client? (Actor)
Action: What will you see as the performance (Behavior)
Condition: Under what circumstance with the client complete the action?
Criteria: What are the standards for success?

Elements	Goal
Who (Actor)	
Action (Behavior)	
Condition	
Measurement or Criteria	
Timeframe	

CHAPTER 8

BOX 8-1 Physical Environmental Considerations

Describe the Environment
What is the best lighting for the intervention? Low, bright, black lights?
What equipment is available? Moving or stationary?
What materials and supplies are available? Paper, pencil, crayons; wipe board and markers?

Groups with Children
Develop a resource list of activities you could use in groups with children.

Theme	Activity	Goals (general areas)	Materials	Resources (e.g., web sites)

CHAPTER 9

TABLE 9-1 Psychosocial Developmental Tasks of Adolescents to Integrate into Group Interventions

Describe the developmental tasks of each stage of adolescence.

PSYCHOSOCIAL DEVELOPMENTAL TASKS OF ADOLESCENCE

The developmental tasks in adolescence accumulate:
- The ability to establishing healthy relationships
- A sense of identify that includes a healthy self-concept and body image, and positive self-esteem
- Gender identification and the capacity for intimacy and expression of one's sexuality
- An occupational identity

Early Adolescence:
In the middle school and early high school, a practitioner will find that adolescents in the groups are:

Middle Adolescence:
In the middle years of adolescence (the high school years), a practitioner is likely to find that the adolescents in the groups are:

Late adolescence:
In the latter years of adolescence (late high school, starting work or college) a practitioner may observe the adolescents in groups are:

BOX 9-1   Group Interventions that Build Social Skills for Social Participation

Define the skills in each category that would help clients build social skills for social participation.

Communication Skills

Interpreting Social Interactions and Situations

Managing Social Interaction and Self-Regulation

Self-Regulation and Expression (Emotions And Cognitive Processes)

TABLE 9-2   Strategies for Working with Adolescents in Groups

Provide examples of how you might use the given strategy (based on MOHO theory) with adolescents:

Strategy	Example in practice
Structure the therapeutic environment to:	.
Validate:	
Identify:	
Give feedback:	
Advise adolescents to:	
Encourage:	
Physically support:	
Coach:	
Negotiate with adolescent concerning:	

MOHO, Model of Human Occupation.

TABLE 9-3   Example of an Individual Psychoeducational Group

Use this template to design a psychoeducational group for adolescents.

PSYCHOEDUCATIONAL GROUP PROGRAM
Title:

Purpose of Group Session:

Goals for Group Session:
By the end of the session group members will be able to:

Materials:

Introduction:

Warm-up (5 to 10 minutes):

Intervention:

Education Session:

Processing—experiential learning component:

Homework:

Conclusion of Group:

BOX 9-3   **Activity Group Taxonomy**

Provide examples of adolescent groups for each type of group.

Type of Group	**Example**
Evaluative	
Task Oriented	
Developmental	
(There are five activity groups in this category and each is structured around abilities of the member based on the developmental level of their psychosocial capacity.)	
■ Parallel	
■ Project	
■ Egocentric	
■ Cooperative	
■ Mature	
Thematic	
Topical	
Instrumental	

BOX 9-4   **A Practitioner's Reflection on Practice Checklist for Groups with Adolescents**

Were the strategies, structure, and group process therapeutically appropriate for adolescents and their goals?

Check those that were present or occurred in the group session.
- ■ Opportunities for experimentation and risk taking within the constraints of a safe, accepting environment
- ■ Participation of most or all members
- ■ Moments of playfulness, fun, and laughter
- ■ Group climate that provide a sense of belonging and was supportive
- ■ Validation of members ideas, feelings, and constructive actions
- ■ Space for independence and personal choice within normative boundaries
- ■ Environmental stressors addressed
- ■ Task demands were appropriate for performance skills
- ■ Group capitalized on skills attained while providing the "just-right" challenge to promote further skill development

- ■ Peer-based learning
- ■ Exploration of roles
- ■ Inclusion of time to express thoughts and feeling
- ■ Age-related social media used
- ■ Group goals met

Group leaders:
- ■ Were clear about rules and expectations
- ■ Were consistent about expectations and followed through on their commitments
- ■ Avoided jargon
- ■ Avoided getting defensive when challenged
- ■ Managed behaviors such as distress, anxiety, or acting out behaviors respectfully (going with resistance and avoiding power struggles)
- ■ Acknowledged successes and constructive behaviors

CHAPTER 10

FORM 10-1   Feedback on Group Experience

Name:
Role in group: Leader, Participant, Observer
Provide feedback on the following items (Be specific and provide examples):
1. Content and interest of the activity
2. Organization of the environment and materials
3. Delivery and therapeutic use of self
4. Temporal awareness
5. Ability to control the group
6. Ability to modify activity to meet individual needs
7. Ability to answer questions
8. Eye contact with participants
9. Materials, organization, preparation
10. Visual aid

FORM 10-2   Self-Evaluation of Group Experience

Leader's Name
1. How well prepared were you?
   a. Were there enough supplies, materials?
   b. Did you feel organized and knowledgeable?
2. How well did you provide directions to the group?
   a. Were you respectful toward members?
   b. Did you clearly describe the steps?
   c. Were written directions or a sample provided?
3. Was the activity interesting?
   a. Was the goal of the group clear?
   b. Did you meet the goal?
4. Overall impression of the group:
5. How did you do at grading and adapting the activity for the different populations?
   a. Was there anybody that was more difficult in the group?
   b. What would do differently?
6. Suggestions for improvement for next time:
7. Summarize your strengths and weaknesses:
8. Ideas:

BOX 10-1   Steps of Group Design

Describe how you would apply each step to a group session.

Steps	Application to Group Session
1. Review individual goals and objectives.	
2. Determine the areas of occupation to be addressed.	
3. Identify present functional levels and necessary accommodations.	
4. Identify group members based on individual needs and goals of group.	
5. Schedule group.	
6. Implement group (describe the group session you would lead).	
7. Document and evaluate session. (How would you evaluate the session?)	

TABLE 10-2   Sample Groups Based on Selected Areas of Occupation

Provide examples of group themes and sessions based on each area of occupation.

Area of Occupation	Sample Group Theme	Session Example
Activities of Daily Living		
Instrumental Activities of Daily Living		
Community Mobility		
Education		
Work		
Play		
Leisure		
Social Participation		

FIGURE 10-2   Process of Group Analysis

Describe how you would apply the process of group analysis by providing an example for each category for one client.

Group Process Category	Example of Application to Specific Client
General condition and population information	
Occupational strengths and weaknesses	
Client factors and body function	
Context of activity	
Teaching and learning activity	
Feedback	

BOX 10-2   Literature Search on Assigned Population

Student:
Date:
Population:

Definition of client factors involved:
Research characteristics of this population in peer-reviewed publications and the Internet.
(Give proper American Psychological Association [APA] reference citations.)
Describe potential occupational limitations faced by members of this population.

Describe some grading and adaptations that would promote successful participation in group activities:
   Adaptations:
   Gradations:
References in APA format

TABLE 10-3 Client Factor Analysis

Use the following form to complete a thorough client factor analysis for a specific activity.

Name:

Activity:

Brief description of activity:

Please describe how each client factor is used in the activity. (Some items may not apply to the selected activity).

Category	Client Factors	X Used	If Used, Describe How It Applies to This Activity (Be Specific)
	Values, beliefs, spirituality		
Specific mental functions Higher level cognitive	Judgment		
	Problem solving		
	Learning		
	Generalization		
	Cognitive Flexibility		
	Metacognition		
	Attention		
	Memory		
	Visual perception		
	Position in space—proprioception		
	Kinesthesia		
	Sequencing complex movement		
	Emotional expression and regulation		
Experience of self and time	Self-concept, self -esteem		
	Body image		
Global mental functions	Orientation		
	Temperament		
	Energy and drive		
Sensory functions	Seeing		
	Hearing		
	Vestibular		
	Taste		
Sensory functions	Smell		
	Touch		
	Pain		
	Temperature and pressure		
Neuromusculoskeletal	Joint mobility UE		
	Joint mobility LE		
	Joint stability (postural control and alignment)		
	Muscle power (primarily UE)		
	Muscle endurance		
	Involuntary movement reactions		

Continued

TABLE 10-3   Client Factor Analysis—cont'd

Category	Client Factors	X Used	If Used, Describe How It Applies to This Activity (Be Specific)
Control of voluntary movement	Fine motor control		
	Gross motor control		
	Bilateral integration		
	Crossing the midline		
	Ocular motor control		
Body functions	Cardiovascular, hematologic, immunologic, and respiratory system functions		
	Voice and speech function		
	Other functions (e.g. digestion)		

LE, Lower extremity; *UE,* upper extremity.

TABLE 10-4   Contexts of Activity

Describe how each context would be used in this activity.
Activity:
Group members:

Context	X Used	Application to This Activity
Cultural		
Personal		
Temporal		
Virtual		
Physical		
Social		

BOX 10-3   Client Factor Analysis

Student:
Date:
Client factor:

Definition of Client Factor:

Summarize at least two peer-reviewed journal articles about this client factor. You may also get information from the Internet (be sure source is reliable). Give proper American Psychological Association reference citations.

Discuss how limitations in this client factor may affect occupational performance.

BOX 10-4   Roles of the Group Leader

Provide examples of the various group leader roles from one group activity session.
Group Activity:
Leader:

Roles	**Examples**
Instructor	
Participant	
Chairperson	
Consultant	
Facilitator	

BOX 10-5 Activity Analysis

Student: Date

Name of activity:
Source of activity (if not original):

Brief description of the activity:

After completing this activity successfully, the participants will have accomplished the following goals or objectives:

Tools and equipment (nonexpendable), cost, and source:

Materials and supplies (expendable), cost, and source:

Space and environmental requirements (room needed, chair and table setup):

Sequence and time required for each step in the activity:

Precautions (sharps, toxins, etc.):

Special considerations (age appropriateness, educational requirements, cultural relevance gender identification, other):

Criteria for successful completion:

Identify special population considerations for this activity. Indicate if the activity would be inappropriate or if the activity would need to be modified for successful participation. Describe these modifications in detail for each of the following populations:
1. Visual deficits (low vision, visual field loss):
2. Motor control deficits (apraxia, dyspraxia, neuromuscular or skeletal issues):
3. Mental functions:
4. Sensory functions:.
In what area of occupation is the activity?
What developmental level is this group (Mosey)?

Mosey A C: Legitimate tools of occupational therapy. In Mosey A, editor: *Occupational therapy: configuration of a profession*, New York, 1981, Raven, pp 89–118.

TABLE 10-5 Grading Rubric for Teaching-Learning Activity

Name:
Activity:
2= excellent; 1 = okay; 0 = poor

Preparation: enough materials, organized	2	1	0
Structure of group: Interesting introduction, clear sequence of steps; nice conclusion	2	1	0
Creativity: Interesting, creative, met goals, novel, appropriate level of difficulty and interest	2	1	0
Therapeutic use of self: voice, humor, speaking skills, professional, engaging, answered questions	2	1	0
Conclusion: Facilitated clean up and conclusion; met time limit	2	1	0
Materials: Written materials professional, neat, and clear; activity materials suitable for project or activity	2	1	0

Comments:

Total points:

BOX 10-6 Feedback on Group Experience

Name:
Role in group: Leader, Participant, Observer
Provide feedback on the following items (Be specific and provide examples):
1. Content and interest of the activity
2. Organization of the environment and materials
3. Delivery and therapeutic use of self
4. Temporal awareness
5. Ability to control the group
6. Ability to modify activity to meet individual needs
7. Ability to answer questions
8. Eye contact with participants
9. Materials and organization, preparation
10. Visual aid

BOX 10-7 Self-Evaluation of Group Experience

Leader's Name:
Group Session:
1. How well prepared were you?
   a. Were there enough supplies, materials?
   b. Did you feel organized and knowledgeable?
2. How well did you provide directions to the group?
   a. Were you respectful toward members?
   b. Did you clearly describe the steps?
   c. Were written directions or a sample provided?
3. Was the activity interesting?
   a. Was the goal of the group clear?
   b. Did you meet the goal?
4. Overall impression of the group:
5. How did you do at grading and adapting the activity for the different populations?
   a. Was there anybody that was more difficult in the group?
   b. What would do differently?
6. Suggestions for improvement for next time:
7. Summarize your strengths and weaknesses:
8. Ideas:

CHAPTER 11

TABLE 11-1 Aging Stereotypes: Anticipated Changes

Describe client factors, functions, traits, or skills and provide examples regarding anticipated changes in older adults.

Client Factor (or Subfactor, Other Function, Trait, or Skill) Examples	Occupational Example of What Is Anticipated
Decreased short-term memory	
Slower movements	
Poor balance	
Hard of hearing	
Cognitive decline	
Sensory changes	

TABLE 11-2 Olfaction and Its Impact on Performance

Provide examples on how olfaction may influence performance and how occupational therapy could help.

Area of Occupation: Specific Activity	Give an Example of How Anosmia or Hyposmia can Affect This Activity	How Could Occupational Therapy Help?
ADL: Eating		
Instrumental ADL: Safety and emergency maintenance		

ADL, Activities of daily living.

TABLE 11-3 Potential Reasons for Decreased ROM or Strength

Provide examples of the reasons for decreased ROM or strength.

Reasons for Decreased ROM or Strength	Example
Disuse	
Strength	
Bandages	
Limited vital capacity	
Disease process	
Trauma	
Pain	
Perception or anticipation of pain	
Edema	
Muscle tone	

ROM, Range of motion.

TABLE 11-4   Factors Contributing to Fall Risk and Potential OT Interventions

Provide examples on potential occupational therapy intervention to reduce fall risk.

Intrinsic Factors	How Could OT Intervention Help?
Muscle weakness	
Poor postural control	
Poor coordination and timing	
Visual perceptual	

Extrinsic Factors	How could OT intervention help?
Uneven floors	
Barriers in the house	
Environmental hazards (e.g., wet, ice, snow areas)	

OT, Occupational therapy.

TABLE 11-5   Cognition, Perception, and Aging

Provide expectations of what may occur as people age and evidence from chapter or research to support this.

Skills, Traits	Expectation of What Would Occur in Old Age	Empirical Evidence (Support For or Against) from Chapter (or Beyond)
Orientation (A & O X 1, 2, 3)		
Energy, Endurance		
Emotional stability		
Motivation		
Attention		
Short-term memory		
Long-term memory		
Prospective memory		
Procedural memory		
Thought functions		
Insight, judgment		
Awareness		
Mental flexibility		
Visual perception		

TABLE 11-6   Grading and Adapting

Activity:
List the steps to the activity and provide an example of how you would change the step for different clients.

Steps	Potential Grading or Adapting (One or More Examples for Each Step as Appropriate)

BOX 11-1 Activity Analysis

Name:

Complete the following activity analysis

1. Name of activity
2. Essential steps (up to 10) including usual time for completion
3. Precautions and contraindications (if any)
4. Age ranges
5. Contextual considerations
6. Activity demands—objects and their properties (typical for activity) tools, materials, equipment
7. Activity demands—space demands
8. Activity demands—social demands
9. Successful outcomes:
10. Degree of being amenable to change (is activity rigid or flexible)
11. Potential transfer of learning—list small to large changes for consideration

Note: Remember there is often more than one right answer for any one section.

BOX 11-2 Activity Analysis: Client-centered

Name:

Activity:

Client Name:

Client Goal being addressed:

1. Name of activity
2. Essential steps (up to 10)
3. Steps to be analyzed (form can be used for one or more applicable steps):
4. Client factors—values, beliefs, and spirituality if applicable
5. Client factors—mental functions
6. Client factors—sensory functions and pain
7. Client factors—neuromusculoskeletal—functions of joints and bones
   a. Which joints are involved?
   b. Mobility required
   c. Muscle power required
   d. Muscle endurance required
   e. Control of voluntary movement
   f. Control of voluntary movement
   g. Mobility—level of mobility required, LE function
8. Is activity amenable to alteration
9. Other applicable body functions (e.g., cardiovascular, hematologic, immunologic, respiratory, voice and speech, digestive, metabolic, endocrine, genitourinary, reproductive, skin and hair and nail functions)
10. Body structures—if applicable see p. 637 OTPF

LE, Lower extremity; *OTPF*, occupational therapy practice framework.

BOX 11-3   Activity Analysis: Cognition, Perception, Sensation Focused

Name:
Client goals addressed in activity:
Cognition, perception, sensation addressed in activity:

1. Name of Activity
2. Essential steps

Specific Examples Related to Activity

3. Client factors—Specific mental functions
   - Insight, judgment
   - Concept formation
   - Metacognition
   - Awareness
   - Cognitive flexibility
4. Client factors—Specific mental functions
   - Attention
   - Initiation, termination
   - Sustained attention
   - Selective attention
   - Alternating attention
   - Divided attention, multitasking
5. Client factors—Specific mental functions
   - Memory
   - Orientation (person, place, time)
   - Immediate memory
   - Short-term memory
   - Working memory
   - Long-term memory
   - Semantic memory
   - Episodic memory
   - Procedural memory
   - Prospective memory
6. Client factors—Specific mental functions
   - Learning
   - Simple 1-2 steps
   - Multistep learning
7. Client factors—Specific mental functions
   - Communication
   - Understanding of written language
   - Understanding of verbal language
   - Expression of written language
   - Auditory expression
   - Expression of nonverbal communication
8. Client factors—Specific mental functions
   - Thought processes
   - Recognition
   - Categorization
   - Generalization
   - Logical, coherent, appropriate thought and awareness of reality
9. Client factors—Specific mental functions
   - Sequencing
   - Sequencing task
   - Sequencing complex movement

Continued

BOX 11-3   **Activity Analysis: Cognition, Perception, Sensation Focused—cont'd**

Specific Examples Related to Activity

10. Client factors—Specific and global mental functions
    - Emotion
    - Coping skills
    - Behavioral regulation
    - Emotional expression, stability
    - Energy, motivation, drive
11. Client factors—Specific and global mental functions
    - Knowledge, skills
    - Demonstration, copying
    - Language
    - Calculations
    - Problem solving
    - Organizing, planning
    - Creating
12. Client factors—sensory functions
    - Vision—acuity
    - Vision—visual fields
    - Vision—fixation
    - Vision—accommodation
    - Vision—saccades
    - Vision—pursuits
    - Hearing—everyday conversation
    - Hearing—background noise
    - Taste functions
    - Smell functions
    - Touch functions
    - Touch functions—stereognosis
    - Touch functions—hot, cold and pain
    - Touch functions—pressure, vibration
    - Proprioception
    - Kinesthesia
13. Client factors—sensory functions—perception
    - Visual perception—item recognition
    - Visual perception—contrast sensitivity
    - Visual perception—form recognition
    - Visual perception—visual closure
    - Visual perception—depth perception
    - Visual perception—visual memory
    - Perception—discrimination of sensory input
14. Client factors—planned movement
    - Execution of learned movement patterns
    - Execution of complex, novel movement patterns

CHAPTER 12

TABLE 12-1 Group Design and Protocol

Therapist's Name: _____

Title of Group

Overall purpose

Sample goals

Time

Optimal size of group

Location

    Directions of location

    Precautions regarding location

    Supervision

Costs

Equipment Needs

Supplies

Sequence of events (include time)

Physical requirements

Precautions and special considerations

Notes

SAMPLE LESSON PLAN

Group members

Group goals

Objectives

Method

Lesson or activity

Conclusion

Notes for next time:

SAMPLE LESSON PLAN

Theme

Goals

Activity

Take home message and incentives

Conclusion

Notes for next time

CHAPTER 13

BOX 13-1 Steps to Ethical Decision Making

Provide an application example outlining the steps to ethical decision making.

Application

1. Gather relevant information.
2. Identify the ethical problem (ethical distress, ethical dilemma, or locus of authority).
3. Use ethical theories or approaches to analyze problem. Who are the other players? Examine AOTA Code of Ethics, Standards of Practice, laws and regulations. Define principles according to Code of Ethics.
4. Explore alternatives.
5. Complete action.
6. Evaluate process and outcome.

Other:

AOTA, American Occupational Therapy Association.
Modified from Purtillo R. Ethical dimensions in the health professions (ed. 4), Bethesda, MD, 2005.

CHAPTER 14

BOX 14-1 Group Task Roles

Identify group members' roles in a task-oriented group and describe behaviors.

Example of Behavior in Group

Initiator-contributor
Information seeker
Opinion seeker
Coordinator
Information giver
Opinion giver
Elaborator
Orienteer
Energizer
Evaluator-critic
Procedural technician
Recorder

TABLE 13-1 Ethical Principles (AOTA 2010)

Principle	Description	Example
1. Beneficence	Occupational therapy personnel shall demonstrate a concern for the well-being and safety of the recipients of their services.	
2. Nonmaleficence	Occupational therapy personnel shall intentionally refrain from actions that cause harm.	
3. Autonomy and Confidentiality	Occupational therapy personnel shall respect the right of the individual to self-determination.	
4. Social Justice	Occupational therapy personnel shall provide services in a fair and equitable manner.	
5. Procedural Justice	Occupational therapy personnel shall comply with institutional rules, local, state, federal, and international laws, and AOTA documents applicable to the profession of occupational therapy.	
6. Veracity	Occupational therapy personnel shall provide comprehensive, accurate, and objective information when representing the profession.	
7. Fidelity	Occupational therapy personnel shall treat colleagues and other professionals with respect, fairness, discretion, and integrity.	

AOTA, American Occupational Therapy Association.
Data from American Occupational Therapy Association: Enforcement procedures for the Occupational Therapy Code of Ethics and Ethics Standards, *Am J Occup Ther* 64(Suppl.):S4-S16, 2010.

BOX 14-2 Group Building and Maintenance roles

Identify group members' roles in a task-oriented group and describe behaviors.

Example of Behavior in Group

Encourager
Compromiser
Harmonizer
Gatekeeper
Standard setter
Group observer or commentator
Follower

BOX 14-3 Individual roles

Identify group members' roles in a task-oriented group and describe behaviors.

Examples of Behavior in Group

Aggressor
Dominator or monopolist
Blocker
Self-confessor
Recognition seeker
Playboy
Help-seeker (help-rejecting
    complainer)
Special interest pleader

BOX 14-5 A Four-Step Intervention Model

Be clear about the description of each step in the intervention model.

Step	Description

Problem
- What are the specific issues in the group?
- Who is involved, what are the behaviors, and how is it impacting other group members and the group process?
- Describe members' roles.

Interpretation
- Provide possible explanations for behaviors.
- Determine the center of the issue.
- Evaluate roles of members.

Intervention
- Consider the identified problem and the proposed theory and the desired outcome of intervention.
- Identify possible approaches.
- Use members' roles and the group's dynamics to intervene whenever possible.

Outcome and Reassessment
- What was the effect of the intervention?
- Identify changes resulting from the intervention process.
- Is there any new information about the group or its members gleaned from the intervention process?
- Identify future actions required.

BOX 14-4 Evaluation of Group Session

Complete an evaluation of the group session by answering the following questions.
- **Were the goals accomplished?** State the outcome and identify your rationale.
- **Was the group successful in helping individuals accomplish their short- and long-term goals?**
- **Was the group content and structure adequate for accomplishing the goals?** Leadership; time and length of meeting; format; sequence, methods, and procedures; media, modalities, techniques employed; norms and behaviors reinforced implicitly or explicitly; methods of reinforcement; and stage of the group
- **Did the structure provide for an "optimal experience" or a "flow state"?**
- **Did the structure allow for new learning or reinforcement of current level of role functioning or occupational performance, or did it reinforce functioning below current level of ability?**

- **Did the structure provide an opportunity for evaluation and feedback regarding the group procedures, process, and member progress?**
- **What changes would you make regarding group goals and structure for the next group, or the next time this group is lead?**
- **Were you as leaders adequately prepared for the group?** Consider time, place, materials, personal knowledge, and physical and emotional environment.
- **How did you function within that role?** Consider how your behavior and position affected the group. What did you do that was effective? What leadership opportunities were missed? What do you think you learned from this group session?
- **Was the group interaction as you anticipated?** What you can identify as a basis for understanding the problems.
- **In the future, what might you do differently as the group leader?** Give rationale.

Adapted from Schwartsberg SL, Howe MC, Barnes MA: *Groups: applying the functional group model,* Philadelphia, 2008, FA Davis Company.

Index

Page numbers followed by *f* indicate figures; *t*, tables; *b*, boxes.

217